Minor Head Trauma

Steven Mandel
Robert Thayer Sataloff
Sarita R. Schapiro
Editors

Minor Head Trauma
Assessment, Management, and Rehabilitation

With 40 Illustrations

Springer-Verlag
New York   Berlin   Heidelberg   London   Paris
Tokyo   Hong Kong   Barcelona   Budapest

Steven Mandel, M.D.
Clinical Professor of Neurology
Jefferson Medical College
Philadelphia, PA 19107, USA

Robert Thayer Sataloff, M.D., D.M.A.
Professor of Otolaryngology
Thomas Jefferson University
Philadelphia, PA 19103, USA

Sarita R. Schapiro, Ph.D.
Director
Behavioral Rehabilitation Services
Jenkintown, PA 19046, USA

Library of Congress Cataloging-in-Publication Data
Minor head trauma / Steven Mandel, Robert Thayer Sataloff, Sarita
    Schapiro, editors.
        p.   cm.
    Includes bibliographical references and index.
    ISBN 0-387-97943-3.—ISBN 3-540-97943-3
    1. Brain damage—Complications.   2. Brain damage—Patients—
Rehabilitation.   I. Mandel, Steven.   II. Sataloff, Robert Thayer.
III. Schapiro, Sarita.
    [DNLM: 1. Head Injuries.   WE706 M666]
    RC387.5.M56   1993
    617.4′81044—dc20
    DNLM/DLC
    for Library of Congress   92-49619

Printed on acid-free paper.

Production managed by Christin R. Ciresi; manufacturing supervised by Jacqui Ashri.
Typeset by Best-set Typesetter Ltd., Hong Kong
Printed and bound by Edwards Brothers, Ann Arbor, MI, USA
Printed in the United States of America.

9 8 7 6 5 4 3 2 1

ISBN 0-387-97943-3 Springer-Verlag New York Berlin Heidelberg
ISBN 3-540-97943-3 Springer-Verlag Berlin Heidelberg New York

Dedication

This book is respectfully dedicated to the late David Rubinstein, M.D., Clinical Professor of Psychiatry, Temple University School of Medicine. Dr. Rubinstein, who also was the father of Dr. Sarita Schapiro, conceived and inspired this text on minor head trauma. The author of more than fifty scholarly publications, Dr. Rubinstein dedicated his life to patient care and medical education. His insights into the problems and needs of patients with signficant head injury led to increased awareness of their plight and the unprecedented interdisciplinary collaboration that resulted in the completion of this book. *Minor Head Trauma* is a modest monument to his sensitivity, dedication, and concern both for his patients and for the scholarly evolution of medical practice.

Steven Mandel
Robert Thayer Sataloff
Sarita R. Schapiro

Preface

Minor Head Trauma is an interdisciplinary text on an important and neglected subject. Minor head trauma often produces clinically important sequelae. However, because many of these aftereffects are subtle and require evaluation that straddles several disciplines, they have not been well recognized, well managed, or well taught by any specialty. This book brings together experts from numerous disciplines and presents the available information on this complex subject comprehensively, but in language easily accessible to interested professionals of any background. The book is intended for physicians, psychologists, physical therapists, speech-language pathologists, nurses, attorneys, and others faced with the challenges of evaluating and treating patients who have sustained minor head trauma.

Chapter 1 provides a succinct overview of the nature and scope of the problem. It presents the definition of *minor head trauma*, a term that implies more significant injury than one might infer from the word *minor*. The authors also point out that minor head trauma is extremely common, and its consequences may be profound. Chapter 2 provides a review of the neuropathology of minor head injury, confirming that significant alterations in brain structure occur, even though they may not always be detectable with the clinical methods in common use. In Chapter 3, an emergency medicine specialist and former neurosurgeon, Dr. Neal Little, reviews the initial, emergency room management of patients with head injury. Chapter 4 highlights the value and importance of radiological imaging, and includes a summary of the potential applications of single photon emission computed tomography (SPECT) and position emission tomography (PET) in the evaluation of minor head trauma patients. Chapter 5 discusses the role of electrophysiological testing in patients who have sustained minor head trauma, providing a useful review of the literature and the authors' clinical experience. Not only routine EEG, but also more esoteric techniques such as brain electrical activity mapping (BEAM) are included.

In Chapter 6, Drs. Schapiro and Sacchetti review the subtleties of neuropsychological diagnosis following minor brain injury. Astute neuropsychological assessment is particularly important in identifying specific sequelae of head injury. The late Dr. David Rubinstein's vast experience in management of psychiatric problems following minor brain injury is crystallized in Chapter 7. Sleep abnormalities are common following head trauma; Chapter 8 reviews the state of the art in sleep assessment and management. Headache is one of the most common and troubling symptoms encountered in American medicine. Chapter 9 reviews the differential diagnosis and complicated treatment of patients with headache following trauma. In Chapter 10, Drs. Sataloff and Spiegel provide a comprehensive review of neurotological evaluation and treatment following minor head trauma. This lengthy chapter discusses hearing loss, tinnitus, vertigo, and facial nerve dysfunction. It includes specific discussion of the latest clinical and technological approaches to diagnosis and treatment.

Temporomandibular joint disorders are also common following minor head trauma and may be responsible for symptoms that could be incorrectly attributed to other organ systems, such as the brain or ear. Chapter 11 reviews the principles of diagnosis and treatment of these disorders. Following minor head trauma, communication deficits are common. Minor head trauma also commonly causes damage to the olfactory system. Evaluation of taste and smell disorders has changed dramatically in the last decade. In Chapter 12, Drs. Spiegel and Frattali summarize current diagnosis and treatment, present a comprehensive review of the epidemiology of this problem, and offer clinically based insights on the practical consequences of olfactory dysfunction. Like other sensory systems, vision may be impaired as a result of closed head injury. In Chapter 13, Dr. Gerner, an experienced neuro-ophthalmologist, reviews the nature and pathogenesis of visual sequelae of head injury. Injuries to the head are often associated with neck injuries; and cervical injury may be responsible for potentially treatable headaches and other symptoms that could be incorrectly diagnosed as incurable consequences of brain injury. The discussion of these problems by neurosurgeon Donald Myers in Chapter 14 is based on the author's vast clinical experience and expert scholarly knowledge of head and neck injury.

Traditional speech-language pathology training may not prepare the therapist for the kinds of treatment needed following minor head trauma. Chapter 15 reviews the speech-language pathologist's role, highlighting the importance of collaboration with other professionals. Chapters 16 through 19 address the complexities of rehabilitation following minor head trauma. By design, these chapters overlap somewhat, and some concepts are presented more than once. However, each chapter addresses the problems from a different professional perspective, highlighting the value and necessity of team management of these patients. Chapter 16 provides an in-depth discussion of problems associated with cognitive function, and extends the concepts put forth by Rhona Paul-Cohen. In Chapter 17, the specific roles of various professionals on the rehabilitation team are described. Chapter 18 highlights the problems faced when patients who have suffered minor head injury attempt to resume normal professional and community activities. These problems and their management are especially important, because if they are not expertly attended to, even minor impairments may become disabilities. In Chapter 19, Dr. Sachs shares the insights of extensive clinical experience in problems faced by families of patients who have suffered minor head trauma and its sequelae. Such an injury can be markedly disruptive, and evaluation and possible treatment of the family are essential to the rehabilitation process.

We offer this text in the hope that it will increase understanding of the problems of patients who have sustained minor head trauma, encourage more diligent attention to their plight in training programs and clinical settings, and inspire new interdisciplinary investigations. Although the existence of this book points out that we know significantly more about minor head trauma than we did even five years ago, a great deal more remains to be learned. It is our sincere hope that additional research will result in equally great scientific and clinical advances in the next five years.

Steven Mandel
Robert Thayer Sataloff
Sarita R. Schapiro

Contents

Contributors

Francisco Batlle, M.D., Resident, Department of Neurosurgery, Jefferson Medical College, Thomas Jefferson University, Philadelphia, PA 19107, USA

Sonia Bermudez, M.D., Professor of Radiology, Jarveriana University, Department of Radiology, Bogota, Colombia

Sanford Davne, M.D., Department of Orthopaedic Surgery, Jefferson Medical College, Thomas Jefferson University, Philadelphia, PA 19107, USA

Karl Doghramji, M.D., Assistant Professor, Department of Psychiatry and Human Behavior, Director, Sleep Disorders Center, Jefferson Medical College, Thomas Jefferson University, Philadelphia, PA 19107, USA

Serge Duckett, M.D., Ph.D., D.Sc., Director and Professor, Alpers Neuropathology Laboratory, Department of Neurology, Jefferson Medical College, Thomas Jefferson University, Philadelphia, PA 19107, USA

Stephane Duckett, Ph.D., Department of Psychology, Bryn Mawr Rehabilitation Hospital, Malvern, PA 19355, USA

Anthony Farole, D.M.D., Associate Professor, Department of Otolaryngology (Dentistry), Jefferson Medical College, Associate Director, Oral and Maxillofacial Surgery, Thomas Jefferson University, Philadelphia, PA, 19107, USA

Mark Frattali, M.S., M.D., CCC-A, Resident, Department of Otolaryngology, Jefferson Medical College, Thomas Jefferson University, Philadelphia, PA 19107, USA

Edward W. Gerner, M.D., Associate Professor, Wills Eye Hospital, Thomas Jefferson University Hospital, Philadelphia, PA 19107, USA

Carlos Gonzales, M.D., Professor of Radiology and Neurosurgery, Director of Neuroradiology, Thomas Jefferson University Hospital, Philadelphia, PA 19107, USA

Mercedes P. Jacobson, M.D., Comprehensive Epilepsy Center, Department of Neurology, The Graduate Hospital, Philadelphia, PA 19146, USA

Lana Liberto, Ph.D., Director, Training and Development, Doylestown Hospital, Doylestown, PA 18901, USA

Neal Little, M.D., F.A.C.E.P., Diplomate, American Board of Emergency Medicine, Clinical Instructor, University of Michigan Medical School, Ann Arbor, MI 48106, USA

Karen Lutz, O.T.R./L, Senior Occupational Therapist, Doylestown Hospital, Doylestown, PA 18901, USA

Donald L. Myers, M.D., Assistant Professor, Department of Neurological Surgery, Jefferson Medical College, Thomas Jefferson University, Philadelphia, PA 19107, USA

Lynn Nash, B.S., O.T.R./L, Senior Occupational Therapist, In-Patient Rehabiliation, Doylestown Hospital, Doylestown, PA 18901, USA

Lori Sadwin O'Leary, B.A., Research Assistant, In Association with Arnold Sadwin, M.D., Philadelphia, PA 19103, USA

Rhona Paul-Cohen, M.S., CCC-Sp, Consultant and Allied Staff Member, Rancocas Hospital, Sunset Road, Willingboro, NJ 08046, USA

Robert W. Rothrock, P.A.C., Coordinator, Chronic Pain Program, Pennsbury Pain Center, Morrisville, PA 19067 USA

David Rubinstein, M.D., F.A.P.A., Clinical Professor of Psychiatry, Temple University School of Medicine, Philadelphia, PA 19140, USA

Thomas Swirsky Sacchetti, Ph.D., A.B.P.P., Diplomate in Clinical Neuropsychology, Clinical Assistant Professor, Department of Psychiatry and Human Behavior, Jefferson Medical College, Philadephia, PA 19107, USA

Paul R. Sachs, Ph.D., Private Practice, Rehabilitation and Neuropsychology, Lower Merion and Norristown, Pennsylvania, Adjunct Faculty Member in the Neuropsychology, Program at Drexel University, Philadelphia, PA

Arnold Sadwin, M.D., Assistant Clinical Professor in Family Practice, New Jersey School of Medicine and Dentistry, Stratford, New Jersey, USA; Chief of Neuropsychiatry, Graduate Hospital, Senior Attending Psychiatrist at the Institute of Pennsylvania Hospital, Senior Staff Psychiatrist at Belmont Hospital, Philadelphia, PA 19103, USA

Donna Sadwin, B.F.A., Art Therapist Specializing in Minor Head Trauma, In Association with Arnold Sadwin, M.D., Philadelphia, PA 19103, USA

Michael R. Sperling, M.D., Associate Professor, Department of Neurology, University of Pennsylvania School of Medicine, Director of EEG Laboratory, The Graduate Hospital, Philadelphia, PA 19146, USA

Joseph R. Spiegel, M.D., F.A.C.S., Assistant Professor of Otolaryngology, Department of Otolaryngology, Jefferson Medical College, Thomas Jefferson University, Philadelphia, PA 19103, USA

Kathryn Tomlin, M.S., CCC/SP, Department of Speech Pathology, Doylestown Hospital Rehabilitation Center, Doylestown, PA 18901, USA

Joyce Zinsenheim, M.D., Assistant Director, Consultation and Liaison Service, Albert Einstein Medical Center, Philadelphia, PA 19141, USA

— 1

Minor Head Trauma: An Overview

Sarita R. Schapiro, Robert Thayer Sataloff, and Steven Mandel

It is estimated that in the United States between 400,000 and 500,000 individuals are hospitalized every year for head trauma (1,2). Hospitalization for minor head injury alone occurs with an incidence of 131 cases for every 100,000 people in the population and accounts for about 60% to 82% of all admissions for head trauma (3). The vast numbers of such patients have led some to label head injury "the silent epidemic" (4). In economic terms, the cost is enormous, estimated to be more than $3.9 billion per year (5). The noneconomic cost to society is even greater, since these injuries often result in significant social and vocational morbidity and increased dependency on family members.

The terms *minor head trauma* and *mild brain injury* are not colloquial, descriptive terms. Rather, they are terms with specific medical definitions. Head injuries are classified as severe, minor (or mild), and minimal. Although authors vary somewhat defining minor head trauma, the term *minor* or *mild* is generally used to refer to individuals who meet the following criteria after a head injury: 1) Glasgow Coma Scale greater than 12 on hospital admission (see Appendix); 2) loss of consciousness, or post-traumatic amnesia, not to exceed 20 minutes; 3) hospitalization less than 48 hours; and 4) no clinical evidence of brainstem or cortical contusion (6). Most authors exclude patients with skull fractures. Post-concussional syndrome is used to refer to the constellation of symptoms that accompany these injuries. They usually include somatic and psychological symptoms such as headache, dizziness, fatigue, diminished concentration,

1

memory impairment, irritability, depression, anxiety, insomnia, hypochondria, hypersensitivity to noise, and photophobia (7). The degree to which these symptoms become manifest and persist depends on several factors, including the pathophysiological mechanisms of the injury, psychosocial factors, and post-injury circumstances.

Debate over the sequelae of minor head injuries has been documented since the 1960s, when discussions regarding post-traumatic symptoms first appeared in the medical literature (8). The debate has centered around whether the symptoms are the result of emotional (i.e., psychogenic) reactions to the trauma, or whether the symptoms represent behavioral manifestations of physical or organic injury to the brain. Anatomic disruption underlying minor head injury often appears insufficient to account for the observed variation in and duration of post-traumatic symptoms (9). The onset of symptoms may be late (i.e., several days or more after the injury), which has been interpreted as suggestive of a psychogenic rather than a physiological process.

Some studies have documented actual damage to the brain following minor head trauma. Gronwall and Wrightson, in 1975, found pathological evidence of microscopic lesions after mild head injury (10), as have other authors, as discussed in Chapter 2. Levin et al. (11) documented a relationship between size and localization of white matter lesions as defined by magnetic resonance imaging and neuropsychological deficits. There is increasing evidence that the pathophysiology after minor head injury may involve a more gradual process than had previously been recognized (12). As Max Feldman reports:

It would appear then that any person who has suffered a head injury, major, minor or minimal, with or without unconsciousness, can be presumed to have an organic basis for such subjective complaints as he may present in respect of headache, giddiness, and "nervousness." Pre-existing emotional disturbances, if claimed to be aggravated by head injury, are to be attributed to the self-same assumed organic brain change. (13)

The problems experienced by victims of mild head injury often are indistinguishable from those found in patients who have sustained more severe head injuries. One cannot assume that there is a linear relationship between the severity of the injury and the severity of ensuing symptoms. Often those who sustain mild head injuries demonstrate more acute distress over their symptoms because they are more aware of their dysfunction and typically hold higher expectations for themselves given the apparent lack of injury severity (14). While the general prognosis for patients following mild head injury has been considered good, the current literature presents increasing evidence suggesting long-term complications for such patients involving cognitive, behavioral, emotional, and vocational disability. In fact, follow-up examinations at three months show that these patients have many of the same problems in memory and task performance as those with severe injuries (4). While most individuals with mild head injuries recover in many ways within the first three months (3), neuropsychological and other sequelae may persist for up to three to five years following injury, resulting in significant social and vocational disability (15). In some cases, sequelae are permanent.

The plight of minor head trauma patients has generally not been appreciated fully by physicians and many related professionals. Because the injuries appear minor (in a colloquial sense), we tend to expect full, rapid recovery. The sequelae of minor brain injury may be subtle and difficult to detect, particularly in the peace and quiet of a medical office. Consequently, the complaints of many patients with significant impairment following head injury have been dismissed as exaggerated, or motivated by concerns related to litigation. Because the problems encountered by these patients may involve so many mental and physical functions, they do not fall neatly into the purview of any one specialty. This has further delayed the development of appropriate diagnostic and therapeutic approaches. Recent scientific advances in understanding the mechanisms of injury have highlighted the naivete of our earlier management and have led the way for important clinical advances. It is now clear that failure to diagnose the cause of common complaints following minor head injury is due generally to lack of expertise on the practitioner's part, rather than to imaginary complaints on the part of the patient.

Interdisciplinary collaboration is paramount in the management of patients following minor head trauma. This book emphasizes the importance of each specialist on the medical team caring for these patients. Collaboration has resulted in great improvements not only in diagnosis and patient rehabilitation, but also in knowledge and understanding for each member of the medical team. Like so many other "new" and "frontier" areas of medicine, enlightened, interdisciplinary management of minor brain injury provides exciting challenges and opportunities for creativity in medicine; and it has proven as gratifying to the clinicians involved in this field as it has to the patients.

References

1. Rimel R, Giordani B, Barth J, Boll T, Jane J: Disability caused by minor head injury. Neurosurgery, 1981; 9:221–228.
2. Rosenthal M: Traumatic head injury: Neurobehavioral Consequences. In Caplan B. (ed): Rehabilitation Psychology Desk Reference. Rockville, MD: Aspen Publishers, 1987; pp 37–63.

3. Levin H, Mattis S, Ruff R, Eisenberg H, Marshall L, Tabaddor K, High W, Frankowski R: Neurobehavioral outcome following minor head injury: A three-center study. J Neurosurg, 1987; 66:234–243.
4. Minor head injury becomes a "silent epidemic." News AFP, 1983; 28(5):345–362.
5. Lynch R: Traumatic head injury: Implications for rehabilitation counseling. Appl Rehabil Counsel, 1983; 3:32–35.
6. Davidoff DA, Kessler HR, Laibstain DF, Mark VH: Neurobehavioral sequelae of minor head injury: A consideration of post-concussive syndrome versus post-traumatic stress disorder. Cogn Rehabil, 1988; 6:8–13.
7. Stevens MM: Post-concussion syndrome. J Neurosurg Nursing, 1982; 14(5):239–244.
8. Trimble MR: Post-traumatic neurosis: From railway spine to the whiplash. Chichester: Wiley, 1981.
9. Alves WM, Coloban AR, O'Leary TJ, Rimel RW, Jane JA: Understanding posttraumatic symptoms after minor head injury. J Head Trauma Rehabil, 1986; 1(2):1–12.
10. Gronwall D, Wrightson P: Cumulative effect of concussion. Lancet, 1975: 2:995–997.
11. Levin HS, Amparo E, Eisenberg HM, Williams DH, High WM, McArdle CB, Weiner RM: Magnetic resonance imaging and computerized tomography in relation to the neurobehavioral sequelae of mild and moderate head injuries. J Neurosurg, 1987; 66:706–713.
12. Povlishock JT, Becker DP, Miller JD, et al.: The morphopathologic substrates of concussion. Acta Neuropathol, 1979; 47:1–11.
13. Feldman M: The post-concussional syndrome: Fact or fancy? South Afr Med J, 1973; 47(46):2247–2248.
14. Bornstein RA, Miller HB, van Schoor JR: Neuropsychological deficit and emotional disturbance in head injured patients. J Neurosurg, 1989; 70:509–513.
15. Edna TJ: Disability 3 to 5 years after minor head injury. J Oslo City Hosp, 1987; 37:41–48.

— 2

The Neuropathology of the Minor Head Injury Syndrome

Serge Duckett and Stephane Duckett

The minor head injury syndrome (MHIS) involves injury to the head which results in a contusion of the brain—without skull fracture or major hemorrhage—followed weeks to months later by debilitating psychiatric manifestations.

About 400,000 persons are treated each year in the United States by physicians for head injuries [1–3]. The vast majority of them (93%) will recover without apparent aftereffects, 2.8% will suffer serious complications, and 1% will die. The rest (3.2%, 12,800) will manifest a variety of psychological problems, presumably associated with a contusion on the surface of the brain, usually in the frontal and temporal area. The neuropathological evidence for MHIS is based on experimental work with laboratory animals and the presence of unexplained old cortical lesions found at autopsy as well as post-mortem findings that can be attributed to coincidental, though separate, lethal lesions. This is a difficult syndrome to diagnose clinically because of 1) the delay of weeks or months that may occur between the injury-causing blow to the head and the earliest mani-festations of psychological changes, and 2) the difficulty in obtaining a clinical history from the patient. In many cases radiological evi-dence—computed tomography (CT) scans and magnetic resonance imaging (MRI)—is unavailable.

MRI is most useful in determining the early tissue changes, results of a localized petechial hemorrhage and edema caused by a contusion on the surface of the cerebral cortex. The CT scan can detect fresh blood earlier than the MRI and is available for early monitoring of the patient upon hospitalization.

MHIS begins with a blow to the head, that is, followed by a brief loss of consciousness lasting from a few seconds to twenty minutes, antigrade and retrograde amnesia, confusion, and, sometimes, precautionary hospitalization for 12 to 48 hours (4). The patient is then released because he appears to have recuperated quickly and there is no evidence of a skull fracture or subdural or subarachnoid hemorrhage. Days to weeks later, there is an onset of progressive neuropsychological changes: lethargy, fatigue, irritability, difficulty concentrating, and forgetfulness, which often result in unpleasant situations at home and at work. Usually there are no other physical neurological symptoms. The following case history is typical (5).

Case: A.T., a 34-Year-Old Woman

A.T. was an intelligent, ambitious, responsible, and successful vice-president of a major advertising firm with a salary of over $100,000 per year. On her way home one night she was involved in a car accident, suffered a mild closed head injury, and was unconscious for 20 minutes. She was taken to the hospital, observed for a few hours, x-rayed, and sent home with the advice to abstain from work for a week or so. Two days later she returned to work—tired and with poor judgment, unable to make proper decisions, forgetful, and increasingly irritable when questioned sympathetically. Her employer reluctantly fired her four months later; six months after that she was fired from a second job. After this she was unemployed and drank heavily. A neurological examination revealed a very capable and intelligent woman with subtle cognitive deficits. A.T. would not accept any position beneath the one she had previously held. She remained unemployed and depressed, and within a year she had two psychiatric hospitalizations.

Pathology

The most common cause of MHIS is a blow to the forehead, as occurs commonly in a car or sports-related accident (6). The mass of the cerebrum moves forward suddenly and the brunt of the pathology occurs in the anterior portions of the frontal and temporal lobes (Figs. 2.1–5). The undersurface of the frontal lobe—the orbital gyri—glides along the bony surface of the anterior fossa (Fig. 2.3), and the roof of the orbit, the crista galli, and capillaries in the crown of the cortex are

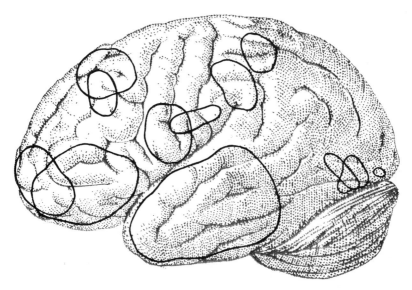

Fig. 2.1. Lateral view of the human brain. The circled areas represent potential areas of cortical injury in MHIS (1). Drawn by Jean-Francois Duckett.

shorn and result in a petechial hemorrhage—the depths of the sulci remain undamaged. The frontal pole may collide with the anterior wall of the skull, or the temporal pole may collide against the lesser wing of the sphenoid bone, causing capillary pathology at the site of impact on the brain. MHIS is rarely caused by a blow across the back of the head causing petechiae on the surface of the cerebellum or occipital lobe. Blows to the head which result in MHIS are never severe enough to fracture the skull or cause a major hemorrhage.

Other forms of limited lesions of the brain without skull fracture or major cerebral hemorrhage caused by trauma have been shown experimentally in animals, but clinico-pathological evidence has not been adequately documented in humans. For example, it has been shown in animals that a minor blow to the head causes herniation of the cingulate or parahippocampal gyri. The brain is suddenly jerked within the skull box, and two parts of the brain—the cingulate and hippocampal gyri—are particularly susceptible because of their presence near the free edges of the meninges—the tentorium cerebelli in the case of the hippocampus, and the cerebral falx in that of the cingulate gyrus (Fig. 2.4). There may be a tortion of the brainstem and cerebellum, resulting in shearing of capillaries and axons within the brainstem.

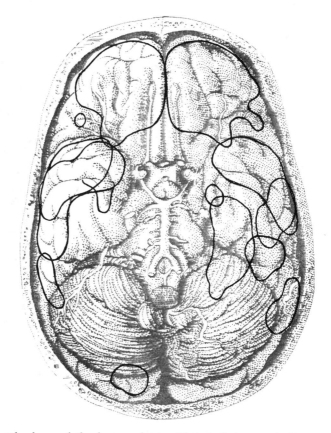

Fig. 2.2. The base of the human brain. The circled areas indicate potential areas of cortical injury in MHIS (1). Drawn by Jean-Francois Duckett.

Histology

The morphological development of a cerebral contusion is the same regardless of the causes. It is a cortical petechia which eventually resorbs, leaving traces of its occurrence, such as gliosis, cyst, and yellow staining. It is often important to establish the time of the lesion for forensic or legal purposes (7–10).

The sequence of histological events following a cortical contusion in humans may be divided into three stages—early, intermediate, and late (7,11). In the early stage (immediately after the injury) the hemorrhage begins and extends into the surrounding cortical areas during the next 24 hours. The edema presents within seconds of the injury and increases in severity over the next few hours, extending the

Fig. 2.3. These drawings illustrate gliding injuries of the cortex. **A**: A section of the normal brain showing the white matter (1), the cortex (2), the meninges (3). and the bone (4). **B**: The arrow indicates a direction of a sudden movement of the brain which results in the brain illustrated in figure 3**C** where the cortical has been injured by the gliding movement of the brain across the bony surface. Drawn by Jean-Francois Duckett.

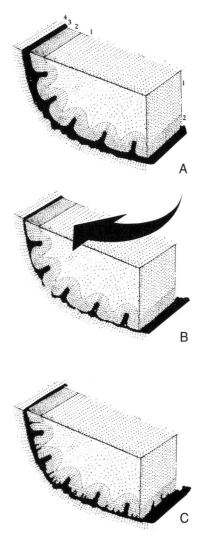

lesion far beyond the hemorrhagic area (12–14). Neurons and other cells in the affected area swell, shrink, and die. Axons swell and balloon with secondary demyelination (15,16). A small number of polymorphonuclear (PMN) leukocytes appear six to eight hours after the hemorrhage and disappear after a few hours. Shortly later, blood-borne monocytes appear in the necrotic tissue and vigorous phagocytose debris (8–10,13,17). The edema disappears by the sixth day and there appears a proliferation of capillaries and gliosis which leads eventually to a scar on the surface of the brain (8–10,18). Intact RBCs remain in the lesion for up to six months (19,20). A few days

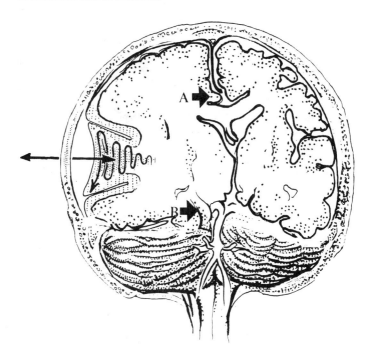

Fig. 2.4. This drawing shows the results of a sudden trauma to the head, namely herniation of the cingulate gyrus beneath the falx cerebri (**A**) and of the hippocampus by the cerebellar tentorium (**B**). Drawn by Jean-Francois Duckett.

after the injury lymphocytes may appear diffusely around blood vessels and remain for years (9,10). Beginning during the intermediate stage, that is, the second week following injury, the capillaries proliferate in situ for about one month, to be slowly replaced by a network of sclerotic tissue and eventually a scar of glial tissue or collagen (21,22). Astrocytic proliferation begins a few days after injury and goes on for months and even years. Gliosis is the dominant factor during the late stages of the contusion. Eventually, at autopsy, the pathologist will find a foci of scarred, cystic, or stained tissue (plaque jaune) which will indicate an old contusion (Fig. 2.5).

Although the characteristic lesion of MHIS is a contusion in the cerebral cortex, the underlying white matter may be involved. In the case of MHIS, the white matter pathology is localized and may be caused by edema associated with the petechial hemorrhage in the cortex, or it may be due to a shearing of axons caused by the abrupt cerebral movement. Silver staining of axons shows these either to be broken or reveals retraction balls at the site of axonal tear associated with secondary demyelination. Important white matter pathology is a

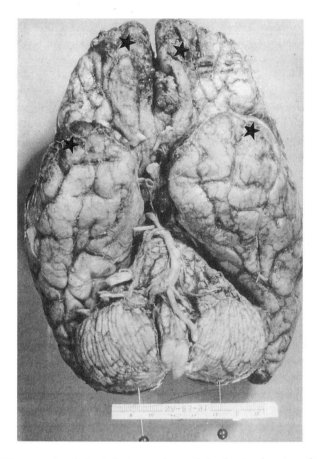

Fig. 2.5. Photograph of the inferior surface of the brain showing the damage to the orbital area of the frontal cortex and temporal pole (indicated by stars) shortly after cerebral trauma.

frequent complication of major head injuries caused by mechanical forces suddenly unleashed by the trauma (8,16,23,24).

Conclusions

There is little information available at present concerning the neuropathologic substratum of (MHIS) because it is not lethal and the clinical manifestations do not warrant a biopsy. The information that is available is based on chance findings in the course of autopsies usually performed years after the MHIS, experimental studies, or presumed pathologic similarities with the much more frequent major head injury syndromes.

Acknowledgments

We thank Mr. Jean-Francois Duckett for allowing us to use his illustrations (Fig. 2.1–4) and Ms. Shirley Sadak for her editorial assistance.

References

1. Courville CB: Pathology of the Central Nervous System. 3rd edition. Mountain View, CA: Pacific Press Publication Association, 1960.
2. Austin EJ: Head trauma in the aged. In Duckett S (ed): Pathology of the Aging Human Nervous System. Philadelphia: Lea & Febiger, 1990.
3. Mandel S: Minor head injury may not be minor. Postgrad Med J, 1989; 85(6):213–220.
4. Plaut MR, Gifford RR: Trivial head trauma and its consequences in a perspective of regional health care. Milit Med, 1976; 141(4):244–247.
5. McMahon RT, Flowers SM: The high cost of a bump on the head. Business Health, 1986; 3:47–48.
6. Gennarelli T: Mechanisms and pathophysiology of cerebral concussion. J Head Trauma Rehabil, 1986; 1(2):23–29.
7. Oppenheimer R: Microscopic lesions in the brain following head injury. J Neurosurg Psychiatry, 1968; 31:299–306.
8. Lindenberg R, Freytag E: The mechanism of cerebral contusions, a pathologic-anatomic study. Arch Pathol, 1960; 69:440–469.
9. Oehmichen M: Timing of cortical contusion. Correlation between histomorphologic alterations and post-traumatic interval. Z Rechtsmed, 1980; 84:79–94.
10. Oehmichen M, Raff G: Zeitabhangige histomorphologische Veranderungen von Rindenprellungsherden nach Contusio cerebri. Beitr Gerichtl Med, 1978; 36:291–294.
11. Povilshock JT, Becker DP, Miller JD, et al.: The morphopathologic substrates of concussion? Acta Neuropathol (Berl), 1979; 47(1):1–11.
12. Langfitt TW, Weinstein JD, Kassell NF: Vascular factors in head injury. Contribution to brain-swelling and intracranial hypertension. In Caveness WE, Walker AE (eds): Head Injury. Philadelphia: Lippincott, 1966; pp 172–194.
13. Nevin NC: Neuropathologic change in the white matter following head injury. J Neuropathol Exp Neurol 1967; 26:77–84.
14. Schroder JM, Wechsler W: Odem und Nekrose in der grauen und weissen Substanz beim experimentallen Hirntrauma. Licht-und elektonen-mikroskopische Untersuchungen. Acta Neuropathol (Berl), 1965; 5: 82–111.
15. Povilshock JT, Becker DP, Cheng CI, et al.: Axonal change in minor head injury. J Neuropathol Exp Neurol, 1983; 42(3):225–242.
16. Strich SJ: Shearing of nerve fibers as a cause of brain damage due to head injury: a pathological study of twenty cases. Lancet, 1961; 2(Aug 26):443–446.
17. Oehmichen M: Mononuclear Phagocytes in the Central Nervous System. Philadelphia: Saunders, 1978.

18. Clark, JM: Distribution of microglial clusters in the brain after head injury. J Neurol Neurosurg Psychiatry, 1974; 463–474.

19. Kennedy JC: Investigations of the early fate and removal of subarachnoid blood. Pacific Med Surg, 1967; 75:163–168.

20. Strassmann G: Formation of hemosiderin and hematoidin after traumatic and spontaneous cerebral hemorrhage. Arch Pathol, 1949; 47:205–210.

21. Corsellis JAN, Brierley JB: Observations on the pathology of insidious dementia following head injury. J Ment Sci 1959; 105:714–720.

22. Baggenstoss AH, Kernohan JW, Drapiewski JF: The healing process in wounds of the brain. Am J Clin Pathol, 1943; 13:333–348.

23. Grcevic, N: Topography and pathogenic mechanisms of lesion in "inner cerebral trauma." Rad Yug Acad Sci, 1982; 402:265–331.

24. Adams JH, Graham DI, Murray OLS, Scott G: Diffuse axonal injury to non-missile head injury in humans: An analysis of 45 cases. Ann Neurol, 1982; 12:557–563.

— 3

Emergency Management of Head Injury

Neal Little

Overview

Head injury is a common occurrence and a serious health problem (1), accounting for 2% of all deaths and 26% of injury deaths reported in the United States (2). Head injury is one of the most significant components in multiple trauma and is among the most serious causes of long-term morbidity. Sixty to seventy percent of all motor vehicle accidents result in some type of head injury. Blunt head injuries rarely occur as an isolated event; there are associated injuries in most cases, the most significant being those to the cervical spine, and the most common being extremity injuries. Associated injuries may be difficult to detect because of the impaired mental status of the head-injured patient. Clinically, the most important historical symptom of head injury is loss of consciousness, because this correlates best, although very roughly, with the forces involved. The duration of both retrograde and antegrade amnesia is the next most important sign in evaluation of patients with head injury who have lost consciousness and subsequently awakened. Whereas the duration of the amnesia is by no means itself an absolute indicator of the degree of CNS injury, it is one of the best rough clinical indicators commonly available of the severity of the head injury.

The spectrum of severity of head injuries is wide. The physician must be able to deal with the most severely head-injured patient and likewise have a systematic approach to diagnosis and treatment of even the most trivial head injury. In this chapter injuries to the

14

Table 3.1. Glasgow Coma Scale.

Patient response	Score
Best eye-opening response	
Opens eyes on own	4
Opens eyes when asked in a loud voice	3
Opens when pinched	2
Does not open	1
Best motor response	
Follows simple commands	6
Pulls examiner's hand away when pinched	5
Pulls body part away when pinched	4
Flexes body inappropriately when pinched	3
Becomes rigid and extended when pinched	2
Does not respond to pinch	1
Best verbal response	
Carries on conversation, oriented to person,	
month, year	5
Confused, disoriented	4
Talks but words make no sense	3
Unintelligible sounds	2
No noise	1

head will be divided into three arbitrary categories. It must be understood that any artificial categorization may not apply to all cases—familiarity with the full spectrum of head injuries is essential for any physician called upon to assess head trauma, and it establishes the context in which minor head trauma is diagnosed and treated. For the purposes of discussion and categorization, head injuries will be defined as severe, moderate, and mild. There have been multiple attempts to classify head injuries by using injury-severity scales. These scales are most useful in retrospective analysis, or when studying large populations, following patients over time, or trying to predict morbidity and mortality on a long-term basis. They are not, however, very useful in the initial evaluation and disposition of individual patients seen in an acute-care setting. The most popular of these scales is the Glasgow Coma Scale (3), which is reproduced in Table 3.1. Although a particular number on the Glasgow Coma Scale is not a determinant of the etiology of the neurologic injury, the scale does emphasize important aspects of the neurologic exam. These are best motor response, eye opening, and verbal response.

Severe Head Injury

For the purposes of this chapter, the term *severe head injury* will be used to indicate trauma that results in a patient who is comatose upon initial evaluation or has a profoundly altered level of conscious-

Table 3.2. Initial exam and stabilization in severe head injury.

Airway, breathing, circulation, cervical spine immobilization, compression of
   hemorrhage
Pupils: best motor response
Establish IV access, x-ray cervical spine, intubate
Secondary screening exam for associated injuries, including peritoneal lavage or other
   study to exclude intra-abdominal bleeding
Secondary more detailed neurologic exam
Pupils: best motor response repeatedly

ness. The most important parts of the neurologic exam are the examination of the pupils and motor response. A summary of the initial exam and stabilization priorities are listed in Table 3.2. Whereas in more traditional textbooks on coma (4) the respiratory pattern has been emphasized as an important sign in localizing the level of involvement of the nervous system, in the setting of severe acute head injury, with the commonly present multiple associated injuries, the respiratory pattern loses its significance for several reasons. Associated injuries may produce a degree of shock or acidosis, pulmonary injury, or severe pain which may so alter the respiratory status as to make its localizing value unreliable. Indeed, 50% of patients with severe head injuries caused by blunt trauma have additional major injuries. Moreover, immediate control of the airway is such an important intervention in the early care of these patients that they are not allowed fully to develop what might be an otherwise unhindered respiratory pattern (5). Control of the airway and ventilation has therapeutic value (6), so the localizing value of the respiratory pattern is less useful in this setting than it is in other cases of coma.

Doll's-eye maneuvers, one of the standard diagnostic tests used in the comatose patient, are likewise not utilized in severely head-injured patients because of the likelihood of concomitant cervical spine injury and the need to maintain cervical immobilization. Cold-water calorics are a safer and far more reliable way to obtain the information gleaned by doll's-eyes maneuvers. Virtually all patients with severe head injury will require a neurodiagnostic study, and it would be unusual for the results of caloric testing to be useful in initial therapeutic decisions. Such information may be useful in determining severity of injury for prognostic reasons, however. In the initial evaluation of such patients, it is obvious that the standard ABC's of acute care must be followed first: that is, management of the airway, assurance of breathing, and guarantee of effective cardiac output. The already damaged brain will not be improved by hypovolemia; and thus fluid restriction, commonly employed in the ongoing management of patients, should not be instituted until effective volume recussitation is accomplished. It cannot be emphasized strongly enough that, in multiple trauma patients, a detailed neurologic exam must at times take second place to the evaluation and treatment of shock or potential shock and blood loss. Once the basics have been taken care of and a quick review of the patient's injuries has been obtained, a rapid screening neurologic exam should be performed.

Pitfalls in Assessing Severe Head Injury

It is worth discussing several potential pitfalls in the assessment of the severe CNS injury. These are listed in Table 3.3. Although in the older literature Cushing's sign was used to correlate with a severe head injury or the presence of an intracranial mass, its presence is a very late and/or unreliable finding with expanding intracranial mass. Moreover, the classic combination of elevated blood pressure and slowed pulse may never be seen with a large intracranial mass (7), or it may be such a late finding that it is useless in directing therapy. Likewise, papilledema is a sign that one should never see in an acute head injury. Many hours (8) and potentially several days are required for papilledema to develop, even in the presence of severe intracranial hypertension (9). While subhyaloid hemorrhages indicate severe intracranial hypertension and occur because of the sudden rapid increase in intracranial pressure, they are rarely found in severe trauma (except rarely in children) and do not occur in patients with minor trauma. Therefore determining their presence is of little value, making examination of the fundus a relatively unimportant part of the neurologic exam in trauma.

There are several purposes served by the initial neurologic screening exam: first, to establish the patients's severity of neurologic injury; second, to obtain a reliable baseline exam; and third, to establish whether the patient has either signs a focal intracranial mass lesion or severe neurologic deficit, which could potentially be due to either lateralized or nonlateralized mass intracranial lesions. Whereas the traditional sign of an expanding mass intracranial lesion—that is, the unilateral dilated and fixed pupil (Hutchinson's pupil) with contralateral hemiparesis—is the most common classic sign of an expanding mass lesion (the tentorial pressure cone), one must also be aware of a less common phenomenon known as "Kernohan's notch" (10). This is

Table 3.3. Pitfalls in severe head injury.

Cushing's sign
Papilledema
Dilated pupil from local trauma
Kernohan's notch

a paradoxical motor sign where one would has a unilateral dilated and fixed pupil with an ipsilateral hemiparesis or hemiplegia. In the traditional uncal herniation or tentorial pressure cone, the patient develops a contralateral hemiparesis because of compression on the ipsilateral cerebral peduncle, which results in contralateral hemiparesis. With Kernohan's notch, the brainstem is pushed to the contralateral side of the tentorium and the contralateral cerebral peduncle and third nerve are then impinged on by the edge of the tentorium, resulting in hemiparesis ipsilateral to the mass, and dilated pupil.

Local trauma to the eye may result in a dilated and fixed pupil, owing to contusion of the ciliary ganglion (11). Usually the presence of a dilated and fixed pupil in the head trauma patient justifiably causes serious concern about an expanding intracranial mass lesion. While local trauma to the eye may be the ultimate diagnosis, it usually is one of exclusion after a diagnostic imaging study has ruled out a hematoma.

Shock is unlikely to result from intracranial injury alone except in the immediate per-terminal state, or as a result of severe concomitant spinal cord injury. Therefore, one should assume initially that shock in the head-injured patient with blunt trauma is due to other injury.

Intracranial Lesions in Severe Head Injury

With severely head-injured patients, one must look for, or try to exclude the presence of, a mass intracranial lesion, that is, a hematoma (see Table 3.4). Approximately 50% of severely head-injured patients will have an intracranial hematoma (12). Epidural hematoma, that is, bleeding into the epidural space, usually occurs from a laceration of the middle meningeal artery (13). This produces arterial bleeding and therefore a rapid change in the patient's neurologic symptoms. The classic history is that of an initial loss of consciousness followed by a lucid interval (14), during which time the patient may either awaken fully or at least show improvement in level of consciousness. This classically is followed by a subsequent rapid

Table 3.4. Etiologies of neurologic deficit in head injury.

Subdural hematoma
Epidural hematoma
Intracerebral hematoma
Cerebral cortical contusion
Brainstem injury
Acute hydrocephalus
Cerebral edema
Intracranial hypertension

deterioration. The initial episode of unconsciousness in head-injured patients is usually due to axial distortion, or twisting of the brainstem from the blow to the head. After a blow to the head, there is a great deal of movement of the brain inside the cranium and twisting motion which distorts the brainstem. This results in temporary cessation of activity in the ascending reticular activating system and/or cerebral cortical structures, and thus there is loss of consciousness. The patient may recover from this, but the injury will have produced a second lesion, which results in bleeding; and the bleeding causes a progression in neurologic signs and symptoms. Most commonly, deterioration ensues rapidly, that is, less than 24 hours after trauma, but in rare cases, onset may be delayed four days or longer. With rapid head CT scanning of the trauma patient one may miss the development of the epidural hematoma, and thus neurologic deterioration subsequent to the initial scan may need to be reevaluated with repeat CT (15).

The more common hematoma seen in patients with severe head injury is a subdural hematoma. There may or may not be a lucid interval that can be recognized in these patients. The pathogenesis of a lesion is usually that of a tearing of the veins which bridge from the cerebral cortex to the venous sinuses in the dura. Movement of the brain inside the skull tears these veins, with a resultant venous bleeding. Because the venous bleeding takes place at a somewhat slower rate, the patients frequently present with a less than catastrophic decline in mental status and level of consciousness. However, large lesions can obviously result in a profound neurologic deficit. It must also be noted, however, that patients who have this tearing of the small veins because of movement of the brain inside the head frequently have concomitant injury to the brain itself, with resultant contusion or laceration of brain substance, so all the deficit may not be due to the hematoma. The treatment, once again, is prompt evacuation of the clot (16). Depending on its size and patient status.

Intracerebral hematomas happen as a result of head injury because of shearing forces in the brain. The brain substance itself has tears in it, with resultant bleeding that dissects along the pathway of the shearing force. This then results in a focal neurologic deficit relative to the brain area involved, and the deficit is usually the result of the combined compressive forces of the hematoma on the brain and the disruption of neural tissue itself. The history of these patients may be similar to that of patients with subdural hematoma; however, it is common for the hematoma to become visible on CT in a somewhat delayed fashion, that is, 6 to 24 hours post-trauma (17). Intracerebral hematoma patients will frequently have focal findings, although many patients have several intracerebral lesions, and thus multifocal findings. The timing of surgery for these patients—if, in fact surgery is done at all—is highly variable. The decision to remove the hematoma is most dependent on size, location, clinical course, and intracranial pressure. Hence, the initial baseline evaluation of the patient will be useful in deciding the course of therapy based on subsequent improvement or deterioration. Even though the patho-physiological events are discussed separately, there may be some component of all of them in any given patient and in different areas of the brain in the same patient. Patients with disruption of neural tissue and/or brain injury may develop diffuse intravascular coagulation [18,19] because of the effect of brain tissue in the bloodstream initiating the coagulation cascade [20].

Patients who are in this category of severe head injury may not have an intracranial mass lesion: approximately 50% will not. Their deficits are due either to brain swelling or a contusion of tissue, injury to the brainstem, or to a process of progressive cerebral edema and elevated intracranial pressure. Sixty to eighty percent of patients with severe head injury will have elevated intracranial pressure [21] (greater than 10 mmHg to 15 mmHg). Edema in the brain, as else-where in the body, tends to beget edema. Once swelling has started, venous congestion and poor venous return occurs, which in turn causes increased venous pressure and more edema. The relationship between intracranial pressure and the partial pressure of carbon dioxide in the blood is such that hypercarbia increases and hypocarbia decreases intracranial pressure. P_{CO_2} is the chief regulator of cerebral blood flow. At relatively low or normal levels of intracranial pressure, modest changes in the P_{CO_2} result in relatively small changes in intracranial pressure.

However, once the intracranial pressure is elevated, changes in P_{CO_2} have dramatic effects on intracranial pressure [22]. This is the rationale for hyper-ventilation of the head-injured patient and also for aggressive airway management. Oxygenation may also be impaired, either from concomitant lung or chest injury or neurogenic pulmon-ary edema [23].

Initial Therapy in Severe Head Injury

There are several ways to control elevated intracranial pressure. As already mentioned, one of the most effective, easiest to establish, and safest methods is that of hyperventilation to reduce the P_{CO_2}. The optimum P_{CO_2} to achieve for lower intracranial pressure is 25 mmHg [24,25]. The next most frequently employed method to lower intra-cranial pressure is the use of osmotic diuretics, the most common of which is mannitol. Glycerol and urea can also be used [26]. The usual dose of mannitol is 0.5 to 1.0 mg/kg, or 12 to 25 g, in the adult [27].

Barbiturates also lower intracranial pressure. The medium- to short-acting barbiturates are most commonly employed for this purpose, and they act in a very rapid and predictable fashion. Though rarely employed, hypothermia (28) is another technique used in the management of severe head injury to lower intracranial pressure and cerebral edema. Consideration of the use of such agents as barbiturates will depend on other treatment priorities and monitoring capabilities. Furosemide has also been used to lower intracranial pressure (29).

The use of potent corticosteroids is no longer as popular as it was in the past. There is considerable controversy (30,31) about whether they have any effect on intracranial pressure (32), traumatic brain edema, or outcome in severe head injury (33). There are certain insults to the nervous system in which steroids seem to be beneficial, but trauma is not one of them. Potent corticosteroids given in the setting of trauma may increase septic complications (34).

At times the management of a patient with a massively elevated intracranial pressure requires the use of an intracranial pressure monitor (35–37). There are no reliable clinical signs of elevated intracranial pressure; and just as with blood pressure, one must have a measurement in order to treat on an active, reliable, and continual basis. If no contraindications exist, some authors suggest that these patients should be placed in a 30- to 45-dealed head-up position to lower intracranial pressure (38,39) but only if adequate hydration exists and wide variations in blood pressure are unlikely (40). These therapeutic aspects are summarized in Table 3.5.

Seizures in the setting of a head injury are common (41). They may happen immediately when the head is struck as a result of a sudden contusion of the cortex and resulting electric discharge. The prognosis is good and the seizure probably only reflects the sudden contusion of the cortex. However, the seizure may be a sign of a subdural hematoma, and the resultant lethargy may obscure neurologic findings. One should at least suspect subdural hematoma in a patient who has had a seizure after head injury. Also, after the seizure, the patient may be unconscious and may have focal neurologic signs that could be due to a mass lesion or the postictal state alone. Patients

Table **3.5.** Initial therapeutic considerations in severe head injury.

Cervical-spine immobilization
Intubation and hyperventilation to $P_{CO_2} = 25$ mmHg
Head up 30 degrees
Maintain perfusion and blood pressure
Consider mannitol 12–25 g IV
Urinary catheter

with head injuries that are most prone to having seizures are those with penetrating injury to the brain either from depressed skull fractures or missile or knife wounds (42). Such patients should have immediate seizure prophylaxis, because if a patient in this category does have a seizure, reliable information as to whether the patient's neurologic status has changed or not will be unavailable. The patient could be obtunded on the basis of a developing mass intracranial lesion. Development of focal neurologic deficits would have the same potential etiology after a seizure. It is therefore much better to prevent a seizure than to worry about the changes that occur after a seizure and to wonder whether they are due to an expanding mass lesion or a postictal state. However, despite seizure prophylaxis, many patients will still experience seizures.

Immediately after a seizure occurs, the usefulness of the neurologic exam in evaluating the patient's progression of signs and symptoms is greatly decreased. Seizures also produce elevation of intracranial pressure and may exacerbate other injuries, such as long-bone fractures. For this reason aggressive seizure management is warranted.

Once the baseline intravenous access, cervical spine stabilization, and compression of obvious hemorrhage have been obtained, management of the patient with severe head injury should include intubation both to protect the airway and to control the Pco_2. Patients with severe head injury require a definitive study to rule out mass intracranial lesion. The study of choice in acute injury is an unenhanced (43) CT scan (44,45). Magnetic resonance imaging may detect more lesions, particularly contusions (46,47), but for the first 24 hours post-injury the CT scan is more sensitive for subdural or epidural hematomas, which are the most important entities to diagnose or exclude with the study because of their surgical implications. Most of the lesions that can be found with MRI and not CT are not specifically treated, and thus are not an initial priority. After 24 hours, MRI is more sensitive for blood and may have a role in the longer-term management of the patient. If CT is unavailable, other studies, such as cerebral angiography, may be acceptable. Nuclear brain scan is relatively useless for the purposes described above. Skull x-rays do not reveal anything that a CT scan would not (48,49), so if one must make plans for a diagnostic test, one should proceed immediately to the CT scan in this category of patient.

One should have obtained the cervical spine series, lateral, AP, and odontoid prior to the CT scan because of the head positioning required for the scan, or one may keep the patient's neck immobilized if proceeding directly to CT prior to cervical x-rays. Initial diagnostic tests are summarized in Table 3.6. Potential complications of severe head injury, which can occur in an immediate or delayed fashion, are listed in Table 3.7.

Table 3.6. Diagnostic tests in severe head injury.

Cervical spine x-rays
CT scan or angiogram
Arterial blood gasses
Baseline CBC, electrolytes, BUN, glucose, coagulation status

Table 3.7. Complications of severe head injury.

Delayed-onset intracranial hematomas, cerebral edema
Meningitis, cerebral abscesses
Hydrocephalus
Neurogenic pulmonary edema
Cardiac arrhythmia
Diffuse intravascular coagulation
Syndrome of inappropriate Antidiuretic hormone secretion
Seizures

Moderate Head Injury

Moderate head injury involves some alteration of level of consciousness short of coma and/or focal neurologic signs. Most patients with minor head injury as defined in this book fall into this category. Concussion, by definition, means transient loss of a neurologic function as a result of trauma, with rapid return to normal. Usually this means loss of consciousness (50), but other temporary losses, such as visual loss, also qualify. One must be sure very early in the evaluation of the patient that mild change in mental status is not due to shock or hypoxia from other injuries. One can never ascribe shock or hypotension to head injury alone, because a person cannot lose enough blood into the brain to cause hypovolemia without dying from intracranial injury long before hypovolemia becomes apparent. Only rare exceptions occur in infants.

One may attribute a patient's altered mental status to intoxicants such as alcohol or other drugs; however, one must be wary in ascribing altered mental status purely to the effects of alcohol in a patient who has had a head injury. This is obviously one of the clinician's most difficult and challenging diagnostic problems. Patients with moderate head injury should be watched closely for progressions of signs that may indicate the development of a mass intracranial lesion. While it is not common for these patients to develop lesions requiring neurosurgical intervention, some do (3% in one study) (51).

In moderate-head-injury patients, skull x-rays may have some usefulness (52–54). A fracture across the middle meningeal groove or venous sinuses would prompt one to be very aggressive in the management of the patient because of the potential for development of intracranial hematoma. Fractures across the sinuses, particularly the frontal sinus, may require management of the sinus injury itself. As with all tests, a negative skull x-ray does not exclude the presence of significant intracranial injury; serial neurologic exams, separated by short intervals, are the most useful methodology. The progression or regression of signs and symptoms will allow for more precise management and facilitate a decision about ordering a CT scan for these patients. Patients progressing rapidly should be considered for a definitive diagnostic test for an intracranial mass lesion and/or preparation for surgery. Some patients with moderate head injury may (55) need to be observed in a hospital setting (56). Although this is an individual decision in each case, several factors would encourage admission: for example, if the patient has a skull fracture (especially across the middle meningeal artery or venous sinuses or basilar skull); if the patient is an infant, an elderly person, or someone unlikely to be observed closely at home (57); or if the patient shows a neurological deficit. Observation is most appropriately done in a hospital with a neurosurgery service.

Objects protruding from the head as a result of penetrating trauma should never be removed. While the foreign body is still lodged in the head it provides tamponade of bleeding vessels. Release of the tampon can cause catastrophic bleeding and deterioration of the patient. Penetrating foreign objects should be removed only in the operating room under controlled conditions.

In the setting of acute trauma, it is frequently impossible to detect CSF rhinorrhea or otorrhea because of the blood that mixes with the CSF from associated facial injuries. It probably occurs more often than it is detected and subsequently seals itself. Intracranial air, is present in 20% of cases (58) of CSF leakage.

Mild Head Injury

In this section the patient with a mild closed head injury will be discussed. A mild head injury involves either no loss of consciousness or a very brief loss of consciousness and a normal neurologic exam. One must also include those without signs or suspicion of penetrating injury to the head or depressed skull fracture. A very common example of this would be a young child with a mild head injury sustained at school brought in by parents for evaluation. The disposition of these patients will obviously depend a great deal on the assessment of the severity of injury and the time lag between injury and examination. In such patients there is nothing more useful than a very thorough neurologic exam. A great deal of reassurance can be communicated to the family by a thorough, professional neurologic exam, testing such things as gait and tandem walking and finger–nose testing. This thoroughness does a great deal more to reassure concerned parties than do such things as skull x-rays. It is important in these patients, as in others, to palpate the head. As a general rule, in children older than two to three years of age, if there is no clinical sign of a skull fracture—that is, no particular spot on the head that is very tender—and none of the other signs that suggest skull fracture—such as CSF rhinorrhea or otorrhea, Battle's sign, or depressed skull fracture—the usefulness of a skull x-ray is extremely limited. There is a large volume of literature concerning the usefulness of skull x-rays in this setting (59–72) and the greater efficacy of CT (73). There is also an abundance of literature suggesting that, in general, x-rays are not useful in the further management of the patient. Of course, there are exceptions to this; however, thorough documentation of a normal exam along with the assurance of a competent neurologic observation is a much more useful disposition for the patient than is detection of an occult skull fracture. A difficult question in these patients is when, if ever, to x-ray. Some of the criteria that are useful are mentioned above in the section on moderate head injury. Several others that might be considered would be a significant injury directly over the region of the frontal sinus which could have resulted in at least an outer-table depressed fracture of the frontal sinus which might require ENT evaluation, or the presence of a ventricular shunt. In very young children, especially if child abuse is suspected, an x-ray of the skull may be useful in selected cases.

Other questions with respect to mild-head-injury patients have to do with how long they should be observed and by whom. As a general rule most of these patients can be discharged from the emergency department. If there is any question about the observer's reliability, the patient may be kept in the emergency department for somewhat extended periods of time, until a reliable observer can be found. In rare instances the patient may need hospitalization for observation. A more significant question is that of admission for all skull fractures. Patients with skull fractures are frequently admitted to the hospital for neurologic observation. However, it is unusual in the patient who has a relatively benign history, normal exam, and a skull fracture not in a "dangerous area" to find progression of neurologic symptoms to suggest developing intracranial mass. Dangerous injuries include fractures across the middle meningeal artery or venous sinus and at times fractures posteriorly in the skull, because posterior fossa hematomas may present with catastrophic suddenness. There is no unanimity among practitioners concerning when and whether some of these patients should be admitted for observation, and an individual decision must be reached concerning each case. Computed tomography scan is probably more cost-effective than admission, and a negative CT reliably predicts that intracranial sequalae will not occur in this category of patients.

Patients who present for evaluation several days or weeks after the initial trauma can also pose a diagnostic dilemma. Common symptoms seen after head injury are headache (74), dizziness, and difficulty concentrating (75,76). By themselves they are not predictors of delayed complications of head injury, that is, chronic subdural hematoma, subdural hygroma, or post-traumatic hydrocephalus. The degree to which these patients require such studies as CT scan is variable. In general, in light of a completely normal, thorough neurologic exam and adequacy and reliability of follow-up, further studies are not in order immediately for most of these patients. Special circumstances may weigh in favor of definitive studies such as CT or MRI, and an individual judgment must be made for exceptions to the guidelines given above. Examples of such special circumstances include impaired coagulation, for example, coumadin (77); preexisting ventricular shunt for hydrocephalus; unreliability of observation or follow-up; or frequency of presentation for evaluation.

Pediatric Head Injury

In cases of very young children with head injury, that is, children under the age of two years, the history and examination should include several factors that would not be considered in an adult. It is rare to find in the history a reliable reporting of neurologic deficits such as weakness, numbness, or double vision. The examination of children is rarely as formal as that of adults. Observation of behavior and normal coordinated motor acts constitutes the majority of the examination. As mentioned in the section on severe head injury, a subhyaloid hemorrhage in children is at times indicative of a sudden rise in intracranial pressure. A sunken fontanel with the child in the sitting position and not crying is the best and most reliable clinical sign that the intracranial pressure is not high. The fontanel is the most sensitive and the earliest sign in children with head injury. Also, because of the open fontanel and the expansion of the intracranial sutures, it is rare to find focal neurologic signs in children even with an expanding hematoma. The history of an expanding hematoma may be a head injury with a sudden loss of consciousness followed by a relatively more alert period, and then subsequent deterioration consisting of such nonspecific symptoms as lethargy, poor feeding, irritability, and then catastrophic respiratory arrest and death. One rarely progresses through the focal findings of unilaterally dilated pupil, focal hemiparesis, etc. This should also make one aware that these signs should not be looked for to assess the severity of head injury. Level of consciousness and arousability remain the most sensitive indicators. Children who have a ventricular shunt for hydrocephalus for whatever reason are more at risk for the development of sudden deterioration from subdural hematoma because they have an additional pressure-release system whereby the brain can shift an enormous amount without development of signs of intracranial mass. When the brain's capacity to shift has been expended, a sudden catastrophic demise occurs. Such patients should be treated as a special category, and more aggressive management is in order.

Because of the nonspecificity of signs of neurological deterioration in young children, one must be assured that if the child is released from the emergency department the observes are competent and concerned and can return the child promptly for reevaluation. Child abuse can take the form not only of direct blows to the head, but also of vigorous shaking, which can produce a subdural hematoma and multiple areas of intracerebral hematomas [78].

Pediatric patients can develop a syndrome of sudden, massively elevated intracranial pressure with increased cerebral blood flow and increased cerebral blood volume [79]. Mannitol is not recommended in this setting because it increases cerebral blood flow [80]. One is more liberal in ordering skull x-rays in children under age one year, because fracture may be present without the clinical criteria already mentioned, and particularly if a shunting tube is in place. Also, children with a very localized force to the head (such as from a hammer) should be x-rayed to detect depressed fracture [81], although CT will detect the fracture if the radiographer is alerted to the specific area in question and does cuts through it.

Other Considerations

A hospital that does not have neurosurgery capability is in a particularly difficult position with regard to all forms of head injury. Patients with severe head injury frequently have other severe injuries, and the timing of transfer to a center with a neurosurgeon becomes an extremely difficult question of judgment. One must try to stabilize the patient hemodynamically and prevent further harm. One must also to some degree diagnose and treat acute injuries; but on the other hand, one cannot take a great deal to assess head-injured patients who will receive definitive care elsewhere. The timing of various interventions in these patients must be determined by the specific circumstances of the injury—the patient's presentation, distance to other hospitals, availability of specialists, etc. As a general rule, if one cannot exclude the development of an intracranial mass lesion and one must send a patient elsewhere for treatment, all speed should be used in the transfer with only the establishment of an intravenous line, stabilization of the cervical spine, assurance of the airway (82), and splinting of suspected fractures. Detection of occult intra-abdominal bleeding is relatively useless in this setting unless it can be dealt with quickly—before the head injury can progress. This is obviously a difficult judgment to make. As discussed above, patients with moderate head injury who will need neurologic observation should not be observed in a setting or on a service that cannot render definitive treatment should the development of a mass intracranial lesion occur.

Summary

The most useful parts of the neurologic exam in patients with head injury are as follows: in the comatose patient the appearance of the pupils, extraocular movements, and best motor response: in patients with moderate head injury, level of consciousness, repeated mental status and pupillary exam, and any drift of the outstretched extremities on the motor exam. The less useful parts of the neurologic exam in the setting of acute injury are examination of the fundus, detailed sensory exams, and tests of reflexes and Babinski's signs (83). Initial therapy in the patient with severe head injury is directed at providing a milieu optimal for recovery of damaged brain and prevention of secondary injury. Control of Pco_2 and Pco_2 and adequate perfusion should be accomplished while provisions for definitive diagnostic modalities, that is, CT scan, are being made. In patients with minor head injury, a thoroughly conducted exam including appropriate imaging and reliable observation are usually all that is in order in the acute management period.

References

1. Anderson DW, McLaurin RL (eds): National head and spinal cord. J Neurosurg, 1980; 53:S1–S43.
2. Sosin D, Sacks J, Smith S: Head injury-associated deaths in the united states from 1976–1986. JAMA, 1989; 262:16, 2251–2255.
3. Teasdale G, Jennett B: Assessment of coma and impaired consciousness, a practical scale. Lancet, 1974; 2:81–84.
4. Plum F, Posner J: The Diagnosis of Stupor and Coma. Philadelphia: Davis, 1980; pp 32–40.
5. Mill JD, et al.: Early insults to the injured brain. JAMA, 1978; 240(pt 5): 439–442.

6. Enevoldsen E, et al.: Autoregulation and CO_2 responses of cerebral blood flow in patients with acute severe head injury. J Neurosurg, 1978; 48: 689–703.
7. Eliasson S, Prensky A, Hardin W (eds): Neurological Pathophysiology. New York: Oxford University Press, 1974.
8. McCrary JA, Smith JL: Neuro-ophthalmological evaluation of the neurosurgical patient. In Youmans J (ed): Neurological Surgery. Philadelphia: Saunders, 1973.
9. Singer HS, et al.: Head trauma for the pediatrician. Pediatrics, 1978; 62(pt 5):819.
10. Weston PAM: Admission policy for patients following head injury. Br J Surg, 1981; 68:663–664.
11. Byrnes D: Head injury and the dilated pupil. Am Surg, 1979; 45(pt 3):139.
12. Becker DP, et al.: The outcome from severe head injury with early diagnosis and intensive management. J Neurosurg, 1977; 47:491–502.
13. Geigy Pharmaceuticals: Head Injury, Principles of Modern Management. Neurol Clin, 1982; 4(3).
14. Cordobes F, et al.: Observations on 82 patients with extradural hematoma. J Neurosurg, 1981; 54:179–186.
15. Borovich B, Braun J, et al.: Delayed onset of traumatic extradural hematoma. J Neurosurg, 1985; 63:30–34.
16. Seelig JM, et al.: Traumatic acute subdural hematoma. N Engl J Med, 1981; 25:304.
17. Soluniuk D, Pitts L, et al.: Traumatic intracerebral hematomas: Timing of appearance and indications for operative removal. J Trauma, 1986; 26:9, 878–794.
18. Van Der Sander JJ, et al.: Head injuries and coagulation disorders. J Neurosurg, 1978; 49(pt 3):357.
19. Miner ME, et al.: Disseminated intravascular coagulation fibrinolytic syndrome following head injury in children: Frequency and prognostic implications. J Pediatr, 1982; 100(pt 5):687.
20. Clark JA, et al.: Disseminated intravascular coagulation following cranial trauma. J Neurosurg, 1980: 52(pt 2):266.
21. Miller JD, et al.: Significance of intracranial hypertension in severe head injury. J Neurosurg, 1977; 47:503–516.
22. Kindt G, Gosch H: Arterial P_{CO_2} effect at various levels of intracranial pressure. In Brock, Dietz (eds): intracranial pressure, experimental and clinical Aspects. Berlin: Springer-Verlag, 1972.
23. Rose J, et al.: Avoidable factors contributing to death after head injury. Br Med J, 1977; 2:616–618.
24. Marshall L, et al.: The outcome with aggressive treatment in severe head injuries. Part 11: acute and chronic barbiturate administration in the management of head injury. J Neurosurg, 1979; 50:26–30.
25. Jones PW: Hyperventilaton in the management of cerebral oedema. Intensive Care Med, 1981; 7(pt 5):205.
26. Levan AB, et al.: Treatment of increased intracranial pressure: A comparison of different osmotic agents and use of thiopental. J Neurosurg, 1979; 5(pt 5):570.

27. Bruce DA, et al.: Resuscitation from coma due to head injury. Crit Care Med, 1978; 6(pt 4):254.
28. Nelson S: Review of therapeutic agents used in head injuries. Curr Concepts Trauma Care, 1977; 1(pt 1):3.
29. Cottrell JE, et al.: Furosemide and head injury. J Trauma, 1981; 21(pt 9): 805.
30. Dick A: The role of steroids in head trauma. Curr Concepts Trauma Care, 1977; 1(pt 1):5.
31. Braakman R, et al.: Megadose steroids in severe head injury: Results of a prospective double-blind clinical trial. J Neurosurg, 1983; 58(pt 3):326.
32. Gudeman SK, et al.: Failure of high-dose steroid therapy to influence intracranial pressure in patients with severe head injury. J Neurosurg, 1979; 51(pt 3):301.
33. Cooper PR, et al.: Dexamethasone and severe head injury: A prospective double-blind study. J Neurosurg, 1979; 51(pt 3):307.
34. DeMaria E, Reichman W, et al.: Septic complications of corticosteroid administration after central nervous system trauma. Ann Surg, 1985; 202:2, 248–252.
35. Marshall L, et al.: The outcome with aggressive treatment in severe head injuries. Part 1: the significance of intracranial pressure monitoring. J Neurosurg, 1979; 50:20–25.
36. Narayan RK, et al.: Intracranial pressure: To monitor or not to monitor? A review of our experience with head injury. J Neurosurg, 1982; 56(pt 5):650.
37. Saul TG, et al.: Effect of intracranial pressure monitoring and aggressive treatment on mortality in severe head injury. J Neurosurg, 1982; 56(pt 4):498.
38. Kenning JA, et al.: Upright patient positioning in the management of intracranial hypertension. Surg Neurol, 1981; 15(pt 2):148.
39. Ropper AH, et al.: Head position, intracranial pressure and compliance. Neurology (NY), 1982; 32(pt 11):1288.
40. Rosner M, Coley I: Cerebral perfusion pressure, intracranial pressure, and head elevation. J Neurosurg, 1986; 65:636–641.
41. Annegers JF, et al.: Seizures after head trauma: A population study. Neurology, (NY) 1980; 30:683–689.
42. Caveness WF, et al.: The nature of posttraumatic epilepsy. J Neurosurg, 1979; 50:545–553.
43. Enhanced computed tomography in head trauma, diagnostic and therapeutic technology assessment. Q&A. JAMA, 1985; 254:23, 3370–3371.
44. Vicario S, et al.: Emergency presentation of subdural hematoma: A review of 85 cases diagnosed by computerized tomography. Ann Emerg Med, 1982; 11(pt 9):475.
45. Gentry L et al.: Prospective comparative study of intermediate field MR and CT in the evaluation of closed head trauma. Am J Roent, 1988; 150:3, 673.
46. Jenkins A, Teasdale G, Hadley M, et al.: Brain lesions detected by magnetic resonance imaging in mild and severe head injuries. Lancet, 1986; Aug 23, 445–446.

47. Hadley D: Magnetic resonance imaging in acute head injury. Clin Radiol, 1988; 39(2), 131–136.
48. Tress BM: The need for skull radiography in patients presenting for CT. Radiology, 1983; 146(pt 1):87.
49. Healy JF, et al.: Computed tomographic evaluation of depressed skull fractures and associated intracranial injury. Comput Radiol, 1982; 6(pt 6): 323.
50. Parkinson D: Concussion. Mayo Clin Proc, 1977; 52:492–496.
51. Dacey R, Alves W, et al.: Neurosurgical complications after apparently minor head injury. J Neurosurg, 1986; 65:203–210.
52. De Campo T, et al.: How useful is the skull x-ray examination in trauma? Med J Aust, 1980; 2(pt 10):553.
53. Phillips L: Emergency services utilization of skull radiography. J Neurosurg, 1979; 4(pt 6):580.
54. Phillips L: Emergency services utilization of skull radiography. J Neurosurg, 1979; 4(pt 6):580.
55. Mendelow AD, et al.: Admission after mild head injury: Benefits and costs. Br J Med, 1982; 285:1530.
56. Fischer RP, et al.: Post concussive hospital observation of alert patients in a primary trauma center. J Trauma, 1981; 21(pt 11):920.
57. Karpman RR, et al.: Observation of the alert, conscious patient with closed head injury. Arch Med, 1980; 37(pt 11):772.
58. Chandler J: Traumatic cerebrospinal fluid leakage. J Otolaryngol North Am, 1983; 16(pt 3):623–632.
59. Leonidas JC, et al.: Mild head trauma in children; when is a roentgenogram necessary? Pediatrics, 1982; 69(pt 2):139.
60. Bligh AS, et al.: Patient selection for skull radiography in uncomplicated head injury: A national study by the Royal College of Radiologists. Lancet, 1983; 8316:1–15.
61. A study of the utilization of skull radiography in 9 accident-and-emergency units in the U.K. Royal College of Radiologists. Lancet, 1980; 8206(pt 2):1234.
62. Jennett B: Skull x-rays after recent head injury. Clin Radiol, 1980; 31(pt 4):463.
63. DeSmet AA, et al.: A second look at the utility of radiographic skull examination for trauma. Am J Radiol, 1979; 132:95.
64. Phillips L: Emergency services utilization of skull radiography. J Neurosurg, 1979; 4(pt 6):580.
65. Masters SJ: Evaluation of head trauma: Efficiency of skull films. Am J Roent, 1980; 135(pt 3):539.
66. Cumins RO, et al.: High yield referral criteria for post-traumatic skull roentgenography. JAMA, 1980; 244(pt 7):673.
67. Phillips LA: Comparative evaluation of the effect of a high yield criteria list upon skull radiography. J Am Coll Emerg Phys, 1979; 83:106.
68. Eyes B, et al.: Post-traumatic skull radiographs. Time for reappraisal. Lancet, 1978; 8080(pt 2):85.
69. Balasubramaniam S, et al.: Efficacy of skull radiography, Am J Surg, 1981; 142(pt 3):366.

70. Larsen KT, et al.: High yield criteria and emergency department skull radiography: Two community hospitals experience. J Am Coll Emerg Phys, 1979; 8(10):393.
71. de Lacey G, et al.: Mild head injuries: A source of excessive radiography? Clin Radiol, 1980; 31(pt 4):32.
72. Masters S, McClean P, et al.: Skull x-ray examinations after head trauma, recommendations by a multidisciplinary panel and validation study. N Engl J Med, 1987; 316:84–91.
73. Baker S, Gaylord G, et al.: Emergency skull radiography: The effect of restrictive criteria on skull radiography and CT use. Radiology, 1985; 156:2, 409–413.
74. Rimel RW, et al.: Disability caused by minor head injury. J Neurosurg, 1981; 9(pt 3):221.
75. Wrightson P, et al.: Time off work and symptoms after minor head injury. Injury, 1981; 12(pt 6):445.
76. Rutherford W: Sequelae of concussion caused by minor head injuries. Lancet, 1977; 8001:1–4.
77. Wintzen AD, et al.: Subdural hematoma and oral anticoagulant therapy. Arch Neurol, 1982; 39(pt 2):69.
78. Raphaely RC, et al.: Management of severe pediatric head trauma. Pediatr Clin North Am, 1980; 27(pt 3):715.
79. Bruce DA, et al.: Diffuse cerebral swelling following head injuries in children: The syndrome of "malignant brain edema." J Neurosurg, 1981; 54(pt 2):170.
80. Bruce DA, et al.: Pathophysiology, treatment and outcome following severe head injury in children. Childs Brain, 1979; 5(pt 3):174.
81. Bruce DA, et al.: The value of CAT scanning following pediatric head injury. Clin Pediatr (Phila), 1980; 19(pt 11):719.
82. Gentleman D, Jennett B: Hazards of inter-hospital transfer of comatose head-injured patients. Lancet, 1981; 8251:853–856.
83. Parrish, R: The significance of babinski signs in children with head trauma. Ann Emerg Med, 1985; 14(4):329–342.

— 4

Imaging of Cranioencephalic Trauma

Carlos F. Gonzalez and Sonia Bermudez

Introduction

In the United States alone there are 400,000 patients each year who seek medical attention because of head trauma. Eighty percent of these patients have injuries that are considered serious (1).

Because of the high costs and significant disability associated with head trauma, these injuries constitute a serious health problem. The criteria for qualification as minor trauma include a Glasgow coma index of 13 to 15, loss of consciousness or failure to respond appropriately in less than 20 minutes, and confusion along with retrograde and antegrade amnesia which requires hospitalization. Fifty percent of patients with minor head trauma develop a post-concussion syndrome with symptoms of headache, dizziness, and neuropsychological deficits. Other, more serious complications of minor head injury are asymptomatic extradural hematomas (2), fatal thrombosis of the basilar artery (3), hemorrhage into preexisting conditions such as fibrous dysplasia (4), and essential thrombocytopenia (5).

New diagnostic techniques such as magnetic resonance imaging (MRI) have shown that, in patients with minor brain injuries, small lesions can occur which are frequently related to the neuropsychological deficits occasionally found in these patients. Imaging studies in this group of patients are oriented toward the early detection of complications. It is important to determine when studies such as computed tomography (CT) or MRI are to be performed. Ideally, CT studies should be done on all patients with head trauma, as this

33

would permit an early and safe discharge of patients whose examination is negative (6).

Feuerman et al. (7) recommended that a CT scan be performed on all patients with minor head injury whenever the Glasgow Coma Scale (GCS) is less than 15 and the patient has either an abnormal mental status or hemispheric neurological deficits. Also recommended was that these patients be admitted for observation, since GCS values of 13 and 14 are associated with intracerebral hematoma and/ or further deterioration. Other investigators, however (8,9), prefer plain film of the skull or EEG in order to identify patients who require further examination by CT.

In 1987, a multidisciplinary panel (10,11) divided head-injured patients into three risk groups according to patient history and physical and neurologic findings. Based on this classification, a protocol was developed which includes the use of CT as well as clinical management procedures. Magnetic resonance imaging, at that time, was not as readily available and was therefore not included in the study.

The first group consisted of low-risk, symptomatic patients. No imaging was recommended for these patients. This decision was based on the results of an extensive follow-up of 5,524 low-risk patients in whom there was no evidence of occult intracranial lesions or later sequels. In the second group, high-risk patients, that is, patients with depressed levels of consciousness, focal neurologic signs, or penetrating injuries, emergency CT examination was performed as soon as possible. If the CT was positive, neurosurgical evaluation was necessary. In the third group, moderate-risk patients, including mildly symptomatic patients, the main recommendation was for prolonged clinical observation. If the symptoms persisted or deteriorated or new symptoms occured, CT was performed.

Imaging Methods

Since 1974, CT examination has been considered the "gold standard" for imaging in the evaluation of head trauma. Computed tomography can answer questions previously unresolved by skull films and angiography. Because of its wide availability, ease of use, and ability to demonstrate edema and blood, CT has reduced the need for unnecessary craniotomy procedures by as much as 58% (12) and continues today as the imaging modality of choice in trauma patients.

Magnetic resonance imaging (MRI) is also of considerable value in trauma owing to its ability accurately to demonstrate non-hemorrhagic lesions such as cortical contusions, diffuse axonal injuries, and brainstem injuries. In comparison to CT, MRI correlates better with pathology. Magnetic resonance imaging has the ability to image the cranial or brain area in multiple planes, has improved contrast resolution, and affords more complete visualization of traumatic lesions (13,14). Magnetic resonance imaging also provides a better understanding of the early effects and late consequences of head injury (15). Because of its ability to detect functionally significant abnormalities, MRI helps greatly in predicting the neuropsychological changes important in the patient's outcome (16).

Plain films of the skull are of limited value in the identification of intracranial injuries because of their inability to allow visualization of intracranial soft tissues. Brain tissue, the ventricular system, and blood have approximately the same attenuation value on plain film and cannot therefore be differentiated. Also, plain films cannot directly demonstrate intracranial lesions such as contusions and hematomas.

Fundamental Physical Principles

A brief discussion of fundamental physical principles is essential in understanding the information obtained with the new imaging modalities CT and MRI.

Computed Tomography

In the CT system, images are the final result of x-ray attenuation passing through the element that is being examined. In contrast with the conventional wide x-ray beam, CT uses a very collimated beam that usually rotates. Instead of conventional film, the receptors are detectors which are extremely sensitive to x-ray attenuation. Both the x-ray beam and the detectors are located in the gantry, a circular structure with a central hole in which the organs to be examined are placed. The gantry aperture determines the slice thickness. The information obtained by the detectors is reconstructed using a computer program and placed as CT numbers in a matrix. Hounsfield numbers, or units (HU), that represent density measurements directly related to the attenuation values of the organ studied are displayed in a wide gray color scale. This fact allows for structures with very close attenuation values to be differentiated. The zero value in CT corresponds to water; the negative value of the scale represents fat and air. On the positive side of the scale are the soft tissues, hemoglobin, calcium, bone, and metals. The normal gray matter, for example, has an attenuation coefficient close to 40 HU and a white matter attenuation coefficent close to 30 HU. Structures with the same CT number of gray matter are usually referred to as "isodense." If the structure has a higher or lower CT number, it is called hyperdense or hypodense. A CT number for extravascular blood (hematoma) varies with the hemoglobin concentration, which depends on the age of the hemorrhage. If bleeding is recent with high hemoglobin concentrations, CT will be very hyperdense with CT numbers as high as 90 HU. This density increases at a linear rate as the hemoglobin concentration increases (17).

Magnetic Resonance Imaging

Magnetic resonance imaging has entirely different principles (17,18). The magnetic resonance effects is observed only in nuclei having a net spin, that is, in nuclei having an odd atomic or mass number. Hydrogen has this property and is abundant in the body. It is, therefore, an excellent biological element sensitive to the magnetic resonance process. Magnetic resonance imaging utilizes an external magnetic field to orient the nucleus in the direction of the external field (longitudinal alignment). Radiofrequency excitation waves perpendicular to the field, on the other hand, cause a displacement away from the longitudinal alignment, resulting in a transverse magnetization. The signal, that is, the voltage induced by this transverse magnetization, can be detected and registered by a coil of wire near the body. The nuclei eventually return to their equilibrium state with a relaxation time constant characteristic of the particular tissue.

Two relaxation constants exist, T1 and T2. T1 is governed by the thermal interactions between the resonating protons and other magnetic nuclei in the environment. As a result of this interaction, energy is lost to the environment and the protons regain their longitudinal magnetization. The relaxation time of T2, on the other hand, is a reflection of the decay of the transverse magnetization owing to the existence of different local magnetic fields within the tissue. The selection of different pulse sequences, that is, different ways of exploiting the radiofrequecy and the transverse magnetization, permits us to obtain images that are T1-weighted or T2-weighted. If an element or tissue has a short T1 and T2 time constant, it will be hyperintense in T1-weighted images (white) and hypointense in T2-weighted images (black). For example, water that has long T1 and T2 time constants is visualized as hypointense (black) in T1-weighted images and hyperintense (white) in T2-weighted images. Paramagnetic substances that interact with protons can further be used, in certain cases, to produce shortening of T1 and T2, resulting in tissue contrast enhancement.

Skull Fractures

Linear Fractures

Visualization of linear fractures alone is no longer critical to the patient's management. Since the most important consideration in head trauma is to determine whether associated brain injuries are present, CT is the best method of imaging. Linear fractures are usually visualized on the scout view or bone window display of the CT scan. Plain film of the skull should be performed in case of doubt. CT is critical in demonstrating a depressed skull fracture and the position of the bone fragments. If the depressed fragment is beneath the inner table of the adjacent calvarium, it is important to determine whether or not it overlies a major dural sinus or the motor cortex. Those fractures associated with intracranial air or foreign bodies, and those that compromise the paranasal sinuses or mastoid cells, are also significant because of the risk of intracranial infection. Knowledge of these facts is of considerable importance in the correct diagnosis and management of the patient.

Basilar Fractures

These fractures usually have a typical clinical picture manifested by hemorrhage behind the tympanic membrane, otorrhea or rhinorrea, subcutaneous hematoma surrounding the mastoid process or the orbits, and compression of cranial nerves. Computed tomography of the base of the skull in these cases should be done using thin contiguous slices and bone reconstructions that allow good visualization of the cranial nerve(s) canals and foraminae.

Intracerebral Lesions (Focal)

Cortical Brain Contusion

Cortical brain contusions are small superficial streaks of perivascular hemorrhage associated with variable amounts of necrosis seen usually at right angles of the crests of gyri (19,20). They generally occur at the site of impact and tend to be multiple, producing a mass effect owing to edema on the adjacent neural tissue. Contusions are located mainly in the frontal and temporal lobes, a fact that can be explained by the shape of the skull, since cortical injury is more likely to occur adjacent to the edges of the inner table of the skull, along the floor of the anterior fossa, petrous, and sphenoid ridges. When the impact is against the stationary head with depression of the calvarium against the adjacent brain tissue, the contusion is referred to as a "coup contusion." When the brain is in motion relative to the calvarium, contusions may occur at a site remote from the point of the initial impact; these are commonly referred to as "contra coup" contusions.

Computed tomography in these patients reveals areas of high density corresponding to contusions that are frequently hemorrhagic and surrounded by a low-density area produced by adjacent edema (Fig. 4.1). The mass effect produced by the edema usually increases by the fourth to fifth day (19,20). Contusions by definition are cortical, but their dimensions may reach 2 to 4 cm. The subacute and late stages of the contusions show progression from an isodense CT appearance to an area of low density representing the final scar. Computed tomography and T1-weighted MRI usually underestimate

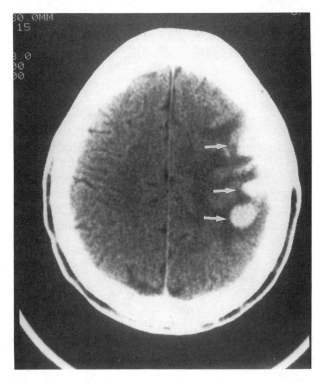

Fig. 4.1. Cortical brain contusion. A 26-year-old woman examined after head injury produced by an automobile accident. *CT scan: axial section.* The examination reveals multiple cortical high-intensity lesions representing hemorrhagic cortical contusions, in the high parietal convexity of the left hemisphere (arrows). Edema of the underlined white matter is visualized.

the true size of the lesions. T2-weighted MR images are significantly more sensitive than T1-weighted images.

In hemorrhagic contusions, MR appearance changes in accordance with the changes in the hemoglobin and in the water present in the lesion (21,22). In the acute stage, deoxyhemoglobin results in shortening of T2. After 3 to 4 days, the conversion of deoxyhemoglobin to methoglobin is visualized as increased signal intensity primarily seen in the T1-weighted images (Fig. 4.2A). Further degradation of the methemoglobin to hemosiderin produces a low signal on T2-weighted images, mainly in the periphery of the hematoma (Fig. 4.2B, arrow). This effect can persist as late as two years after the initial trauma.

The subcortical gray matter contusions that involve the thalamus and lentiform nucleus represent a small percentage of traumatic brain lesions. However, the severity of the neurologic impairment caused by these lesions is serious and the patient usually dies shortly after injury. Hemorrhagic lesions are apparently produced by the rupture of multiple small perforating arterial vessels.

Parasagittal contusions are commonly produced by acceleration of the head without direct impact. They are usually bilateral and symmetric, and are seen in babies in the so-called shaken baby syndrome or in whiplash in adults.

Brainstem Lesions

Patients with these lesions often have severe impairment of consciousness. Usually other traumatic conditions, such as diffuse axonal injuries, are also present. It is important to differentiate between primary and secondary brainstem lesions.

In the primary lesions, torsion forces occurring at the time of injury produce direct impingement of the tentorial edge or clival bone fragment upon the brainstem (23). Rotational acceleration of the head in the lateral direction also occurs (24,25). The patients usually experience immediate and sustained loss of consciousness, abnormal brainstem reflexes (pupillary light oculocephalic and oculovestibular), and respiratory dysfunction. In the secondary brainstem lesions, supratentorial mass effect with subsequent herniation are the causes of the patient's symptoms, which consist of an initial lucid interval with subsequent deterioration of consciousness.

The anatomic distribution of the lesions is also different. Primary lesions are located in the dorsal and dorsolateral aspects of the brainstem and frequently are accompanied by other indirect signs of injury, such as rotation and displacement of the brainstem, and effacement

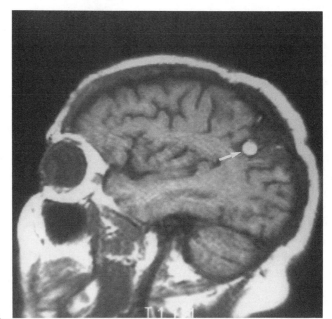

A

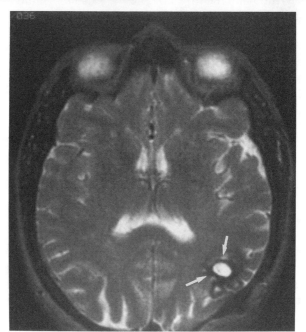

B

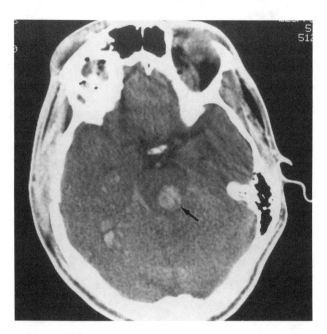

Fig. 4.3. Brainstem hemorrhagic lesion. A 28-year-old male comatose after head injury following a motorcycle accident. *CT scan: axial section.* The examination performed at the level of the brainstem reveals a well-defined, rounded, posteriorly located high-density brainstem hemorrhagic lesion (arrow). Blood is also seen in the ambiens and subtentorial cisternal.

of the adjacent cisterns. Secondary lesions are more commonly found in the ventral paramedian and ventrolateral aspects of the brainstem.

Since CT is quite insensitive to edema and other changes in this area, it is useful mainly in the detection of hemorrhagic lesions (Fig. 4.3). On MRI, brainstem lesions are visualized as areas of low signal intensity in the brainstem. On T2-weighted images, old lesions show atrophy, either focal or diffused (Fig. 4.4). Magnetic resonance imaging, however, is far more sensitive in this location because of its

←————————————————————————

Fig. 4.2. Cortical brain contusion. A 16-year-old boy after a head injury sustained in a diving accident. **A**: *MRI—sagittal T1-weighted image* a few days after the injury. The examination reveals a rounded, well-defined, high-intensity hemorrhagic lesion (methahemoglobin) in the left parietal convexity surrounded by a mild degree of edema (arrow). **B**: *MRI—axial T2-weighted image* taken three weeks after the injury in the same patient. The examination reveals the previously described area of hyperintensity in the left parietal convexity (arrow) surrounded by a halo of hypointensity, representing degradation of the methahemoglobin to hemosiderin.

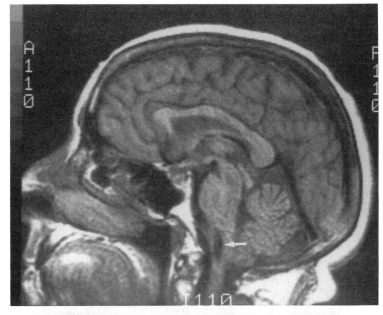

A

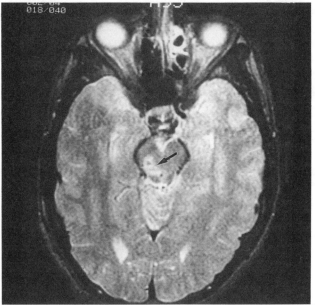

B

Fig. 4.4. Post-traumatic brainstem lesion. A 17-year-old male following CPR car accident. **A**: *MRI-sagittal T1-weighted image*. The examination, performed several weeks after the injury, shows an elongated, well-defined, low-intensity lesion in the upper brainstem (arrow). **B**: *MRI: axial T2-weighted image* of the same patient reveals a high-intensity area in the posterolateral portion of the upper brainstem (arrow), corresponding to the same traumatic brainstem lesion. The patient never recovered from the coma.

better contrast resolution and the absence of significant posterior fossa artifacts.

Intraparenchymal Hematomas

Injuries of vessels (arteries, veins, or both) and laceration of the cortex are usually the cause. A contusion, however, may also result in a homogenous, more confluent intracerebral hematoma, most commonly found in the frontal and temporal lobes.

Although the majority of the hematomas are visualized in the first examination, some may have a delayed appearance. This frequently occurs after surgery for the removal of other traumatic lesions, mainly subdural hematomas.

In the acute phase of the hematoma, the CT appearance consists of a homogenous, well-defined, high-density focus usually surrounded by a small hypodense zone owing primarily to adjacent edema (Fig. 4.5). During the healing of the hematoma, there is a stage in the evolution where neovascularity is present. Ring enhancement following the intravenous injection of contrast media may therefore be seen after the first week of the injury. This enhancement has been known to persist for as long as six to seven weeks. Since hematomas resolve by lysis, they usually leave a residual cavity that later in the process is visualized on CT as a focus of hypodensity associated with focal ventricular dilatation and cortical atrophy. Intracerebral hematomas are readily seen on CT (19).

The products of degradation of hemoglobin have paramagnetic effects, and therefore are responsible for the variable appearance of hemorrhage in accord with its evolution (22). Products of degradation include oxyhemoglobin, deoxyhemoglobin, methemoglobin, and the hemosiderin. Magnetic resonance imaging is extremely sensitive in the characterization of hemorrhagic lesions as well as in determining their age. Oxyhemoglobin and deoxyhemoglobin have a negligible MR effect. The free methemoglobin on the other hand has an important MR effect by producing mainly a T1 shortening and, in minor grade, T2 shotening. Hemosiderin produces an important T2 shortening. In the hyperacute intracranial hemorrhage, extravascular blood has a very similar appearance to intravascular blood; in T1 and T2 images, it appears isointense with the nervous tissue. In subacute hemorrhage (three days to three weeks old) there is red cell lysis and formation of methemoglobin and hemosiderin. The methemoglobin reaches its maximum concentration three to four days after the bleeding. In the early subacute period, the methemoglobin is recognized as a hyperintense "halo" in the T1- and T2-weighted images (Fig. 4.6). In the late subacute period, the entire hematoma becomes

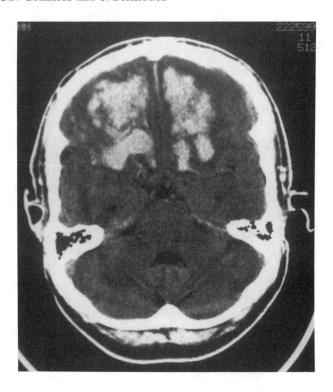

Fig. 4.5. Intracerebral hematoma. A 22-year-old female after head injuries produced by a fall during ballet dancing. *CT of the brain axial sections.* The examination reveals large diffuse areas of increased density involving both frontal lobes, representing large intracerebral hematomas.

hyperintense in T1- and T2-weighted images. The conversion to hemosiderin begins at the periphery of the hematoma and can be recognized early in the T2-weighted images. The associated edema produces a hypointense zone around the hematoma in T1-weighted images and hyperintense zone in T2-weighted images. In old hemorrhages, the partial reabsorption of the clot decreases the size of

Fig. 4.6. Intracerebral hematoma. A 17-year-old male with multiple brain traumatic lesions. **A**: *MRI—sagittal T1-weighted image.* The examination reveals multiple cortical and subcortical hemorrhagic lesions in the left frontal-parietal region. The lesions show a halo of hyperintensity felt to represent methahemoglobin in subacute trauma (arrows). **B**: *MRI—axial T2-weighted images* showing the same changes visualized in the T1-weighted images (arrows).

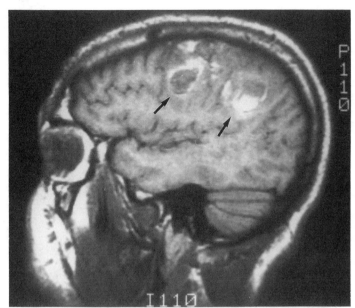

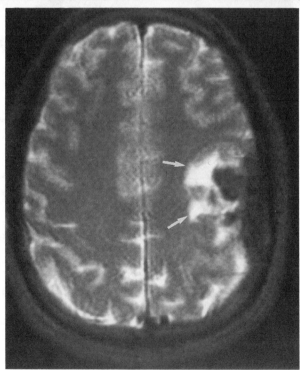

the hematoma and the edema effect as well. Methemoglobin can persist for a long time, with hemosiderin being more apparent. The images are then hyperintense in T1- and T2-weighted images with a well-formed peripheral hypointense halo owing to the hemosiderin. Hemosiderin can be seen on MR imaging of resolved hematomas as a hypointense ring surrounding the CSF residual collection.

Intraventricular Hemorrhage

This occurs with both minor and severe head trauma. Prior to the advent of CT, intraventricular hemorrhage was considered a rare

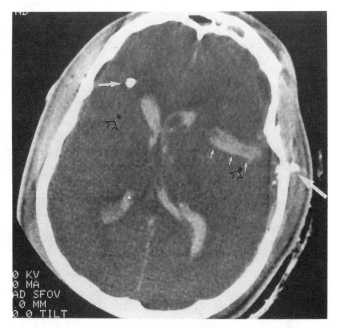

Fig. 4.7. Gunshot injury to the brain. A 36-year-old male shot in the head. *CT of the brain, axial section.* The examination reveals multiple bone and metallic fragments seen in the left temporal region. A significant amount of soft tissue swelling is noted. The bullet tract on the brain is visualized as a well-defined linear area of increased density representing blood in the left frontal temporal region (small closed arrows). There is also a significant amount of blood in the ventricular system that is significantly shifted from left to right due to brain edema. Part of the bullet is seen in the left temporal bone (large closed arrow) and anterior to the right frontal horn (small closed arrow). Multiple punctate areas of low density representing air (open arrows) are visualized in the brain parenchyma of both cerebral hemispheres.

occurrence. Now it can be seen in 2% to 3% of all patients with head trauma, but it is not necessarily associated with a poor prognosis (26) (Fig. 4.7). If the hemorrhage is massive, it could result in severe hydrocephalus, and drainage is then advised (18). Intraventricular hemorrhages are usually associated with other contusions or hemorrhages present in the subcortical or subependymal areas.

Computed tomography easily detects any minor or large intraventricular hemorrhages, which appear as high-density areas and are seen within the ventricles (Fig. 4.7). This collection usually disappears rapidly after the injury in comparison with the evolution of the other types of intracranial hemorrhage (18,29). Magnetic resonance imaging is useful mainly in the detection of associated lesions.

Penetrating injuries

The most common penetrating injury is the gunshot wound. The intracranial lesions produced by a gunshot wound are mainly related to the velocity of the bullet. Low-velocity bullets leave multiple bone and metallic fragments associated with foci of necrosis and hemorrhage (Fig. 4.7). High-velocity bullets leave a well-defined tract of parenchymal damage, usually producing severe damage as a result of centrifugal forces. The penetration of this injury can be determined by the presence of pneumocephalus. However, pneumocephalus may be also due to fractures involving the nasal sinuses or the mastoid cells (27).

Intracranial Lesions (Diffuse)

Shear Lesions—Diffuse Injuries of the Axon

These lesions, also known as shear lesions, are due to the rotational forces occurring during severe trauma. Mostly affected are the deeper areas of the brain where the strongest forces are applied. With the development of new imaging techniques such as MRI, these lesions are now easily identified and have become the most common type of traumatic primary lesion visualized (45.2%) (13,14). The patients in this group usually have a history of unconsciousness at the moment of impact, indicating that the magnitude of the rotational force is great enough to reach the mesencephalon.

Patients with diffuse brain injury can be divided into two types: (I) those who die immediately and (II) those who survive somewhat longer. In group I, petechial hemorrhages are seen in frontal and temporal white matter. In group II, small tears and hemorrhages in midline structures such as the corpus callosum, pons (rostrus), cerebral white matter, and brainstem are also seen. The lesions are smaller than 1 cm, without significant brain swelling, and correspond to ruptures of axons in the cerebral white matter which later evolve to demyelination. The difference between patients in grades I and II is degree rather than type of injury.

The CT examination is not the most accurate method of identifying shear lesions, even though the use of high resolution can be useful (28). On CT, small and discrete areas of hemorrhage without mass effect can be seen in the white matter of frontal and temporal lobes, corpus callosum, and brainstem. Magnetic resonance imaging, however, is more accurate. The lesions are seen as hypointense areas on the T2 sequences (hemosiderin) with central areas of hyperintensity (Fig. 4.8). Peripheral lesions tend to be smaller. They are usually ovoid to elliptical with a long axis parallel to the direction of the nerve bundles. The most typical locations are the corticomedullary interface and the large white matter fiber bundles (corona radiata, corpus callosum [Fig. 4.9], and internal capsule). The majority of callosal lesions are found in the splenium (13,14).

Edema

Acute cerebral swelling after trauma has been demonstrated by CT. The cause is not especially clear (19–23). Most likely, it is due to increased blood volume or increased brain fluid in the form of edema caused by loss of autoregulation of the cerebral vasculature. The traumatic stimulus, or the systemic reactions such as hypercarbia or hypotension, may be the events that initiate the changes resulting in

---→

Fig. 4.8. Diffuse axonal traumatic injury. A 36-year-old male who suffered a severe traumatic injury to the brain six months before examination. **A:** *MRI—axial T2-weighted image.* The examination taken at the level of the brainstem reveals a well-defined small area of hypointensity at the level of the left quadrigeminal plate (arrow). These changes represent an old traumatic hemorrhagic lesion in this region containing hemosiderin. **B, C:** *MRI— axial and coronal T2-weighted images* of the same patient showing multiple hypodense areas in the right thalamic and upper brainstem areas (arrows). These changes represent old shear injuries produced by the previous trauma containing hemosiderin. **D:** *MRI—coronal T2-weighted section* of the brain of the same patient showing bilateral lesions in the parietal lobes consistent on a central area of hyperintensity surrounded by area of hypointensity (hemosiderin) (arrow). These lesions are good examples of multiple old axonal lesions. There is also hydrocephalus and cortical atrophy.

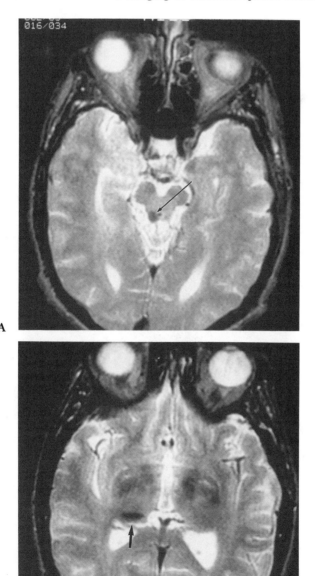

A

B

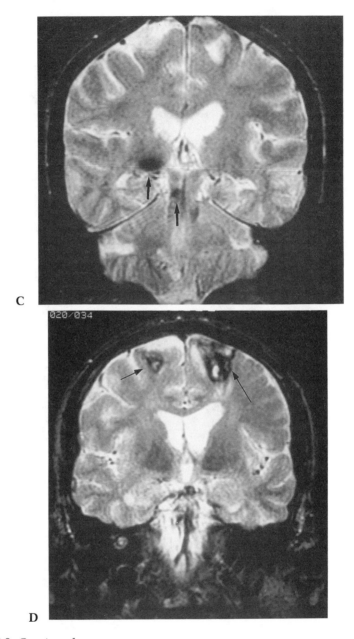

C

D

Fig. 4.8 *Continued*

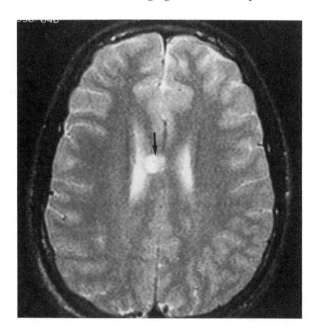

Fig. 4.9. Diffuse axonal traumatic injury. A 17-year-old boy following a motocycle accide. *MRI—axial T2-weighted spin echo section* taken at the level of the corpus callosum. A well-defined centrally located traumatic lesion is seen in the central portion of the corpus callosum (arrow). Lesions in this region are frequently seen in diffuse axonal traumatic lesions.

cerebral edema. Edema is the most common CT finding on pediatric head trauma. Although the majority of these patients do not die, autopsies of those who do reveal diffuse white matter damage and axonal injuries.

The most common CT appearance of edema is a decrease in the size of the ventricles and CSF space without an obvious intra-axial or extra-axial lesion. If the edema is significant, the compression is sufficient to cause non-visualization of the ventricular systen and subarachnoid cisterns. Sometimes it is difficult to evaluate the ventricular size without knowing the size of the ventricle for each patient before the trauma; thus the diagnosis can be made only in retrospect. Low-density zones with attenuation values less than that of white matter have been described and can be due to infarcts secondary to the trauma. CT findings of small ventricles and compressed cisterns are nonspecific and can also be observed in hyponatremia and brain death owing to ischemia of both hemispheres (18). Occlusion of the third ventricle and basal cisterns in severe craniocephalic trauma has been considered a poor prognostic factor (29) because it suggests significant intracranial pressure.

Extra-Axial Lesions

Epidural Hematomas

These lesions are blood collections located between the dura and the cranial vault. Since the dura is firmly attached to the skull at sutures, these hematomas are usually well localized and have a lenticular or biconvex shape. Epidural hematomas are not commonly associated with intraparenchymal damage. They are frequently seen in the temporoparietal region and are usually due to the rupture of meningeal artery branches. Occasionally they are seen in continuity with a skull fracture owing to bleeding of the spongiosa. Clinically, there is a history of rapid onset of symptoms because of the mass effect produced by the accumulated blood, with compromise of the level of consciousness and neurologic signs of cerebral herniation. Early diagnosis is important to the outcome of the patient, who usually needs emergency surgical evacuation of the hematoma (19–23).

Computed tomography is without question the most effective noninvasive diagnostic method available to demonstrate blood collection. The lesion in the acute stage usually appears as a well-defined biconvex, hyperdense collection (Fig. 4.10). Occasionally a hypodense central zone called the "swirled lucency" may be seen, representing active bleeding (the unclotted blood is less dense than clotted blood). Epidural hematomas are not commonly associated with underlying brain damage, although sometimes cortical infarctions originate because of the compressive effects of the hematoma on adjacent cortical vessels. The changes seen in MRI are similar to those seen in CT.

Subdural Hematomas

Although the acute and chronic subdural hematomas are blood collections located between the dura and the arachnoid membrane, they are in fact very different lesions.

Acute Subdural Hematoma

These lesions are fresh blood collections that usually originate from contusions or lacerations of the main cortex, with rupture of middle cerebral artery vessels and bleeding in the arachnoidal and dural tissue. These arteries are located on the convexities of the temporal frontal and parietal lobes. The subjacent brain damage associated with the acute subdural collection is usually significant. There is no

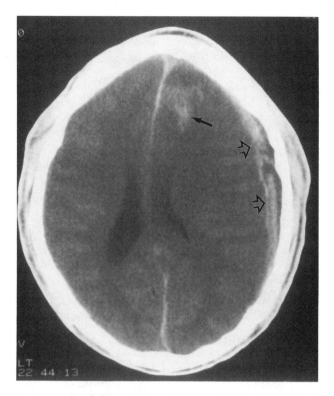

Fig. 4.10. Acute epidural hematoma. A 22-year-old male following direct trauma to the brain on the left. *CT scan: axial section.* The examination, done ten days after the injury, reveals a well-defined area of increased density compressing the underlying brain (open arrows) Shifting of the midline structures, mainly the ventricular system due to significant amount of edema, is visualized. An intracerebral hemorrhagic contusion is seen also in the right frontal region (arrow).

definite evidence of acute subdural collections' becoming chronic subdural hematomas in their evolution. The onset of the symptoms occurs immediately after severe trauma and is usually associated with a significant compromise in the level of consciousness.

Computed tomography on the first examination usually shows a hyperdense biconcave collection of blood associated to a large intracerebral mass effect owing to parenchymal damage and edema (Fig. 4.11). After a period of one week or more, the collection becomes isodense or hypodense to gray matter in accordance with the changes on the hemoglobin and the mixing of the blood with cerebrospinal fluid. The most common location of acute subdural hematomas is in the frontoparietal convexities, although they may occasionally be found in the interhemispheric fissure, mainly in children or in

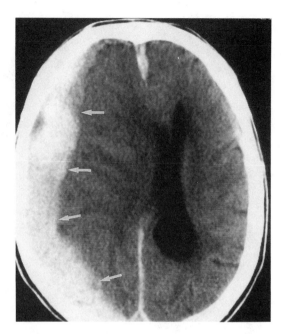

Fig. 4.11. Acute subdural hematoma. A 15-year-old male seen after a severe motorcycle accident. *CT scan: axial sections.* The examination reveals a large, well-defined collection of blood compressing the underlying brain in the right hemisphere (arrows). Shifting of the ventricular system owing to significant blood collection and marked edema is visualized. The patient died shortly after the accident.

adults with significant brain atrophy. In MRI, acute subdurals are hypodense in T2-weighted images and have a significant mass effect resulting from edema.

Chronic Subdural Hematoma

These hematomas start as slow effusions of blood into the subdural space, usually owing to rupture of bridging veins. They usually occur in patients with brain atrophy in areas where the bridging veins are more vulnerable to traumatic tearing. Patients who have had previous rupture of these vessels are prone to recurrent leaking after minor traumas. This fact explains the presence of layers of varying densities often seen in the same collection. In older patients, chronic subdural hematomas are usually associated with minor trauma. Included in the clinical symptoms are memory and behavior changes which may be apparent only weeks to months after the injury. Usually there is no impairment of the level of consciousness and the patients complain only of headaches or changes in mental state.

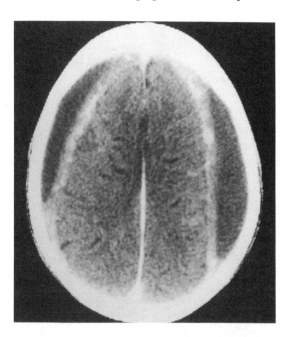

Fig. 4.12. Chronic subdural hematoma. A two-year-old boy with progressive deterioration after the placement of a shunt tube in the ventricular system for the treatment of hydrocephalus. *Enhanced CT scan: axial section.* The examination reveals bilateral subdural hypodense collections compressing the underlying brain. Enhancing of the subdural membrane and cortical brain is seen. Bilateral chronic subdural hematomas are sequently seen after shunting procedures.

Computed tomography of chronic subdural hematoma shows a biconcave or crescent-shaped collection whose density can be correlated with the age of the subdural collection. The subacute subdural (7–12 days) hematoma usually appears isodense, whereas the chronic hematoma (more than 22 days) is usually hypodense. After administration of intravenous contrast, enhancement of the membrane surrounding the hematoma and displacement of the contrast enhanced cortical blood vessels are seen (Fig. 4.12). In recurrent subdural hematomas, the blood elements tend to gravitate toward the dependent portions of hematoma, thus forming a fluid level in which more dependent and denser areas correspond to an aggregate of blood cellular elements.

Magnetic resonance imaging demonstrates well (30,31) the shape and mass effect of the subdural collection and allows determination of its approximate age. The evolution of subdural hematomas follows the same stages of the intraparenchymal hemorrhage; however, chronic hematomas do not have the hemosiderin-related hyper-

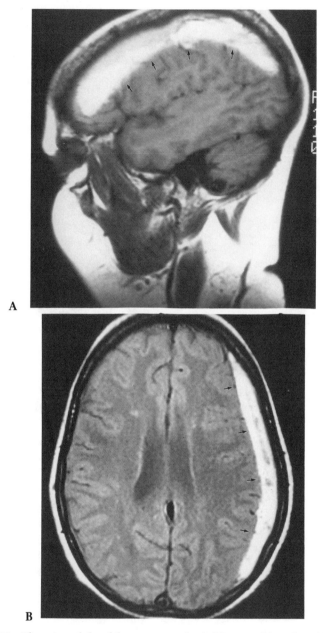

Fig. 4.13. Chronic subdural hematoma. **A:** A 30-year-old male with progressive headaches after head injury. *MRI: sagittal T1-weighted image.* The examination reveals a well-defined, cresent, hyperintense subdural collection of blood in the left convexity (arrows). Minimal damage of the underlying brain is seen. **B:** *MRI: axial T2-weighted image* of the same patient. The same changes are visualized (arrows).

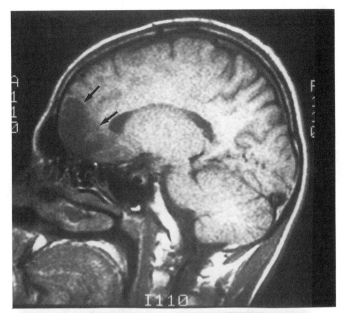

A

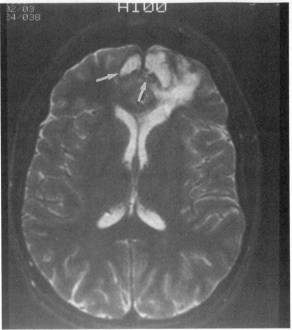

Fig. 4.14. Focal atrophy. A 48-year-old female with a previous history of trauma. **A**: *MRI—sagittal T1-weighted image.* Examination reveals an ill-defined area of decreasing density in the frontal region corresponding to a previous frontal contusion (arrows). **B**: *MRI—axial T2-weighted spin echo section.* The examination reveals bilateral frontal hypodense area corresponding to the old contusion (arrows). An area of decreased intensity seen behind the left contusion represent residual edema. Note the compensatory dilation of the left frontal horn.

intensity seen in the intraparenchymal bleeds. Acute hematomas are hypointense in T2-weighted images. Early subacute collections have a peripheral hyperintensity in T1-weighted images (Fig. 4.13); they may also have a central hypointensity on T2. Late subacute collections are hyperintense on both T1 and T2. Finally, in the chronic phase the collections are iso- or slightly hypointense in T1 with membranes or layers seen inside the collection. This MRI appearance may be explained by the dilution of methemoglobin and hemosiderin, probably owing to the absence of a blood-brain barrier (31). Compared to CT, MRI has a superior ability to detect subdural collections, which are seen as isodense on CT.

Subarachnoid Hemorrhage

Subarachnoid hemorrhage is a nearly constant feature in patients who have cortical brain contusions, and is frequently present in blunt injuries. It is usually associated with other brain lesions and by itself does not produce changes in the level of consciousness. In these patients, CT may reveal diffuse hyperdensity of the basilar cisterns and in the falx. Blood in the convexities is usually not visualized owing to the adjacent hyperdense calvarium. Visualization of subarachnoid hemorrhage on MRI is difficult (32).

Basal subdural hematomas which are usually fatal are found in people with alcohol intoxication and with a head trauma of the skull base. The mechanism responsible is frequently rupture of the wall of the vertebral or basilar artery.

Secondary Brain Damage

A secondary injury implies that the lesion is due to compression or ischemia which presents 24 to 72 hours after trauma. Brainstem injuries, hemorrhagic and non-hemorrhagic, and cerebral infarcts are the most common secondary brain injury.

Cerebral Infarcts

These lesions are the most common complication seen the first week after trauma and usually result from compromise of the arteries of the circle of Willis owing to secondary herniation of the brain (18). Other causes of infarction are emboli originating in fractures of long bones and venous sinus thrombosis. On CT the appearance of these infarcts is similar to those resulting from other causes: a well-defined hypodense area with a typical vascular distribution. Infarcts produced by venous sinus thrombosis usually follow the distribution of the occluded sinus, i.e., thrombosis of the superior sagittal sinus produces bilateral parasagittal hemorrhage infarcts.

Infection

Infection must be considered a complication of craniocephalic trauma. This complication is usually present in open injuries and in trauma produced by bullets and, rarely, following surgical procedures (18). Epidural empyemas and intracerebral abscesses, which can originate from a parenchymal contusion or hematoma, are recognized as hypodense areas that share "ring" enhancement, following intravenous injection of contrast media. Extra-axial empyemas are suspect when the membranes of the extra-axial collection enhance after the intravenous contrast injection.

Sequelae

Focal or Generalized Cerebral Atrophy

In the area of traumatic lesions are common sequelae of compressive extra-axial collections. In the areas of intraparenchymal hematomas or contusions, gliosis or cicatricial tissue is usually present. This is manifested as well-defined hypodense areas usually associated with adjacent ventricular enlargement (Fig. 4.14).

Hydrocephalus

Active, or normal pressure, hydrocephalus (NPH), is usually related to the subarachnoid hemorrhage associated with trauma. However, these complications develop in only 1% to 6% of all patients with head injuries. Sometimes it is difficult to differentiate between active hydrocephalus and atrophic changes in the white matter. Magnetic resonance imaging or isotope cisternography could be useful in these particular situations. On the other hand, ventricular dilatation may be the only change observed after trauma in the severely neurologically comprised patient.

Leptomeningeal Cyst, "Growing Fracture," Traumatic Carotid Cavernous Fistula, and CSF Rhinorrhea

All these conditions can be late sequelae of vault fractures. Leptomeningeal cysts are due to CSF leakage secondary to a dural rupture. Fractures of the cranial base are usually the cause of carotid cavernous fistula, manifested as enlargement of the cavernous sinus and ingurgitation of the ipsilateral ophthalmic vein. When a cranial base fracture involves the cribiform lamina, a CSF fistula may occur. In this case, CT examination is very important to demonstrate the exact location of the fracture and sometimes a contrasted cisternography is necessary to determine the exact location of the leak.

Imaging in Mild to Moderate Head Injury

The abnormalities described in the previous sections are found in head trauma in general, and do not always apply to minor head injuries. They are, however, included in this chapter, since many of them may be found following mild head trauma but to a minor degree. Since axonal injury seems to be found most frequently, consisting of morphopathological changes associated with minor to moderate brain injury, it is unlikely that these microscopic changes can be dectected by CT or MRI (33); however, larger lesions are identified by MRI. In general, mild injuries are rarely associated with abnormal CT, whereas MRI seems to be more sensitive. Most of the changes visualized so far on MRI have been located in the white matter and, in the past, have been confused with artifacts or attributed to ischemic changes in the elderly or subclinical multiple sclerosis in the younger. Jenkins et al. (37) in a more detailed study of this subject found that the patients with deep lesions have superficial lesions as well, a fact that correlates better with the usual contusions observed in more severe injuries. Levin et al. (34,37), demonstrated also that the location of lesions in the brain following minor trauma closely correlates with the distribution of contusions found in patients suffering from severe trauma. For example, the frontal and temporal regions are more commonly affected. These studies also demonstrate a significant correlation between the severity of impact (degree of altered consciousness), the location of the lesions, and the results of neurobehavioral tests performed after trauma. Also, improvement of specific neurological dysfunctions paralleled the resolution of the MRI abnormalities found in these patients.

Infrequently, mild injuries in children may be followed by a deterioration that is preceded by a lucid or symptom-free period. In some cases this deterioration is manifested by diffuse brain swelling on CT or MRI. Obliteration and narrowing of the ventricular system and obliteration of the basal cysterns are usually observed (38). The origin of cerebral swelling in children is a matter of great controversy, with regard to both its nature and clinical significance. Two current theories are available to explain these changes. One attributes them to a vascular cause that is a cerebral vasodilation (38,39), the other holds that cerebral swelling is only a manifestation of diffuse post-traumatic edema (40,41). The overwhelming majority of children with mild head trauma, however, rapidly return to normal function. Although intracranial hematomas are very rare, CT scans are usually performed to rule them out.

Dynamic Imaging Studies

Although the value of new dynamic imaging studies such as positron emission tomography (PET) and single photon emission computed tomography (SPECT) in patients with minor head trauma has not been fully clarified, it is important to be aware of these tests and their possible applications.

Positron emission tomography is a technique which permits imaging of the rates of biological processes, essentially allowing biochemical examination of the brains of patients in vivo. Positron emission tomography utilizes emission tomography with a tracer kinetic assay method employing a radiolabeled, biologically active compound (tracer) and a mathematical model describing the kinetics of the tracer as it is involved in a biological process. Positron emitters such as ^{11}C, ^{13}N, ^{15}O, and ^{18}F can be used as tracers. The tissue tracer concentration measurements needed by the model are provided by the PET scanner.

Positron emission tomography following head injury has not been investigated as thoroughly as other imaging modalities, including CT, MRI, and SPECT (discussed below). However, as Jamieson et al. point out, PET adds another dimension to our understanding of the brain, by demonstrating metabolic alterations (42). Positron emission tomography quantitates local tissue distribution of radioactive tracers that are distributed throughout the brain according to function. Commonly measured functions include local cerebral glucose metabolism, cerebral blood flow, cerebral oxygen utilization, and cerebral blood volume. Langfitt and co-workers compared CT, MRI, and PET in the study of brain trauma (43). Although they studied only a small number of patients, they found that PET showed metabolic distrubances that extended beyond the structural abnormalities demonstrated by CT and MRI, and missed by xenon 133 measurement of cerebral blood flow. Although much additional research is needed to determine the appropriate uses of PET in head trauma, and to interpret meaningfully the abnormalities observed, PET appears sensitive to dysfunctions following injury that are not detected by more commonly available studies.

Humayun studied local cerebral glucose abnormalities in patients with cognitive impairments following minor head trauma (44). The authors used fluorodeoxyglycose 18 with PET imaging in three patients and three matched controls. The patients were studied between three and twelve months following injury, and all had abnormalities in attention and recent memory documented by neuropsychological testing. Computed tomography, MRI, EEG, and drug screens were negative at the time of the PET scanning. The closed-head-injury group showed significantly decreased metabolic rates for glucose in the medial temporal, posterior temporal, and posterior frontal cortices, as well as in the left caudate nucleus. Glucose metabolism was significantly increased in the anterior temporal and anterior frontal cortices. These PET studies suggest that patients with deficits following closed head injuries have regional metabolic brain abnormalities indicative of altered neuronal function detectable by PET, despite the absence of abnormalities on CT, MRI, or EEG.

As its name indicates, SPECT is also a form of emission tomography. It utilizes a technique that detects single photons one at a time, rather than positron-induced photon pairs like the photons detected with PET. Also like PET, SPECT uses a radioactive tracer introduced intravenously. Emission computed tomography provides images that are not nearly as sharp as transmission CT. One particularly useful technique involves the use of technitium 99m HM-PAO (Tc-99m HM-PAO), a lipophilic chemical microsphere that crosses capillary walls freely. Within the brain, it is converted to a hydrophilic form that cannot leave the brain. Only a portion of the TC-99m HM-PAO is converted, with the remainder diffusing back into the bloodstream. The amount cleared by back-diffusion depends on blood flow. Abdel-Dayem and co-workers compared Tc-99m HM-PAO SPECT with CT following acute head injury (45). Single photon emission CT had the following advantages: 1) it reflected perfusion changes; 2) it was more sensitive than CT in demonstrating lesions; 3) it demonstrated lesions at an earlier stage than CT; 4) and it was helpful in separating lesions with favorable prognosis from those with unfavorable prognosis. Roper et al. also compared Tc-99m HM-PAo SPECT with CT in 15 patients with acute closed head injury (46). They also found that SPECT can detect focal disturbances of cerebral blood flow that are not seen on CT. They observed that SPECT distinguished two types of contusions: those with decreased cerebral blood flow, and those with cerebral blood equal to that of the surrounding brain. Bullock et al. found SPECT useful in mapping blood-brain barrier defects, including delayed blood-brain barrier lesions, in 20 patients with acute cerebral contusions and 4 with acute subdural hematomas (47). Ducours and co-workers found SPECT abnormalities in nine out of ten patients with normal transmission CT following craniofacial injury (48). Oder et al. suggested that SPECT may help to improve outcome prediction in patients with persistent vegetative state following severe head injury (49); and Morinaga used SPECT to demonstrate regional brain abnormalities in six patients with hyponatremia following head injury. The abnormalities observed on SPECT improved when the hyponatremia improved (50).

Although extensive additional research and clinical experience are needed to clarify the roles of functional imaging studies, it appears likely that they may be useful to document abnormalities following minor head trauma. As Duffy observed, "brain-imaging procedures, such as the CT scan, the PET (positron emission tomography), and NMR (nuclear magnetic resonance) and BEAM [brain electrical activity mapping] represent different windows upon brain function. They provide separate but complementary information" (51).

References

1. Mandel S: Minor head injury may not be "minor." Postgrad Med, 1989; 85(6):213–225.
2. Servadei F, Faccani G, Roccella P, et al.: Asymptomatic extradural haematomas. Results of a multicenter study of 158 cases in minor head injury. Acta Neurochir, 1989; 96(1–2):39–45.
3. Sproge E, Jakobsen S, Falk E: Fatal thrombosis of the basilar artery due to a minor head injury. Forensic Sci Int, 1990; 45(3):239–245.
4. Kurokawa Y, Sohma T, Tsuchita H, et al.: Hemorrhage into fibrous dyplasia following minor head injury. Effective decompression for the ophthalmic artery and optic nerve. Surg Neurol, 1989; 32(6):421–6.
5. Eliamel MS, Rugman FP: Extradural hematoma associated with essential thombocythaemia in a child after a relatively minor head injury. Br J Acc Surg, 1989; 20(4):236–7.
6. Ros SP, Ros MA: Should patients with normal cranial CT scans following minor head injury be hospitalized for observation? Pediatr Emerg Care, 1989; 5(4):216–18.
7. Feuerman T, Wackym PA, Gade GF, Becker DO: Value of skull radiography, head computed tomographic scanning and admission for observation in cases of minor head injury. Neurosurgery, 1988; 22(3):449–53.
8. Liguori G, Foggia L, Buonaguro A, et al.: EEG findings in minor head trauma as a clue for indication to CT scan. Childs Nervous System, 1989; 5(3):160–2.
9. Servadei F, Ciucci G, Morichetti A, et al.: Skull fracture as a factor of increased risk in minor head injuries. Indication for a broader use of cerebral computed tomography. Scanning Surg Neurol, 1988; 30(5):364–69.
10. Masters SJ, McClean PM, Arcarese JS, et al.: Skull X-ray examinations after head trauma. Recommendations by a multidisciplinary panel and validation study. N Engl J Med, 1987; 316(2):84–91.

11. Thornbury JR, Master SJ, Campbell JA: Imaging recommendations for head trauma. A new comprehensive strategy. Am J Roent, 1987; 149(4):781–83.
12. Quencer RM: Neuroimaging and head injuries: Where we've been/where we're going. Am J Roent, 1988; 150(1):13–18.
13. Gentry LR, Godersky JC, Thompson B, et al.: Prospective comparative study of intermediate field MR and CT in the evaluation of closed head trauma. Am J Roent, 1988; 150(3):673–682.
14. Gentry LR, Godersky JC, Thompson B: MR imaging of head trauma: Review of the distribution and radiopathologic features of traumatic lesions. Am J Roent, 1988; 150(3):663–72.
15. Hadley DM, Teasdale GM, Jenkins A, et al.: Magnetic resonance imaging in acute head injury. Clin Radiol, 1988; 39(2):131–139.
16. Wilson JT, Wiedman KD, Hadley DM, et al.: Early and late magnetic resonance imaging and neuropsychological outcome after head injury. J Neurol, Neurosurg, Psychiatry, 1988; 51(3):391–396.
17. Villafana TH: Physics and instrumentation: CT and MRI. In Lee SH, Rao KC (ed): Cranial Computed Tomography and MRI. 2nd edition. New York: McGraw Hill, 1987, chap 1.
18. Grossman B: Magnetic Resonance Imaging and Computed Tomography of the Head and Spine. Baltimore: Williams and Wilkins, 1990; chaps 1–3, 7.
19. Dolinskas C: Intracranial trauma. In Gonzalez CF, Grossman B, Masdeu J (eds): Head and Spine Image. New York: Wiley Medical, 1985.
20. Bostrom K, Helander CG: Aspects on pathology and neuropathology in head injury. Acta Neurochir (Suppl) 1986; 36:51–55.
21. Hesselink J, Dowd C, Healy M, et al.: MR imaging of brain contusions: A comparative study with CT. Am J Roent, 1988; 150:1133–1142.
22. Gomori JM, Grossman RI, Goldberg HI, Zimmerman RA, Bilaniuk LT: Intracranial hematomas: Imaging by high field MR. Radiology, 1985; 157:87–93.
23. Zimmerman RA: Infratentorial trauma. In Taveras JM, Ferrucci JT (eds): Neuroradiology and Radiology of the Head and Neck. Philadelphia: Lippincott, 1986; 3(68):1–5.
24. Gentry LR, Godersky JC, Thompson BH: Traumatic brain stem injury: MR imaging. Radiology, 1989; 171:177–187.
25. Gennarelli TA, Thibault LE, Adams JH, Graham DI, et al.: Diffuse axonal injury and traumatic coma in the primate. In Dacy RG Jr, Winn HR, et al. (eds): Trauma of the Central Nervous System. New York: Raven Press, 1982; 169–193.
26. Christie M, Marks P, Liddington M: Post-traumatic intraventricular hemorrhage: A reappraisal. Br J Neurosurg, 1988; 2:343–350.
27. Walker F, Vern B: The mechanism of pneumocephalus formation in patients with CSF fistulas. J Neurol, Neurosurg Psychiatry, 1986; 49:203–205.
28. Wilberger JE Jr, Rothfus WE, Tabas J, et al.: Acute tissue tear hemorrhages of the brain: Computed tomography and clinicopathological correlations. Neurosurgery, 1990; 27:208–213.

29. Colquhoun IR, Burrows EH: The prognostic significance of the third ventricle and basal cisterns in severe closed head injury. Clin Radiol, 1989; 40(1):13–16.
30. Sipponen JT, Sepponen RE, Sivula A: Chronic subdural hematoma: Demonstration by magnetic resonance. Radiology, 1984; 150:79–85.
31. Fobben ES, Grossman RI, Atlas SW, et al.: MR characteristics of subdural hematomas and hygromas at 1.5 T. Am J Neurosci Res, 1989; 10:687–693.
32. Bradley WG Jr, Schmidt PG: Effect of methamoglobin formation on the MR appearance of subarachnoid hemorrhage. Radiology, 1985; 156:99–103.
33. Oppenheimer DR: Microscopic lesions in the brain following head injury. J Neurol Neurosurg Psychiatry, 1968; 31:299–306.
34. Jenkins A, Teasdale G, Hadley MDM, MacPherson P, Rowan JO: Brain lesions detected by magnetic resonance imaging in mild and severe head injuries. Lancet, 1986; 2:445–446.
35. Levin HS, Larrabee GJ: Disproportoinate decline in visuospatial memory in human agin. Soc Neurosci Abstr, 1983; 9:918.
36. Levin HS, Amparo EG, Eisenberg HM, Williams DH, High WM Jr, McArdle CB, Weiner RL: Magnetic resonance imaging and computerized tomography in relation to the neurobehavorial sequelae of mild and moderate head injuries. J Neurosurg, 1987; 66:706–713.
37. Levin HS, Eisenberg HM, Amparo EG, Williams DH, High WM Jr, Croffored MJ: Depth of parenchymal lesions visualized by magnetic resonance imaging in relation to level of consciousness after closed head injury. Paper presented at the American Association of Neurological Surgeons Meeting, April, 1988, Canada.
38. Zimmerman RA, Bilaniuk LT, Bruce DA, Dolinskas C, et al.: Computed tomography of pediatric head trauma: Acute general cerebral swelling. Radiology, 1978; 126:403–408.
39. Bruce DA, Sutton LN, Schut L: Acute brain swelling and cerebral edema in children. In de Vlieger M, de Lange SA, Beks JWF (eds): Brain Edema. New York: John Wiley, 1981; pp 125–145.
40. Clasen RA, Guariglia P, Stein RJ, Pandolfi S, Lobick JJ: Histopathology and computerized tomography of human traumatic cerebral swelling. In Baethmann A, Go KG, Unterberg A (eds): Mechanisms of Secondary Brain Damage. New York: Plenum, 1986; pp 29–45.
41. Clasen RA, Penn RD: Traumatic swelling and edema. In Cooper PR (ed): Head Injury. 2nd ed. Baltimore: Williams & Wilkins, 1987; pp 285–312.
42. Jamieson D, Alavi A, Jolles P, Chawluk J, Reivich M: Positron emission tomography in the investigation of central nervous system disorders. Radiol Clin North Am, 1988; 26(5):1075–1088.
43. Langfitt TW, Obrist WD, Alavi A, et al.: Computerized tomography, magnetic resonance imaging, and positron emission tomography in the study of brain trauma. Preliminary observations. J Neurosurg, 1986; 64(5):760–767.
44. Humayun MS, Presty SK, Lafrance ND, et al.: Local cerebral glucose agnormalities in mild closed head injury patients with cognitive impairments. Nucl Med Commun, 1989; 10(5):335–344.

45. Abdel-Dayem HM, Sadek SA, Louris K, et al.: Changes in cerebral perfusion after acute head injury: comparison of CT with Tc-99m HM-PAE SPECT (published erratum appears in Radiology, 1988; 167(2):582; Radiology, 1987; 165(1):221–226.
46. Roper SN, Mena I, King WA, Schweitzer J, Garrett K, Mehringer CM, et al.: Analysis of cerebral blood flow in acute closed-head injury using Tc-99m HM-PAO SPECT and computed tomography (published erratum appears in J Nucl Med, 1991; 32(11):2070; J Nucl Med, 1991; 32(9):1684–1687.
47. Bullock R, Statham P, Patterson J, et al.: The time course of vasogenic oedema after focal human head injury—evidence from SPECT mapping of blood brain barrier defects. Acta Neurochir Suppl (Wien), 1990; 51:286–288.
48. Ducours JL, Role C, Guillet J, et al.: Cranio-facial trauma and cerebral SOECT studies using N-isopropylio-amphetamine (^{123}I) Nucl Med Commun, 1990; 11(5):361–367.
49. Oder W, Goldenberg G, Podreka I, et al.: HM-PAO-SPECT in persistent vegetative state after head injury: prognostic indicator of the likelihood of recovery? Intensive Care Med, 1991; 17(3):149–153.
50. Morinaga K, Hayashi S, Matsumoto Y, et al.: CT and ^{123}I-IMP SPECT findings of head injuries with hyponatremia. No To Shinkei, 1991; 43(9):891–894.
51. Duffy FH, Burchfiel JD, Lombroso CT: Brain electrical mapping (BEAM): A method of extending the clinical utility of EEG and evoked potential data. Ann Neurol, 1979; 5:309–321.

— 5

The Electroencephalogram in Minor Brain Injury

Mercedes P. Jacobson and Michael R. Sperling

EEG Basics

The EEG is a graphic recording of the brain's electrical currents. Developed by Berger in 1929, the EEG is generated by the cerebral cortex and modulated by subcortical nuclei. The EEG is an important aid in classifying and describing seizure disorders [1]. The EEG can be helpful in other clinical settings including the assessment of cerebral function in coma [2], and intoxication, and the identification of pathognomonic features of infectious disorders such as herpes encephalitis, subacute sclerosing panencephalitis or Jakob-Creutzfeldt's disease [3]. The EEG can be diagnostic in certain physiologic disturbances such as metabolic encephalopathy [4] and has an adjunctive role in the evaluation of dementia. It may also be useful in some patients who have sustained minor head trauma.

Electrophysiology

The EEG displays the electrical fields of the brain and their change over time. The electrical fields of the brain are generated primarily by the cortical pyramidal cells. The charge on each cell behaves as a dipole. The thalamus functions by synchronizing the cortical cells, thereby providing the rhythmicity we see in the EEG. To obtain a picture of overall brain activity, 21 electrodes are placed on the scalp according to the international 10–20 system. (Fig. 5.1) This system

INTERNATIONAL (10-20) ELECTRODE PLACEMENT

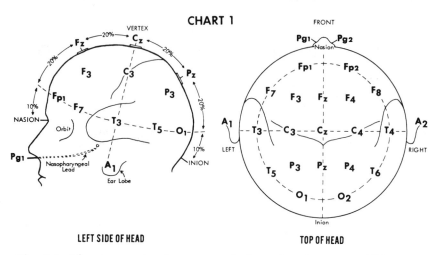

Fig. 5.1. The international system of electrode placement. This sytem assures adequate sampling of all cortical regions and permits comparision of EEGs performed in different laboratories.

assures standard electrode placement and allows comparison of EEGs performed in different laboratories. Each electrode position is determined by specific landmarks on the head, head circumference, and neighboring electrode position. Montages are used to display the electrical activity. Montages allow comparison of the electrical activity between two electrodes and display of such activity on paper. Different montages can represent the activity in different ways. For example, a given montage may help us define an abnormality over the temporal lobe that might not be as well visualized in another format.

An EEG is recorded by a registered technologist according to the criteria of the American EEG Society. A skilled technologist is critical to insure the quality of the tracing, identify potential sources of artifact during the recording and to maintain an optimal recording environment. The electrodes on the left side of the brain are marked with odd numbers. Those on the right are labeled with even numbers. Additional electrodes may also be used, including eye movement monitors and an electrocardiogram (EKG) lead. The electrical signals from the brain are weak. Amplifiers are used to produce the recording that we regard as the routine EEG. Unfortunately, this system will also pick up various artifacts including muscle, EKG, eye movement and electrical interference from any 69 cycle power source.

The EEG machine may have from 8 to as many as 32 channels. Ideally, at least 16 channels should be used to sample all brain regions adequately. The EEG must be recorded for at least 20 minutes. Following acute head injury, maximal wakefulness should be studied. If seizures are suspected, sleep is often necessary to identify epileptiform features. Given the brief nature of the test, most laboratories capture stage I and II sleep, but not stages of sleep. Hyperventilation and photic stimulation are activation procedures and are routine in an initial EEG unless otherwise contraindicated.

In normal wakefulness in an adult the background activity will include the following:

1. The alpha rhythm: This posterior dominant rhythm appears over the occipital, parietal and posterior temporal regions. This rhythm has been likened to an idling rhythm of the quiet, resting brain. It is symmetric in frequency but may show amplitude asymmetry. It is reactive to eye-opening. This rhythm appears in the first 3–4 months of life but reaches normal adult frequency in mid-childhood. Typically the normal frequency of the alpha rhythm is greater than 8.5 Hz. After age of 60 the alpha frequency may slow but should remain in the normal range. It may be absent in a minority of normal subjects. An alpha rhythm is considered abnormal with the following characterisitics:

   Frequency asymmetry >1 Hz.
   Frequency less than 8.5 Hz in an adult in maximal wakefulness
   Right-sided amplitude >50% of left-sided amplitude
   Right-sided amplitude <25% of left-sided amplitude
   Absence of reactivity to eye opening or stimulation

2. In wakefulness, a Mu rhythm may be present in the central regions. This is an alpha frequency (7–12 Hz) rhythm and has an arched shape. Mu is considered the resting rhythm of the sensori-motor cortex (5). Its amplitude attenuates with movement of the contralateral limb or to the suggestion of movement.

3. A small amount of low-amplitude beta activity is seen from the frontocentral regions. This activity is typically less than 20 uV. Medications can enhance beta activity, especially barbituates and benzodiazepines. Concentration or cognition may also increase beta activity.

As an individual becomes drowsy a number of changes are seen in the EEG. These include attenuation of amplitude and slowing of frequency of the alpha rhythm, and an increase in the beta activity followed by the vertex activity and positive occipital sharp transients of sleep (POSTS). The majority of benign but epileptiform-appearing variants appear in drowsiness or early sleep. These include temporal wicket rhythm, rhythmic midtemporal theta of drowsiness, small

Table 5.1. Normal variants.

Posterior slow waves of youth
Paradoxical alpha
Slow or fast alpha variants
Alpha squeak
lambda waves
temporal theta of the elderly

sharp spikes (also known as benign epileptiform transients of sleep), and "14 & 6" positive spikes.

Normal activity in stage II sleep includes vertex sharp and slow waves, sleep spindles, K-complexes and POSTS. Slow wave sleep (stages III–IV) is characterized by increasing amounts of delta activity. For further information the reader is referred to one of several standard texts (6,7).

Clinical Utility

The EEG is most often used to define abnormalities in individuals with epilepsy. For some individuals with epilepsy the EEG may be the only abnormal neurodiagnostic test. An EEG can be *diagnostic* if a seizure occurs during the tracing. Typically, the EEG just provides the footprints that direct the clinician to the correct diagnosis. These footprints include spikes and sharp waves (Fig. 5.2). These transients disrupt the background and may be accompanied by aftergoing slow waves. These abnormalities are localized in partial epilepsy or widespread n generalized epilepsy. They are not always seen on a routine tracing. An initial tracing may yield epileptiform abnormalities in 50% to 60% of cases with the yield increasing to 85% after the third tracing (8).

EEG and Minor Closed Head Injury

Our knowledge of the EEG in minor closed head injury (mCHI) has been derived from a few studies of large numbers of patients performed in the 1940s. Patients were evaluated somewhat differently at that time: the Glasgow coma scale (GCS) had not been devised and neuro-imaging was rudimentary. EEG was much less sophisticated, artifact was extremely difficult to manage, and three- or six-channel machines were standard. Finally, many rhythms which are now recognized as normal were considered pathological 50 years ago.

Only one early study (9) focused primarily on patients with mCHI in the hyper-acute period (< one hour) following injury. This inves-

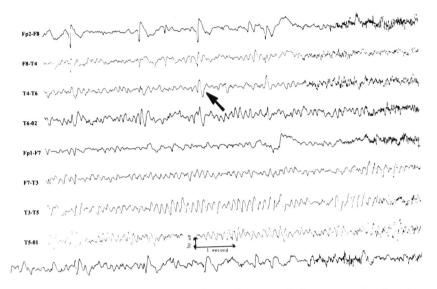

Fig. 5.2. EEG showing frequent right mid-temporal sharp waves and spikes (arrows). This abnormality is often seen in patients with partial epilepsy.

tigator (Dow) also studied the evolution of EEG changes with follow-up studies. The EEG was most abnormal in the first 30 minutes following an injury. The likelihood of identifying an abnormality dropped off significantly after 24 hours. An initially abnormal EEG typically became normal in a brief interval following the trauma. In the hyper-acute stages a patient could be normal by clinical exam but mild changes might be seen on EEG. Acutely, an individual who is confused or drowsy may be expected to have an abnormal EEG. In addition, patients who were clinically abnormal on exam demonstrated more marked changes in their EEGs than those without neurologic deficits (9,10). The acute EEG was not as good a predictor of an individual's ability to return to work as was the clinical assessment. It is to be noted that some of the individuals in both of these early studies had more serious injury than mCHI.

While the vast majority of tracings obtained following mCHI are normal, there are some expected changes in the acute phase. An individual who is drowsy at the time of the recording will have a tracing consistent with the lighter stages of sleep. There may be a mild degree of generalized slowing of all background frequencies. Stimulation of the patient should produce an alerting response (11). An individual who is awake and alert may demonstrate slowing of the alpha rhythm. The alpha rhythm may remain within the normal range and the slowing may not be identified unless follow-up tracings are obtained (12,13).

When Is an EEG Part of the Initial Evaluation of Minor Brain Injury?

EEG is not needed of the vast majority of people with mCHI who can be rapidly assessed by clinical exam and appropriate imaging techniques. Some may be difficult to evaluate owing to concomitant systemic injury, intoxication, preexisting neurologic or psychiatric conditions, or a language barrier. There may be concerns that a seizure precipitated the injury. When the patient can not be adequately evaluated because of he factors cited above, or if the mental status exam is inconsistent with mild head injury, an EEG may assist in diagnosis.

An EEG performed in the first 24 to 48 hours following injury may be abnormal in the absence of brain injury. An EEG obtained at this time may reflect the effects of multiple medications, including benzodiazepines, muscle relaxants, and narcotics (14). Alcohol intoxication may produce theta in the waking EEG (15). In addition, many patients admitted to hospitals in urban centers wait a considerable length of time for evaluation and admission. Such patients are often sleep deprived and anxious. These features may also be apparent in the recording.

EEG and Post-Concussive Syndrome:

What is the role of EEG in evaluation of post-concussive syndrome following mCHI? Patients report multiple complaints, including cognitive impairment and vertigo. Epilepsy is not part of this constellation of symptoms. The majority of patients have normal EEGs following mCHI and individuals with symptomatic complaints following mCHI are no different. The hyperacute EEG changes noted immediately after injury are not predictors of this syndrome. A single EEG, obtained months after the insult, cannot certify traumatic brain injury. It is to be noted, however that a normal EEG cannot disprove post-traumatic injury (11,14,16).

EEG and Seizures

The EEG may be abnormal if seizures have occurred. The interictal EEG may demonstrate spikes or paroxysmal slow waves. These discharges are often accompanied by generalized or focal slowing (17). If a seizure is captured during the recording, ictal discharges can be documented. A tracing obtained a day or so after a seizure may show fewer or no epileptiform abnormalities.

Changes in the EEG Over Time

An EEG may reveal unexpected findings. Sometimes these findings can be clarified with a careful review of the history and medication list. The transitory nature of the abnormality may also help to sort the matter out. Early investigators observed that post-traumatic abnormalities in the EEG abated over time. This was seen in the hyperacute studies by Dow as well as in tracings obtained over a longer period of time from individuals with more serious neurologic deficits [18]. In some cases, serial EEGs demonstrated a progressive normalization of the EEG. However, when epilepsy occurred many months or years after injury, epileptiform abnormalities could later be identified in the EEG [14]. There are no recent studies which follow epileptiform changes in the EEG. However, early studies suggested that if a focal, paroxysmal abnormality was identified in the EEG immediately following head trauma and the abnormality did not change over a period of three months, the abnormality antedated the injury [19,20].

Special Populations

Children

Children with mCHI may have EEG abnormalities more frequently than adults despite an intact neurologic examination. These abnormalities may persist for weeks to months. "Irritative features" such as sharps or spike and wave discharges are much more common in children than adults [14]. Occipital slow waves may also be seen in the first several days following injury [11]. Generalized spike and slow-wave complexes may appear. This infrequent finding probably represents the expression of an inherited trait and hence predates the injury [21].

Epilepsy Patients

Patients with epilepsy are at increased risk for head trauma. In a series of 811 unselected patients admitted for head trauma, 1.7% suffered head trauma because of a pre-existing seizure disorder; and patients with seizure disorders were a disproportionate part of all admissions to hospital with head trauma [22]. Although there are no prospective studies to confirm this, retrospective studies of patients with either severe or milder brain injury have suggested that epilepsy may be exacerbated by head trauma. Adults with a remote history of childhood epilepsy also seem to be more vulnerable to seizures following head trauma [23].

The Elderly

The elderly may suffer mCHI as the result of an acute cardiovascular or cerebrovascular event. Hence the EEG may reflect two processes that cannot be distinguished by EEG alone. In addition, an elderly person with apparently intact neurologic capacities may have suffered prior subclinical stroke or other neurologic disease which may be apparent on the EEG. Most importantly, the elderly are at increased risk for subdural hematoma (SDH) with relatively mild head trauma. CT or MRI are the tests of choice in evaluation of SDH. Occasionally SDH presents as a subtle change in cognition and an EEG is ordered. Prior to the development of CT, the EEG of SDH was called "the great imitator" (24). Acutely, generalized or lateralized delta activity can be seen. Rarely, periodic lateralizing epileptiform discharges are seen. More typically there is an amplitude asymmetry with a reduction of amplitude affected and depression of activity on the affected side. The alpha rhythm is *lower and slower* on the affected side. Subacute and chronic SDHs produce similar reductions in amplitude as well as focal delta activity.

Alcoholics

Alcohol intoxication alters the GCS by approximately one point (25) but can produce significant effects on the EEG including an increase in the background theta activity in wakefulness. Alcoholics are at increased risk for SDH. Hence a persistent asymmetry should raise concerns about possible subdural hematoma on the side with lower amplitude. An EEG obtained during a period of alcohol withdrawal may also show other abnormalities (26). Lastly, individuals with chronic alcoholism are exposed on recurrent head traumas, hence, an EEG obtained after relatively mild head trauma may also demonstrate evidence of prior injury.

Conclusions

For a small proportion of patients, the EEG may provide useful diagnostic information following minor head trauma. For most individuals the EEG is not needed for acute diagnosis as clinical examination and neuro-imaging studies are sufficient. It does not predict outcome after mCHI, particularly for the post-concussive syndrome. A single abnormal EEG obtained days or months after mCHI can not conclusively establish presence or absence of brain injury in the presence or a normal neurologic exam.

COMPUTERIZED EEG and Brain Electrical Activity Mapping (BEAM)

What Is Computerized EEG Mapping?

Computerized EEG (CEEG) is derivved from digitization of the raw (analog) EEG. With this technique, various characteristics of the EEG can be displayed in a topographic map. This map enables us to view the EEG in a format that resembles CT and MRI. Mapping can provide a better picture of the spatial relationships of EEG activity. However, the map is an artificial construct of the curved cortical surface and can distort dipole representation. Hence, the data generated by the map are dependent on the mathematical asumptions upon which it is constructed (27).

How to Generate CEEG

Various characteristics of the EEG can be examined with CEEG. These include frequency analysis, coherence analysis, correlation analysis and power spectrum analysis (28). Commercial programs are available to do this. Amplitude maps displaying various frequency bands are most commonly used and are often refered to as brain electric activity mapping or BEAM (Fig. 5.3).

Before the data can be computer analyzed, the raw EEG must be obtained and reviewed. While computers have may important capabilities in processing EEG, they do not readily identify artifact, and artifact can produce spurious results in computer-analyzed maps. A registered technologist must should perform the test. At the time of data collection a list of all current and recent medications should be recorded (as should recreational drugs). The technologist should note whether the patient has been sleep deprived prior to the study. The electroencephalographer who reviews the data will note artifacts in the background which can confound the results. For example, the computer will misinterpret muscle artifact as beta activity and eye movement as frontal delta. Normal variants in the background EEG can also affect the map. At least three artifact free epochs should be used to generate the quantitative record. Any abnormality identified in the record should be reproducible: that is, seen on more than one occasion. Like conventional EEG, there should be a physiologic field of distribution for any given abnormality. An individual map is interpreted in comparision to a normative database. Thus, if errors are made in software design, generation of the database, or in collecting the individual CEEG, misinterpretation of the results is possible. A

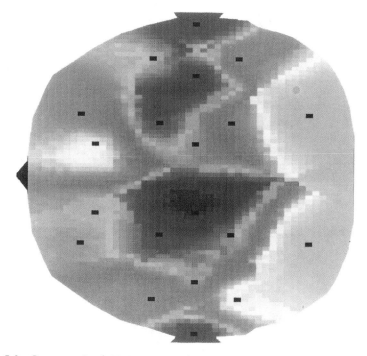

Fig. 5.3. Computerized EEG topographic map of alpha frequency activity. Note the prominence of this activity in the occipital region, where the alpha rhythm normally appears.

report of the EEG should accompany the EEG map, and the technique used to collect the data must be clearly stated (29).

Defining Normal

Computerized EEG was used initially in populations of patients with psychiatric disease. Large groups of patients were compared to control groups without known psychiatric or neurologic disease. Defining the limits of normal became important. Techniques such as neurometrics outlined and compared various groups of patients with different disorders. Multivariate analysis was used to improve specificity and sensitivity. This method was useful in determining that two populations are indeed different. However, as a diagnostic method, the approach could not determine if an individual suffered from a specific illness (30).

Clinical Utility

Despite its shortcomings, computer analyzed EEG may provide new information insome particular situations. In addition, in restricted applications, one can obtain valuable data with relatively few electrodes. Compressed spectral analyzed EEG (CSA-EEG) can identify abnormalities in individuals following stroke as well as those with prior transient ischemic attacks (TIAs) only. These findings can help differentiate among groups at risk for stroke (31). Quantitative EEG can be of use during intraoperative monitoring of carotid endarterectomy (32). In severe closed head injury, compressed spectral array EEG is as good a predictor of outcome as the Glasgow Coma Scale or the neurologic exam (33). This may be especially important in the ICU setting for patients requiring paralyzing agents. CSA-EEG does not appear to be a good predictor for outcome following brainstem stroke. For patients with hepatic encephalopathy a grading scale has been applied to the CSA data which does correlate with prognosis (34). In the evaluation of epilepsy CSA can outline a region of focal slowing which may accompany an epileptic focus (Nuwer). The actual spike can be studied by this technique although CEEG has not proved to be superior to conventional visual analysis. Hence, CSA-EEG may be a useful tool following serious head injury, in the ICU and perhaps also in the operating room.

What Is the Role of CEEG in mCHI?

From what we know about EEG changes in mCHI, we know that they may be subtle. The EEG may demonstrate subtle, transient changes following mCHI with initial slowing of the alpha rhythm although it remains within the range of normal. Hence, in order to study the effects of mCHI one would want to study individuals in a temporal (longitudinal) fashion following mCHI and to compare the findings to individuals without history of mCHI. Finally, one would search for predictive findings which might identify individuals at risk for post-concussive sequelae.

Unfortunately, there are only a handful of studies which include this population. In a prospective study of 26 consecutive patients admitted to the hospital with mCHI, Montgomery (35) found a modest increase in background theta on initial CSA-EEG. This theta disappeared on follow-up studies six weeks later. The theta activity did not correlate with likelihood of post-concussive symptoms. Thatcher (36) examined 162 patients admitted to hospital with head trauma. While the majority of these patients had GCS score suggesting much more serious injury, some had scores of 12 to 15. These investigators found that CSA-EEG was of some use in predicting the likelihood of disability at one year. Phase analysis proved to be a better predictor than GCS score or Brainstem Auditory Evoked Response (BAER) in assessing disability at one year. EEGs were obtained 1 to 21 days following injury. The CEEG generated from these recordings were compared to those of age-matched controls. While these results are interesting, their value in patients with mCHI remains uncertain. In addition, given the transitory nature of EEG findings in mCHI, a 1–21 day interval in recording the CEEG may fail to capture early abnormalities; and hence valuable observations may be overlooked. In a comparative study of amateur boxers, soccer players, and track and field athletes. CSA-EEGs of the three groups were not statistically different. However, this study demonstrated a statistically significant difference in the incidence of mildly abnormal routine EEGs between the boxers and the other athletes. In other words, CSA-EEG was less sensitive than conventional EEG in discriminating a population with multiple mild or minimal brain injuries from a control group (37).

Summary

In the study of mCHI, CEEG remains a research tool. It cannot be used to diagnose injury, guide management, predict outcome, or offer prognosis for individual patients. It can only produce a probability that a given individual resembles or differs from a specific cohort. Hence, at this writing results of CEEG have no proven applicability to individuals with the post-concussive syndrome.

Post-Traumatic Epilepsy

Seizures or suspected seizures following head trauma require careful attention and evaluation. The questions that patients have regarding post-traumatic seizures are typically those that anticipate the future. Will I ever have another one? Can you eliminate them? Is antiepileptic drug therapy needed and if so, for how long? Before we can answer these questions, we need to be certain that history and ancillary testing help support a diagnosis of seizure or epilepsy. A seizure is a clinical event characterized by alteration of behavior or consciousness caused by an abnormal electrical discharge in the brain. Epilepsy is the disorder of recurrent, unprovoked seizures. Thus, a single seizure is not epilepsy and may not always portend the development of epilepsy.

Post-traumatic epilepsy is most strongly associated with severe head injury. Consequently, the majority of large studies reviewing the risk of epilepsy and natural history of post-traumatic epilepsy have focused on individuals with severe head trauma. Confounding interpretation of the literature, the authors have sometimes used the terms *epilepsy* and *seizures* interchangeably. Additionally, seizures following head trauma have been divided into immediate, early and late periods. Unfortunately, these terms are defined differently in various studies.

Pathophysiology

The pathophysiology underlying seizures reflects ongoing cerebral response to trauma. Seizures in the immediate post-traumatic period (minutes) may arise from global disturbances of cerebral dysfunction and are not always indicative of structural injury. Early seizures, occurring in the first week following injury (38) may be caused by acute neuronal injury and exacerbated by deposition of blood. Late seizures, appearing after weeks to mothers, are thought to arise from other pathophysiological processes. Penfield and Jasper were the first to postulate the concept of a ripening scar which gives rise to late epilepsy (39). Histologically, the epileptic focus arises from a cortical injury which develops into a cicatrix with cell loss and gliosis. Chronic hemosiderin deposits are an additional irritant (40). Synaptic reorganization may also contribute to the development of post-traumatic epilepsy (41).

Seizure Types

Immediate seizures may be generalized or focal. In contrast to *early* seizures, immediate seizures do not appear to increase risk for later epilepsy. Focal features such as unilateral motor activity, eye deviation, or Todd's paralysis, are identified in 50% to 75% of early seizures. Sixty percent of early seizures begin within 24 hours of injury. Status epilepticus is more common in children than adults and has been reported in rare cases following mCHI. Late seizures may be of any type except absence attacks. Focal features may be identified in up to 80% of these cases. Temporal lobe seizures are rarely seen in the acute phase but may comprise up to 20% of late seizures (42). Despite the later development of epilepsy 20% to 40% of individuals will have normal EEGs after the onset of epilepsy (14,43,44).

Table 5.2. Risk factors for epileptic seizures and epilepsy after nonmissle head trauma.

Early seizures
    Intracranial hemaotma
    Focal neurological signs
    Posttraumatic amnesia >24 hours
    Any neurological signs
    Depressed skull fracture
    Subarachnoid hemorrhage
    injury before 5 years of age
    Linear skull fracture
Late seizures
    Intracranial hematoma
    Early seizures
    Depressed skull fracture
    Posttraumatic amnesia >24 hours
    Injury after 16 years of age

Adapted from 40.

Large epidemiologic studies suggest that the risk of post-traumatic epilepsy for all patients regardless of severity is between 5% to 10% (45,46,47) Specific types of injury have a much higher probability of subsequent epilepsy. These include intracerebral hematoma, depressed skull fracture, amnesia lasting more than 24 hours and the presence of focal neurologic signs. In the setting of severe head trauma early seizures increase the risk of later epilepsy.

Natural History of Post-Traumatic Epilepsy

The relative risk for developing epilepsy following moderate to severe closed head injury is greatest in the first year, decreases in years two through five, and is similar to the general population after five years (46,47,48). Many of the early investigators in this field postulated that later seizures are more highly associated with the development of epilepsy, however, Jennett demonstrated that early seizures increased the risk for subsequent epilepsy [49]. This held true in the setting of mCHI (45). Most patients who will have seizures have them within the first 12 months following trauma (46,47) and the majority will have had them by four years (45). Most of patients will achieve good seizure control and many will ultimately be seizure free in the years following trauma (14,43,46). A minority of patients will go on to develop refractory epilepsy. Frequent seizures in the first months following trauma are associated with persistent, refractory epilepsy. Multifactorial genetic components may influence the appearance of post-traumatic epilepsy: some individuals are inherently more susceptible to developing epilepsy than others. The EEG is not a reliable predictor of post-traumatic epilepsy. Some patients with refractory seizures will have normal or nonfocal EEGs. Finally, epileptiform abnormalities may not be identified in the EEG until after an individual has developed epilepsy (14).

Large Studies Which Include mCHI

An initial review of 1,000 cases of head trauma established that early seizures following mCHI were rare. However, in this study of both children and adults, early seizures carried a 1% to 2% risk of subsequent seizures or epilepsy (47). A retrospective study of 2,747 patients, followed for 28,176 patient-years, included 1,640 individuals with mild head trauma. Mild head trauma was defined as head trauma without fracture and with loss of consciousness or post-traumatic amnesia lasting less than 30 minutes. Patients with pre-existing epilepsy or multiple brain injuries were excluded. The incidence of early or immediate seizures following mCHI was small for both children and adults. However, children younger than age five had a small increase in relative risk of seizures in the immediate post-traumatic period. In this study, neither early nor immediate seizures increased relative risk for epilepsy. Hence, mild CHI did not significantly alter relative risk for late epilepsy in children or adults (47). Similar conclusions regarding the more benign prognosis of early seizures in the pediatric population following minor head trauma have been reviewed by others (50). This contrasts with an earlier retrospective review of hospital admissions for "trivial" injury in children less than sixteen years of age. Trivial injury was defined as head trauma without loss of consciousness, post-traumatic amnesia, depressed fracture or hematoma. Twenty-five percent of these children went on to develop epilepsy (51). Because this is a selected population, these results may not be generally applicable.

The prognostic implications for early seizures following mCHI may not be fully resolved, but most studies suggest that they are benign. Given the incidence of epilepsy in the general population (1% to 2%) the incidence of epilepsy following mCHI is not different than that of the general population (47,52).

In studies of severe head trauma, prophylactic phenytoin use has been shown to be effective in preventing early seizures (53,54). However, antiepileptic drugs (AEDs) have not proven effective in preventing late post-traumatic seizures for this group of patients. AEDs are not indicated for prophylactic use following uncomplicated mCHI. When a solitary, immediate or early seizure occurs following mCHI treatment is usually not required. Careful observation and neurologic assessment in the coming weeks are the mainstays of therapy. However, certain medical conditions such as fracture or cardiopulmonary compromise might lead one to prescribe a brief course of therapy.

Monitoring

After mCHI some individuals report episodic light-headedness, depersonalization, transient confusion or loss of contact with reality. While these features suggest complex partial seizures, they are rarely caused by epilepsy. A multidisciplinary approach with long-term EEG monitoring and neuropsychological evaluation can help define and treat these events.

Conclusions

Minor closed head injury was initially shown to produce a small increase in risk for subsequent epilepsy. This has not been borne out by subsequent studies which excluded individuals with previous seizures or head trauma. Younger children are at increased risk for early seizures following mCHI. However, mCHI has not been proven to cause epilepsy in this age group.

Summary

The utility of EEG in the management and prognosis of mCHI is at present limited. The EEG can be helpful when the mental status examination does not fit with history and other diagnostic data or if circumstances prohibit a thorough neurologic examination. Unfortunately, there are no pathognomic EEG features for minor brain injury. The EEG does not predict the post-concussive syndrome or subsequent epilepsy. Research must be done to define the role of CEEG in mCHI; at present, it has no proven utility. Given the tremendous potential of computers for data reduction and analysis, we can hope that new diagnostic and prognostic measures will be developed that will be applicable to individuals rather than populations.

References

1. Daly DD: Epilepsy and syncope In Daly DD, Pedley TA (eds): Current Practice of Clinical Electroencephalography, 2nd ed. New York: Raven Press, 1990 Chapter 10, pp 263–334.

2. Rae-Grant AD, Barbour PJ, Reed J: Development of a novel EEG rating scale for head injury using dichotomous variables. EEG Clin Neurophysiol 1991; 79:349–357.
3. Kiloh LG, McComas AJ, Osselton JW, Upton ARM: Infective and noninfective encephalopathies In: Clinical Electroencephalography, 4th ed. London: Butterworths, 1987; pp 165–197.
4. Markand ON: Electroencephalography in diffuse encephalopathies. Neurophysiology 1984; 1:357–407.
5. Schoppenhorst M, Brauer F, Freund G, Kubicki S: The significance of coherence estimates in determining cerebral alpha and mu rhythms. EEG Clin Neurophysiol 1980; 48:25–33.
6. Niedermeyer E, Lopes da Silva F (eds): Electroencephalography: basic principles, clinical applications, and related fields. Baltimore: Urban & Schwarzenberg, 1987.
7. Daly DD, Pedley TA (eds): Current Practice of Clinical Electroencephalography, 2nd ed. Raven Press New York: 1990.
8. Ajmone-Marsan C, Zivin LS: Factors related to the occurrence of typical paroxymal abnormalities in the EEGs of epileptic patients. Epilepsia 1970; 11:361–381.
9. Dow RS, Ulett G, Raaf J: Electroencephalographic studies immediately following head injury. Am J Psychiatry 1944; 101:174–183.
10. Williams D: The Electro-encephalogram in acute head injuries. J Neurol Psychiatry 1944; 4:107–130.
11. Stockard JA, Bickford RG, Aung MH: The electroencephalogram in traumatic brain injury. In: Vinken PJ, Bruyn GW, (eds): Handbook of Clinical Neurology. 1974; vol 23, pp 317–367.
12. Meyer-Mickeleit RW Das Elektroenzephalogramm nach gedeckten Kopfverletzungen. Dtsch Med Wochenschr 1953; 1:480–484.
13. Koufen K, Dichgans J: Haufigkeit und ablauf von traumatischen EEG-Veranderungen und ihre klinischen korrelationen. Fortschr Neurol Psychiatry 1978; 46:165–177.
14. Courjon J, Scherzer E: Traumatic disorders. In Magnus O (ed): Handbook of EEG and Clinical Neurophysiology Amsterdam: Elsevier, Clinical EEG part B 1972; vol 14.
15. Glaze DG: Drug Effects In Daly DD, Pedley TA (eds): Current Practice of Clinical Electroencephalography. 2nd ed. New York: Raven Press, 1990; pp 489–512.
16. Bernad PG: Neurodiagnostic testing in patients with closed head injury. Clin Electroencephalogr 1991; 22:203–210.
17. Stone JL, Ghaly RF, Hughes JR: Electroencephalography in acute head injury J Clin Neurophysiol 1988; 5:125–133.
18. Williams D: The Electroencephalogram in chronic post-traumatic states. J Neurol Psychiatry 1941; 4:131–146.
19. Gibbs FA, Weigner WR, Gibbs EL: The electroencephalogram in post-traumatic epilepsy. Am J Psychiatry 1944; 100:738–749.
20. Kiloh LG, Osselton JW: Clinical Electroencephalography. London: Butterworths 1961; p 125.
21. Hughes JR: The medicolegal EEG In Hughes JR, Wilson WP (eds): The EEG and Evoked Potentials in Psychiatry and Behavioral Neurology. Boston: Butterworth Publishers, 1983; pp 365–367.

22. Hauser WA, Tabaddor K, Factor PR, Finer C: Seizures and head injury in an urban community. Neurology 1984; 34:746–751.
23. Jennett B: Epilepsy after nonmissile head injuries. 2nd ed. Chicago: Yearbook Medical Publishers, Inc. 1975.
24. Fischer-Williams, M: Brain tumors and other space-occupying lesions In: Niedermeyer E, Lopes da Silva F (eds): Electroencephalography: basic principles, clinical applications, and related fields. Baltimore: Urban & Schwarzenberg, 1987; pp 250–252.
25. Young B: Sequelae of head injury In: Wilkins RH, Rengachary SS (eds): Neurosurgery. New York: McGraw-Hill, 1985; pp 1688–1693.
26. Victor M, Adams RD, Collins GH: The Wernicke-Korsakoff Syndrome: A clinical and pathological study of 245 patients, 82 with post-mortem examinations. Philadelphia: F.A. Davis, 1971; p 32.
27. Perrin F, Bertrand O, Giard MH, Pernier J: Precautions in topographic mapping and in evoked potential map reading. J Clin Neurophysiol 1990; 74:498–506.
28. Lopes da Silva FH: A critical review of clinical applications of topographic mapping of brain potentials. J Clin Neurophysiol 1990; 74:535–551.
29. Nuwer MR: The development of EEG brain mapping. J Clin Neurophysiol 1990; 74:459–471.
30. John ER, Prichep LS, Fridman J, Easton P: Neurometrics: Computer-assisted differential diagnosis of brain dysfunctions. Science 1988; 239:162–168.
31. Van Huffelen AC, Poorvliet DCJ, Van der Wulp CJM: Quantitative electroencephalography in cerebral ischemia. Detection of abnormalities in "normal" EEGs. Prog Brain Res 1984; 62:3–25.
32. Ahn SS, Jordan SE, Nuwer MR: Computerized EEG brain mapping. In: Moore W (ed) Surgery for cerebrovascular disease. New York: Churchill Livingstone, 1987; pp 275–280.
33. Karnaze DS, Marshall LF, Bickford RG: EEG monitoring of clinical coma: The compressed spectral array. Neurology 1982; 32:289–292.
34. Van der Rijt CCD, Schalm SW, de Groot G, de Vlieger M: Objective measurement of hepatic encephalopathy by means of automated EEG analysis. EEG and Clin Neurophysiol 1984; 57:423–426.
35. Montgomery EA, Fenton GW, McClelland RJ, MacFlynn G, Rutherford WH: The psychobiology of minor head injury. Psychol Med 1991; 21:375–384.
36. Thatcher RW, Cantor DS, McAlaster R, Geisler F, Krause P: Comprehensive predictions of outcome in closed head-injured patients. The development of prognostic equations. Ann N Y Acad Sci 1991; 620:82–101.
37. Haglund Y, Persson HE: Does Swedish amateur boxing lead to chronic braion damage? 3. A retrospective clinical neurophysiological study. Acta Neurol Scand 1990; 82:353–360.
38. Jennett WB: Early traumatic epilepsy. Lancet 1969; 1023–1025.
39. Penfield W, Jasper H: Epilepsy and the Functional Anatomy of the Human Brain. Boston: Little, Brown, 1969; pp 896.

40. Engel J: Seizures and Epilepsy. Chapter 8 Epileptogenesis Salem: FA Davis, 1989; pp 221–234.
41. Sutula TP: Experimental models of temporal lobe epilepsy: new insights from the study of kindling and synaptic reorganization. Epilepsia 1990; 31(Suppl 3):S45–54.
42. Jennett B: Early traumatic Epilepsy. Arch Neurol 1974; 30:394–398.
43. Jennett B: EEG prediction of post-traumatic epilepsy. Epilepsia 1975; 16:251–256.
44. Bricolo A: Electroencephalography in neurotraumatology. Clinical Electroencephalography 1976; 7:184–197.
45. Jennett B: Epilepsy After Nonmissible Head Injuries. 2nd ed. Chicago: Yearbook Medical Publishers, Inc., 1975.
46. Caveness WF, Meirowsky AM, Rish BL, Mohr JP, Kistler P, Dillon JD, Weiss GH: The nature of posttraumatic epilepsy. J Neurosurg 1983; 50:545–553.
47. Annegers JF, Grabow JD, Groover RV, Laws ER, Elveback LR, Kurland LT: Seizures after head trauma: A population study. Neurology 1980; 30:683–689.
48. Phillips G: Traumatic epilepsy after closed head injury. J Neurol Neurosurg Psych 1954; 17:1–10.
49. Jennett B: EEG prediction of post-traumatic epilepsy. Epilepsia 1975; 16:251–256.
50. Rosman NP, Oppenheimer EY: Posttraumatic epilepsy. Pediatr Review 1982; 3:221–225.
51. Jennett B: Post-traumatic epilepsy In: Laidlaw J, Richens A (eds): A Textbook of Epilepsy. New York: Churchill Livingstone, 1982; pp 155–194.
52. Perr IN: Medico-legal aspects of post-traumatic epilepsy. Am J Psychiatry 1960; 116:981–992.
53. Young B, Rapp RP, Norton JA, Haack D, Tibbs PA, Bean JR: Failure of prophylactically administered phenytion to prevent late posttraumatic seizures. J Neurosurg 1983; 58:236–241.
54. Temkin NR, Dikmen SS, Wilensky AJ, Keihm J, Chabal SC, Winn HR: A randomized, double-blind study of phenytoin for the prevention of post-traumatic seizures. N Engl J Med 1990; 323:497–502.

— 6

Neuropsychological Sequelae of Minor Head Trauma

Sarita R. Schapiro and Thomas Swirsky Sacchetti

Research on the neuropsychological manifestations of mild head injuries has grown rapidly in the past decade. Mild head injury is being understood increasingly as a serious health and economic problem (1–3). In a classic study, Rimel et al. (1981) reported that after three months, mildly head-injured patients reported a number of persistent symptoms, including headache and memory problems (4). A third of these patients who had been employed prior to their injury had not returned to work. Furthermore, it has been reported that 25% of children sustaining closed head injury show morbidity within five years of their injury (5).

The natural recovery rate for individuals following mild head injury is unknown (6). There is considerable variability, which appears to be associated with a number of factors. These include age, intelligence, previous head injuries, and a history of psychiatric or drug abuse problems (7,8). The persistence of neuropsychological symptoms for months and sometimes years after a mild head injury has been documented repeatedly in the literature (9–11).

Cognitive Dysfunction Following Mild Head Injury

Neuropsychological assessment of individuals following minor head injury has consistently demonstrated a number of cognitive and behavioral deficits that may interfere with the person's ability to function. These typically include problems with attention and concentration, initiation and planning, judgment and perception, learning and memory, speed of information processing, and communication. There is a great deal of variability in the extent to which these functions may be compromised following minor head injury. The most commonly reported neuropsychological sequelae are problems with attention/concentration, short-term memory, and speed of processing information (12).

Attention and Concentration

Difficulties with attention and concentration are among the most common cognitive deficits following minor head injury (1,2,13–15). In a study by Hugenholtz et al., patients were found to demonstrate significant attentional deficits three months following a mild concussion in the absence of any apparent neurological problems (1). Patients typically experience difficulties sustaining attention or concentrating on a task over time. There are complaints of difficulty following a conversation, concentrating on reading, or focusing on a television program.

The difficulties experienced with attention can be obvious or subtle. Often the problems are difficult to detect in a structured, one-to-one situation with an examiner or therapist. However, the problems become more apparent when the individual is required to attend to information in a more natural environment. One reason for this involves the inability of these patients to shift attention effectively from one task to another or to deal effectively with distractions. Difficulties experienced in this regard appear to be associated with impairment in the internal regulatory system (16).

Another context in which attentional problems are encountered involves social interactions. If the patient is engaged by a given individual directly in a conversation, there may be no difficulty sustaining attention. However, if there is more than one person talking, or if the topic being discussed is not considered particularly relevant to meet the person's individual needs, there may be increasing distractibility. Comments by the individual may become tangential. The individual often is unaware of the tangentiality of his comments. He may appear egocentric, self-centered, or selfish to others. Consequently, the symptoms associated with attentional deficits result in complications involving social relationships with family members, co-workers, and friends. Friendships may dissolve because of the brain-injured person's difficulty in maintaining reciprocity in communication.

Initiation and Planning

Disorders involving initiation and planning often manifest themselves in the lack of initiative demonstrated by individuals following minor head injury. Often this is misinterpreted as a psychiatric problem (i.e., depression) when, in fact, it represents a cognitive manifestation of the injury. There is difficulty carrying out goal-directed activity. Behavior that typically would be performed in the context of taking another step toward achieving a goal is fragmented. The individual has difficulty understanding part-whole relationships in daily situations and does not function from the perspective of appreciating a means to an end with respect to a particular set of tasks. For example, preparing for an anticipated event such as a family gathering or a doctor's appointment that may involve obtaining specific information or completing a number of preliminary tasks will be extremely difficult. The individual must rely on the assistance of family members in order to facilitate preparation.

This behavior has been described in the literature as a state of psychological inertia, because the steps necessary to carry out a complex action are not present. Typically, the individual responds literally according to instructions that come from the environment. This reaction is quite different from that observed when the symptom is associated with a psychiatrically based inertia. In the latter situation, the individual will respond to instructions from the environment by becoming irritated or belligerent [14].

Subtle deficits involving initiation and planning often become manifested in problems with organization. Executives and others involved in administrative duties may appear less organized. They have difficulties shifting set from one task to another. These patients often have difficulty considering more than one factor or variable at a time when trying to understand a particular problem. Consequently, there is often difficulty establishing priorities, or sorting relevant from irrelevant information. It is difficult for them to establish a planning strategy that is appropriate for achieving work-related goals.

Similar kinds of difficulties with organization are apparent in the daily home environment. Disorganization pervades the living space if there is no one else to structure the environment. One woman who held a responsible position as a clinical social worker lived alone and complained of the lack of organization she lived with in her apartment. She described stacks of old newspapers, some over a year old, which remained in her living room floor for months. In spite of her awareness of the problem, she seemed unable to solve it by simply picking up the papers and throwing them out.

Difficulties with initiation and planning typically have been associated with frontal lobe dysfunction (17). They are found to occur in conjunction with a variety of other symptoms that cluster around frontal dysfunction, including impaired capacity for self-control, defective problem-solving and mental flexibility, and problems with initiative, motivation, and regulation of behavior.

Impaired Judgment and Perception

Realistic self-appraisal may be compromised in patients following head injury. In the minor-head-injury population, this deficit often takes the form of an exaggerated awareness and hypersensitivity to one's loss of prior function and integrity. This is in contrast to the moderate or severely head-injured population, where there is pervasive lack of insight or awareness of the extent to which the cognitive deficits exist (14).

Patients may become depressed in response to this loss of function. In addition to the manifestations of the subtle physical injury, this heightened awareness of their own deficits results in a considerable degree of psychologic distress (18,19). As time passes, the patient's distress may increase. In individuals with minor head injuries, the lack of objective evidence for their dysfunction leads many injured individuals to fear that they are "going crazy" (20). Family members and friends also tend to deny the person's disability and expect that they should be able to function as they did prior to the injury. This, in turn, serves to increase the individual's heightened sensitivity and preoccupation with his own dysfunction, since the reaction from others serves to invalidate the individual's self-perception. Patients tend to become increasingly isolated and socially withdraw in order to avoid confrontation or expectations of others which cannot be met.

Disorders in perception also become manifest in the individual's difficulty understanding the intentions of others. One minor-head-injured patient insisted that any referral to another specialist for consultation represented an attempt by his family to abandon him and to "put him away" in a hospital forever.

Perceptual disturbances also are apparent at a purely cognitive level with respect to basic skills. Frank perceptual distortions often are apparent on psychometric tests. These may involve visual, verbal, or sensory-perceptual deficits (17,21). The individual may experience difficulty with figure-ground discrimination and analysis of visual, verbal, or tactile/kinesthetic information. This finding tends to compound the inability to perceive information accurately in daily situations or in a social context, and the patients' reactions are distorted further.

Learning and Memory

The most common cognitive symptom observed following head trauma involves impairment in learning and memory functions (22–25). There exists an extensive literature that describes the various forms of amnesia observed in patients following traumatic brain injury. Disturbances with memory and learning have been attributed to ischemic damage involving the hippocampal regions (26).

In minor head trauma patients, memory disturbances typically involve inability to recall new information, while long-term recall of prior knowledge remains essentially intact. Patients typically experience difficulty consolidating new memories. Learning curves with repeated trials for assimilating new information are flat, showing little learning across repetitions. Often patients experience significant problems retrieving newly learned information on their own. That is, they may be unable to recall new information spontaneously. However, when these patients are given opportunities to recognize the new information from a series of choices, they have less difficulty identifying the material correctly.

Difficulties with learning and memory often are observed when there has been a delay between the time the new information was presented and when retrieval is necessary. This typically is the case in daily situations, when one is expected to recall information that was presented earlier in the day or sometime in the recent past. Patients often complain of "forgetfulness," difficulty recalling telephone messages, forgetting what they were doing prior to an interruption, forgetting to turn off the stove or oven after cooking, or difficulty recalling relevant details of a conversation. These types of memory problems can lead to significant interference in daily functioning from both a cognitive and interpersonal perspective. It may lead to argumentative behavior with family members, because the injured person denies having been told a specific detail or having witnessed a particular event and maintains this position with conviction.

Speed of Information Processing

Disorders in speed of information processing are common among head-injured patients. This refers to the head-injured person's difficulty in quickly registering incoming information, in the rapid cognitive processing of the material, and/or in rapid output. Consequently, these individuals often miss pertinent information and misperceive the essence of incoming stimuli. They are slow in carrying out the simplest tasks (e.g., writing their name) and require a considerable degree of patience from family members. Interpersonal discomfort often develops in these circumstances, because of the inordinate amount of time patients require to complete the most basic tasks. Problems with speed of processing represent a common long-term symptom following minor head trauma (15,27–29). Yarnell and Rossie studied a group of 27 patients who suffered from minor whiplash injury following a motor vehicle accident (30). None were more than initially "dazed" from the accident, yet all individuals tested neuropsychologically were found to demonstrate cognitive dysfunction involving vigilance, selective attention, memory, mental stamina, and cognitive flexibility.

It has been found that speed of information processing has a profound impact on general adaptation and social adjustment. Patients who are slow to process information typically withdraw from social interaction in order to avoid catastrophic reaction. They prefer to remain in a simple and predictable environment, as opposed to one that is complex and unpredictable. It is common for these patients to avoid social gatherings, even family functions, and to avoid going to unfamiliar settings.

Communication

Disorders in communication may be aphasic or nonaphasic. Typically, injury to the left, or dominant, hemisphere can result in frank aphasic symptomatology. Such injuries are apparent even several months post-injury, when anomia and word-finding problems persist.

Nonaphasic problems in communication are apparent in some patients. These involve verbal expansiveness, tangentiality during conversational speech, and the use of peculiar words or phrases. Expansiveness refers to the observation that some brain-injured patients simply talk too much, which often creates problems with friends and relatives. They seem to have difficulty knowing when to stop and give others a turn to speak. People tend to become irritated by the head-injured individual and prefer to avoid interacting with him/her. Verbal expansiveness has correlated with frontal lobe dysfunction (31). It frequently is seen with disinhibition.

Tangentiality in communication is another common manifestation of nonaphasic language disorders in patients following minor head injuries. At a literal level, these patients have no difficulty producing syntactically and grammatically correct verbalizations. However, they lack the conceptual and logical awareness to discriminate between essential and nonessential information. Irrelevant information often is incorporated into their productions. Furthermore, conceptual confusion is common, as evidenced in problems with word selection, loose connection of words and ideas, impaired abstract reasoning, and a tendency to stray from the main idea (14).

Another manifestation of a nonaphasic language problem is a tendency to produce peculiar phraseology. Patients may use words in a grammatically unusual fashion. For example, one patient would refer to the concept of age as "number," by saying, "What number am I?" when inquiring about his own age.

Emotional Sequelae of Minor Head Trauma

Personality change is commonly observed following minor head trauma. When there is a preexisting personality disturbance, a head injury can trigger an emotional imbalance with resultant prolongation or exaggeration of these symptoms. The pre-concussion personality coupled with the psychological effects of the trauma are significantly related to the severity of the post-concussion symptoms (11,12,18,32,33). Consequently, prognosis is directly influenced by pre-injury personality variables.

It is becoming increasingly accepted that the symptoms associated with the post-concussion syndrome result from a combination of physiologic and psychogenic factors (32–34). Furthermore, the psychological factors associated with the injury have a direct effect on prognosis. Emotional disturbance appears to increase with duration of disability following the injury (11,32). Bornstein et al. (34) studied 125 patients who had sustained work-related injuries and were continuing to receive worker's compensation benefits. Significant main effects were found on the Minnesota Multiphasic Personality Inventory (MMPI) for the degree of neuropsychological deficit on the Depression, Psychasthenia, and Schizophrenia scales. The authors concluded that the higher levels of neuropsychological deficit were associated with greater personality disturbances.

Stern et al. (35) have suggested a distinction between the psychological manifestations following mild and severe head injuries. They reported that two to three years following the injury, patients with mild injuries exhibited characteristics of an "extroversion" dimension (i.e., they were narcissistic, overdemanding, and could not delay gratification). In contrast, the severely head-injured group was described as high on the "introversion" dimension (i.e., they were passive, apathetic, dependent, and had low self-esteem).

There are a number of symptoms which characterize the emotional changes typically observed following mild traumatic brain injury. These include reduced frustration tolerance, increased regression and dependence, depression, somatization, and denial.

Reduced Frustration Tolerance

Perhaps the most common complaint involving personality change in patients following minor head trauma is increased irritability. These individuals blow up over the slightest provocation and have little patience for the frustration encountered in the daily environment. Family members often describe them as moody, argumentative, and always "on edge." They have difficulty adjusting to change and do not cope well in new, unfamiliar, or unexpected situations. This, coupled with their cognitive difficulties, exacerbates their deficits and adds to their disability. In new situations, these patients become easily overwhelmed. Other emotional reactions may become manifest, including increased anxiety or depression.

Increased Regression and Dependency

Patients typically become doubtful of their performance and indecisive in situations that require any risk to their personal integrity or responsibility. They become increasingly fearful of any further loss and prefer to avoid any situation in which they have experienced failure but in which they consistently were successful pre-injury. One administrator who directed public works for a county office and administrated hundreds of thousands of dollars in annual budgets as part of her job prior to her minor brain injury became fearful of managing her personal household budget subsequent to her injury. She avoided paying her bills regularly for fear of failure, despite her awareness that procrastination and avoidance led to an exacerbation of the problem. Her boyfriend began to take charge of her personal budget, and she became increasingly dependent on him to assume this administrative role for her. O'Hara (36) describes how families of these patients typically reinforce their "learned helplessness" by assisting the patient in avoiding any further risk-taking and by assuming responsibility for them.

Depression

This symptom cluster often is associated with failure of early diagnosis. The patient is confused by what is happening but has recognized that the "old" or pre-injury self is absent or diminished (36). There is a preoccupation with the awareness of loss of pre-injury functioning levels, and the patient appears to be in mourning over this loss. The perseveration which typically is characteristic of their cognitive style further exacerbates their preoccupation with loss of functional integrity.

Since there rarely is corroboration for their subjective symptoms on physical examination or radiographic studiess, these patients often fear that they are "going crazy," because their symptoms remain invalidated by many medical professionals (20). As time passes and their disability continues, self-esteem continues to decline and the distress level increases.

Increase in depressive symptomatology also results in increased isolation and withdrawal. Patients make consistent efforts to avoid exposure and further failure. They will choose to remain at home rather than attend social gatherings or even receive guests in their familiar home environment.

Somatization

Physical symptoms may become exaggerated and replace acknowledgment of emotional distress. Patients will obsess on seeking methods for pain reduction rather than focus on feelings associated with the injury. Preoccupation with pain medication and with other therapeutic interventions such as relaxation training and pain management techniques becomes paramount. These individuals typically demonstrate pre-injury personality profiles characterized by limited insight. There may be a delayed exacerbation of physical symptoms (e.g., headache, dizziness, chronic pain) in the absence of corroboration from medical diagnostic tests (36).

Psychotic Disintegration

This symptom cluster, although rarely reported in the literature, has been described (37). It typically is characterized by escalating depression, paranoia, and suspiciousness. Fragility of ego functioning is apparent, which often requires psychotropic medication or even hospitalization. These patients demonstrate poor eye contact, pervasive lack of initiation, and extreme withdrawal. Isolated cognitive functions may remain intact on neuropsychological testing. However, these individuals are extremely dysfunctional. One such patient is Joe, a 35-year, old area supervisor for a fast food chain, who appeared in a catatonic-like stupor approximately 30 months following a traumatic injury including minor brain injury. Computed tomography scans of the brain obtained shortly after the injury revealed only soft tissue swelling in the right frontal region. His neuropsychological profile revealed general intellectual functioning within the Mentally

Deficient range on the Wechsler Adult Intelligence Scale-Revised (WAIS-R). While Joe demonstrated only mild impairment on measures of sensory-perceptual functions, he showed marked impairment in fine-motor tasks. Higher-level cognitive skills involving speech and language, visual-motor integration, nonvisual psychomotor problem-solving, and memory for new information were severely impaired. Furthermore, his academic achievement skills, which represented recall of old information, were at the first percentile for individuals his age.

Joe was treated psychiatrically as an outpatient with regularly scheduled psychotherapy and pharmacotherapy. Two years later, he was reevaluated neuropsychologically. Significant changes were noted, suggesting notable improvement in all areas of neuropsychological functioning. On reevaluation, he demonstrated Average to High Average general intellectual functioning, with Superior visuospatial problem-solving skills. While his social-emotional profile continued to suggest significant psychopathology, his cognitive functioning was well within normal expectations on measures of memory, reasoning, and problem-solving; psychomotor problem-solving; and speech and language skills. Academic achievement levels had resumed to only slightly below expectations. Mild impairment persisted only with respect to fine-motor speed, spatial recall, and restricted spontaneous speech.

Joe continued in psychiatric treatment and began participation in an interdisciplinary cognitive rehabilitation program involving neuropsychology, occupational therapy, and speech-language therapy twice per week. After six months, plans were initiated to have Joe return to college, where he intends to complete a bachelor's degree in education.

Neuropsychological Sequelae in the Elderly

Most minor head injuries in the elderly population result from falls and pedestrian accidents (24). There typically is a change in functional status following these injuries. They require increased family involvement and community support. A majority of elderly patients experience a change in living arrangements, decreased mobility, and a notable disruption in the ability to carry out activities of daily living (ADL).

Assessment of neuropsychological functioning status in elderly head-injured patients is complicated by the lack of adequate normative data beyond 74 years of age for most tests. Thus, an especially important component in evaluation of this population is the structured interview of family members and the patient. This provides essential information regarding changes in medication, diet, daily care, socialization, driving, and other activities of daily living.

Minor Head Trauma in Children

Although clinical investigations of the effects of minor head injury in children have been reported, longitudinal studies have yet to be performed. Therefore, knowledge regarding the formulation of the effects of minor head injury in children is tentative. While most of these injuries appear to be the result of automobile accidents in children under 15 years of age, domestic falls account for a significant proportion (27%) (38).

It has been incorrectly assumed that children recover more easily from minor brain injury than adults. The evolving literature is consistent in demonstrating, to the contrary, that these injuries can have severe and devastating effects on a child's subsequent development and family relationships.

The differences in recovery rates between adults and children are not understood fully. Levin et al. (25) propose that a number of anatomical and physiological features of the developing brain can lead to a different outcome of head injury in children when compared to that in adults. These include greater flexibility of the child's skull to absorb traumatic forces, shallow cerebral convolutions composing the cortex which may contribute to brain stem injury, more oculovestibular and pupillary defects, increased probability of diffuse injury to white matter, and delayed neurologic deterioration.

All children who sustain minor head injury require medical attention and observation. The developmental level of the child at the time of injury is of critical importance in understanding the effects and impact of the problem. The immediate short-term and long-term effects of minor head trauma in children appear to be related to the developmental level of the child at impact. However, one cannot assume a linear relationship between the nature of the injury and its effect on the subsequent developmental progress of the child. That is, a mild injury may result in significant and devastating effects on the child's development.

Research on the residual effects of head trauma in children has reported contradictory findings. This appears to be related to the differences in the focus of the study. Some have used physical recovery as the criterion to be evaluated, while others have focused on the cognitive and behavioral manifestations of the injury on subsequent development. Bruce et al. (39) examined physical recovery using the Glasgow Coma Scale as the dependent variable and found that 90% showed good recovery following moderate head trauma. Their findings have fostered the view that children tend to recover with little difficulty following head trauma. However, a more recent comprehensive study by Winogron et al. (40) examined the neuropsychological performance of groups of head-injured children and found distinct deficit patterns among mild, moderate and severely injured children. These findings have been corroborated by other researchers (41–43). A summary of the salient findings is as follows:

- Functional morbidity may be present in the absence of physical sequelae.
- Head injuries sustained in early childhood disrupt the development of functional systems (44).
- The older the child is at the time of injury, the more the deficits resemble those seen in adults (45).
- It is common to observe behavioral difficulties, and post-traumatic psychopathology is reported in some cases (46).
- Significant differences in intelligence tests, right and left sides of the body, and sensory losses may or may not be present (47).
- Decline in school achievement and deteriorated self-concept are common sequelae (5).
- Social maladjustment is common, characterized by destructiveness, tempter outbursts, delinquency, and overactivity (48).

Overall, the literature supports the view that minor head injury in children can have devastating effects on their development and family relationships. The notion that children recover readily from minor head injury has not been supported in the literature, particularly that which has studied the cognitive, personality, social, and adjustment processes. In fact, there is increasing evidence suggesting that some children experience significant long-term consequences. Longitudinal studies are needed to evaluate these effects in greater detail.

Recovery

The prognosis for patients who have sustained minor head injuries may be independent of acute severity of injury or degree of physical injury (49). Financial compensation also may not necessarily be an issue when considering the long-term effects of these injuries, since impairments may continue in patients where a claim has been settled, or where no claim has been made (50).

It is becoming more apparent that as time passes and disability continues, patients become increasingly distressed psychologically. This appears to be related to the person's growing awareness of their cognitive difficulties and their dysfunction. In turn, as self-esteem and perception of self-efficacy decline, the individual becomes more withdrawn. There is an increase in symptoms associated with depression (34). Pre-injury personality weaknesses and poor coping strategies often are exacerbated by the stress associated with recovery (19).

Long-term quality of survival may be independent of severity of injury. Even three to five years post-injury, mildly head-injured patients may demonstrate impaired functioning and a high incidence of unemployment in previously employed individuals (49). Effects of age on degree of neuropsychological and vocational morbidity are not striking. Furthermore, compensation does not appear to be an issue that can predict return to work (13,50,51).

It is hypothesized that one explanation for the long-term neuropsychological sequelae of minor head injury is related to the persistence of psychogenic factors that exacerbate functioning levels after the organic factors involved in the injury have resolved. Often psychological factors may interfere with resolution of symptoms in some patients and stimulate the production of new symptoms in others (52).

It has been concluded that the disability associated with minor head injury constitutes a major public health problem. Treatment of the neuropsychological sequelae of minor head injuries must take into account the physical, cognitive, and psychosocial manifestations of the injury. Treatment programs must be multifaceted, involving the patient, the family, and often employers or other community personnel who are directly involved in the patient's daily activities. A combination of cognitive rehabilitation, individual supportive psychotherapy, and pharmacotherapy is necessary for management of the patient's individual treatment needs. Additional support services through occupational therapy, speech pathology, and physical therapy are integrated into an interdisciplinary treatment program that addresses the patient's deficits in the context of his or her neuropsychological functioning status.

The patient's family plays an integral role in treatment of the neuropsychological sequelae of the injury. Family education is essential to assist relatives in understanding the nature and extent of the patient's difficulties and how they will become manifest in daily activities. Furthermore, family members can facilitate recovery by providing the support patients need in their familiar home environment to practice newly re-learned skills and compensatory strategies without reinforcing overdependency on others.

School personnel and employers become critical adjuncts to the treatment process. Consultation with appropriate staff often is incorporated into the treatment program, for reasons similar to those that apply to family members. Special modifications can be appropriate in the school or work environments to promote the patient's success in that setting.

Assessment of Neuropsychological Functions

The particular test or test battery used to assess brain functioning in the mildly head-injured patient is chosen in response to the referral question(s). A question such as Does this individual have memory impairment related to the mild head injury? is highly specific and may require a relatively brief screening battery consisting of memory tests. Often those working in a research setting advocate the use of a limited battery of this type (53). However, clinicians are often asked to deal with more difficult diagnostic considerations. A referral question such as Are this individual's cognitive symptoms related to organic brain damage or to depression and/or secondary gain? requires a more comprehensive battery of tests. Often the neuropsychologist is asked for prognostic information, that is, When will the individual be able to return to work? or for recommendations regarding treatment—What can be done to rehabilitate this individual? Such referral questions obviously required a careful evaluation of the strengths as well as the weaknesses in brain function, as well as a thorough evaluation of emotional and psychosocial factors.

A comprehensive evaluation of brain function should assess the following areas: attention/concentration, initiation/planning, motor/sensory skills, visual perception, learning and memory, language, speed of processing information/reaction time, and complex problem-solving. In addition, a measure of general intellectual functioning is needed to develop a picture of the individual's functional abilities before the injury. A neuropsychologist may be a proponent of one of the "fixed" batteries currently in widespread use or may choose to develop a "flexible" battery which is specifically designed to address a particular referral question and/or a specific neurologic problem. The two most popular fixed batteries are the Halstead-Reitan Neuropsychological Battery (54) and the Luria-Nebraska Neuropsychological Battery (55). Most experts would agree that the use of either of these batteries without the addition of supplemental tests would be inadequate to assess the most prominent deficits associated with head injury, including slowed speed of information processing, short-term memory, and difficulties with attention/concentration. The most commonly reported tests for use in flexible batteries or to supplement a fixed battery in the evaluation of mild head injury are summarized in Table 6.1. Sources for these test materials can be found in Lezak (17).

Table 6.1. Commonly used neuropsychological tests.

Intelligence
  Wechsler Adult Intelligence Scale—Revised (WAIS-R)
  Peabody Picture Vocabulary Test (PPVT)
Attention/concentration
  Digit Span Subtest of WAIS-R
  Symbol Digit Modalities Test (SDMT)
  Paced Auditory Serial Addition Test (PASAT)
  Continuous Performance Tests
Memory/learning
  Wechsler Memory Scale (WMS)
  Wechsler Memory Scale—Revised (WMS-R)
  Rey Auditory Verbal Learning Test
  California Learning Test
  Benton Visual Retention Test
Language
  Boston Naming Test
  Controlled Oral Word Association Test
  Speech Sounds Perception Test
  Wide Range Achievement Test
  Token Test
  Boston Aphasia Screening Exam
Visuo-perceptual
  Rey Complex Figure Test
  Hooper Visual Organization Test
  Benton Judgment of Line Orientation
  Raven's Matrices
Motor/sensory
  Finger Oscillation Test
  Purdue Pegboard
  Grooved Pegboard
  Reitan-Klove Sensory-Perceptual Evaluation
Complex cognitive processes
  Trailmaking Test
  Category Test
  Tactual Performance Test
  Wisconsin Card Sorting Test
Personality
  Minnesota Multiphasic Personality Inventory—Revised (MMPI-R)
  Millon Clinical Multiaxial Inventory—II (MCMI)
  Symptom Checklist—90 (SCL-90)

The accurate assessment of brain function following mild closed head injury depends not only upon the judicious selection of tests given the particular referral question, but also on the clinical skill of the neuropsychologist in the interpretation of the test results. Interpretation is open to two types of error. A false-positive interpretation incorrectly attributes a low test score to organic brain damage, whereas a false-negative interpretation incorrectly labels an individual as unimpaired when, in fact, he or she does have organic brain damage. There are two primary reasons for false-negative errors. An individual with superior levels of premorbid functioning may score within the unimpaired range on testing, although the performance clearly indicates a deterioration attributable to brain damage. Also, the particular battery of tests may be lacking in tasks which are especially sensitive to the pathophysiological effects of mild head injury. For example, complex tasks of sustained attention and concentration which last more than 20 minutes, thereby tapping into a "fatigability" factor, are seldom used and are inadequately normed (56). The false-negative scenario is aptly described by a neurosurgeon, a co-author of the Levin et al. (53) study of mild head injury. The subject of this study, who sustained a head injury, fell into the "normal" range on neuropsychological tests soon after the injury, although he reported a subjective impairment in his memory functioning up to three years following the head injury.

The false-positive error, an error of "overinterpretation," can result from an overemphasis of a few low test scores while the majority of scores fall in the normal range. False-positive errors may be due to the failure to account adequately for an individual's low premorbid ability, or the presence of a long-standing lesion which is unrelated to the head injury. A careful developmental history, including an examination of school and work records, is often helpful in avoiding this type of interpretive error. One may falsely rely upon inadequate norms to make a determination of "abnormality." This is particularly true in the case of older head-injured adults, who are likely to experience normal age-related changes in brain function, but for whom adequate age appropriate norms often fail to exist.

The presence of psychological symptoms such as depression and anxiety can often masquerade as organically based deficits. Given the prevalence of depressive and other psychologically based reactions to the trauma, the possibility of depression or "pseudodementia" should always be carefully evaluated by means of objective personality testing, interview material, test-taking style, and the pattern of cognitive deficits apparent upon formal neuropsychological testing (57,58). Of course, issues of malingering or secondary gain are important considerations in all cases, but especially where litigation is involved. Malingering refers to a conscious of deliberate effort on the part of the patient to appear "impaired." The symptoms can be turned on or off at will. Secondary gain refers to an unconscious process, one outside of the person's awareness, in which unmet emotional needs are being partially satisfied as long as the person has the symptoms in question. Although there is a lack of organic basis for the symptoms in both cases, the distinction is important from a diagnostic and treatment perspective.

A careful history/clinical interview, as well as objective personality testing, are essential in the determination of the psychological factors which may be contributing to the patient's symptom. In cases of malingering, inconsistencies in the patient's history and guarded or suspicious test-taking behavior should alert the clinician to this possibility. A tendency to "fake bad" or exaggerate one's complaints may be gleaned from objective personality tests, such as the MMPI-R. Symptom-validity testing has also been used in the detection of malingering (59). This approach consists of tasks in which only "yes" or "no" answers are possible, and in which a chance performance would result in an approximately 50% accuracy rate. A significantly poorer performance (i.e., one significantly worse than chance) suggests a deliberate effort on the patient's part to appear impaired. Initial research suggests that, although this technique may strongly suggest that symptoms are fabricated, malingering cannot be ruled out in the event of plausible or near-chance results.

Secondary gain is often considered in cases of litigation, in which the "gain" may be financial. However, other gains should be considered in the evaluation of mild head injury based on the individual's personality. An individual with strong dependency needs may be unconsciously using the symptoms to avoid the demands and responsibilities of adult life. An individual with a histrionic personality may be satisfying needs for attention and caring from a spouse, family, and/or the medical system.

Thus, interpretation of neuropsychological testing requires much more than simple quantification of test performance and use of appropriate norms. The results must be considered in the context of the individual, including educational, family, and medical history, test-taking attitude, personality, and issues of secondary gain. It is often helpful to examine the pattern of test scores within the entire battery of tests. Inconsistencies or test performances, which are difficult to interpret based on established principles of brain functioning, are suggestive of a non-organic contribution to the symptom picture. The careful examination of the individual's neuropsychological functioning over the course of time is also helpful in this regard. For example, an individual who shows improvement of memory functioning three months post-injury and deterioration of the same function one year later is most likely impaired owing to psychological factors.

In summary, the particular battery of tests used to assess neuropsychological sequelae of mild head injury depends on the referral question(s). In addition to assessing the major areas of cognitive functions, including attention, concentration, initiation and planning, motor/sensory skills, visual perception, memory, language, speed of processing information, and complex problem-solving, a neuropsychological assessment also evaluates emotional and personality functioning. The results must be considered in light of the patient's premorbid intellectual and psychosocial functioning, with careful attention to the possible role of malingering and/or secondary gain. Future research is needed to assess the sequelae of mild head injury with increasingly easily refined testing instruments, such as computer-administered testing, which is particularly promising in areas of fatigability, distractibility, and reaction time. Large-scale collaborative studies also will be needed to address the influence of age, IQ, previous head injuries, and premorbid psychological problems on the course of neuropsychological symptoms over time.

References

1. Hugenholtz H, Stuss DT, Stethem BA, Richard MT: Neurosurgery, 1988; 22(5):853–858.
2. Barth JT, Macciocchi S, Giordani B, Rimel R, Jane J, Boll TJ: Neuropsychological sequelae of minor head injury. Neurosurgery, 1983; 13:529–532.
3. Edna TH: Disability 3–5 years after minor head injury. J Oslo City Hosp, 1987; 37:41–48.
4. Rimel R, Giordani B, Barth J, Boll T, Jane J: Disability caused by minor head injury. Neurosurgery, 1981; 9:221–228.
5. Klonoff H, Low MD, Clark C: Head injuries in children: A perspective five-year follow-up. J Neurol, Neurosurg Psychiatry, 1977; 40:1211–1219.
6. Conboy TJ, Barth J, Boll TJ: Treatment of rehabilition of mild and moderate head trauma. Rehabil Psych, 1986; 31(4):203–215.
7. Alterman AI, Tarter RE: Assessing the influenceconfounding subject variables in neuropsychological research in alcoholism and related disorders. Int J Neurosci, 1985; 26:75–84.
8. Miller E: Recovery and Management of Neuropsychological Impairments. New York: John Wiley & Sons, 1984.
9. Posthuma A, Wild U: Use of neuropsychological testing in mild traumatic head injuries. Cog Rehabil, 1988; 22–24.
10. Davidoff DA, Kessler HR, Laibstain DF, Mark VH: Neurobehavioral sequelae of minor head injury: A consideration of post-concussive syndrome versus post-traumatic stress disorder. Cogn Rehabil, 1988; 8–13.
11. Levin HS, Eisenberg HM: Post-concussional syndrome. Curr Ther Neurol Dis, 1987; 2:193–196.
12. Alves WM, Colohan AR, O'Leary TJ, Rimel RW, Jane JJ: Understanding post-traumatic symptoms after minor head injury. J Head Trauma Rehabil, 1986; 1:1–12.
13. Rimel R, Giordani B, Barth J, Boll T, Jane J: Disability caused by minor head injury. Neurosurgery, 1981; 9:221–228.
14. Prigatano GP, Fordyce DJ: Cognitive dysfunction and psychosocial adjustment after brain injury. In Prigatano GP (ed): Neuropsychological

Rehabilitation after Brain Injury. Baltimore: Johns Hopkins University, 1986.

15. Gronwall D, Wrightson P: Delayed recovery of intellectual function after minor head injury. Lancet, 1974; 605–609.

16. Binder LM: Persisting symptoms after mild head injury. A review of the postconcussive syndrome. J Clin Exp Neuropsychol, 1986; 8(40):323–346.

17. Lezak MD: Neuropsychological Assessment (2nd ed). New York: Oxford University Press 1983.

18. Slater EJ: Does mild mean minor? J Adolesc Health Care, 1989; 10:237–240.

19. Novack TA: Daniel MS, Long CJ: Factors related to emotional adjustment following head injury. Int J Clin Neuropsychol, 1984; 6:139–142.

20. Gouvier WD: Quiet victims of the silent epidemic: A comment on Dlugokinski. Am Psychol, 1986; 41:484.

21. Sohlberg MM, Mateer CA: Introduction to Cognitive Rehabilitation, Theory and Practice. New York: Guilfor, 1989.

22. Schacter DL, Crovitz HF: Memory function after closed head injury: A review of the quantitative research. Cortex, 1977; 13:150–176.

23. Gade GF, Young RF: Minor head injury. Prim Care, 1984; 11(4):667–679.

24. Levine MJ: Issues in neurobehavioral assessment of mild head injury. Cogn Rehabil, 1988; 14–19.

25. Levin HS, Benton AL, Grossman RG: Neurobehavioral consequences of closed head injury. New York: Oxford University Press, 1983.

26. Graham DL, Adams JH, Doyle D: Ischemic brain damage in fatal non-missile head injuries. J Neurol Sci, 1978; 39:213–234.

27. Barth JT, Macciocchi SN, Giordani B, Rimel RN, Jane JA, Boll TJ: Neuropsychological sequelae of minor head injury. Neurosurgery, 1983; 13(5):529–533.

28. Stuss DT, Ely BA, Hugenhaltz H, Richard MT, LaRochell S, Poiries CA, Be I: Subtle neuropsychological deficts in patients with good recovery after closed head injury. Neurosurgery, 1981; 17(1):41–47.

29. Gronwall D, Wrightson P: Memory and information processing capacity after closed head injury. J Neurol, Neurosurg Psychiatry, 1981; 44:889–895.

30. Yarnell PR, Rossie GV: Brain injury. 1988; 2(3):255–258.

31. Halstead WC: Brain and Intelligence. Chicago: University of Chicago Press, 1947.

32. Elia JC: The post concussion syndrome. Ind Med, 1972; 41:23–31.

33. Lishman WA: Physiogenesis and psychogenesis in the "post-concussional syndrome." Br J Psychiatry, 1988; 153:460–469.

34. Bornstein RA, Miller HB, van Schoor JT: Neuropsychological deficit and emotional disturbance in head-injured patients. J Neurosurg, 1989; 70:509–513.

35. Stern JM, Melamed S, Silber S, et al.: Behavioral disturbances as an expression of severity of cerebral damage. Scand J Rehabil Med, 1985; 12:36–41.

36. O'Hara C: Emotional adjustment following minor head injury. Cogn Rehabil, 1988; 26–33.

37. Kay T: Minor head injury: An introduction for professionals. Framingham, MA: National Head Injury Foundation.
38. Jennett B, Teasdale G: Management of Head Injuries. Philadelphia: Davis, 1981.
39. Bruce DA, Schut L, Bruno LA, Wood JH, Sutton LN: Outcome following head injury in children. J Neurosurg, 1978; 48:679–688.
40. Winogron HW, Knights RM, Bawden HN: Neuropsychological deficits following head injury in children. J Clin Neuropsychol, 1984; 6:269–286.
41. Brink JD, Imbus C, Woo-Sam J: Physical recovery after severe close head trauma in children and adolescents. J Pediatr, 1980; 97:721–727.
42. Levin HS, Eisenberg HM: Neuropsychology outcome of closed head injury in children and adolescents. Child's Brain, 1979; 5:281–292.
43. Gulbrandsen GB: Neuropsychological sequelae of light head injuries in older children six months after trauma. J Clin Neuropsychol, 1984; 6:257–268.
44. Luria A: Higher Cortical Functions in Man. New York: Basic Books, 1966.
45. Golden CJ: Luria-Nebraska Neuropsychology Battery: Children's Version. Los Angeles: Western Psychological Services, 1987.
46. Shaffer D, Chadwick O, Rutter M: Psychiatric outcome of localized head injury in children. In Outcome of Severe Damage to the Central Nervous System (CIBA Foundation Symposium 34). Amsterdam: Elsevier Excerpta Medica, 1975.
47. Knights RM: Problems of criteria in diagnosis: A profile similarity approach. Ann N Y Acad Sci, 1973; 205:124–131.
48. Flack J, Malmros R: A long-term follow-up study of children with severe head injury. Scand J Rehabil Med, 1972; 4:9–15.
49. Uzzell BP, Langfitt TW, Dolinskas CA: Influence of injury severity on quality of survival after head injury. Surg Neurol, 1987; 27:419–429.
50. Merskey H, Woodforde JM: Psychiatric sequelae of minor head injury. Brain, 1972; 95:521–528.
51. Wrightson P, Gronwall D: Time off work and symptoms after minor head injury. Injury, 1980; 12:445–454.
52. Rutherford WH, Merrett JD, McDonald JR: Symptoms one year following concussion from minor head injuries. Injury: Br J Accident Surg, 1979; 10(3):225–230.
53. Levin HS, Mattis S, Ruff RM, Eisenberg HM, Marshall LF, Tabbador K, High WM, Frankowski RF: Neurobehavioral outcome following minor head injury: A three-center study. J Neurosurg, 1987; 66:234–243.
54. Reitan RM, Wolfson D: The Halstead-Reitan Neuropsychological Battery: Theory and Clinical Interpretation. Tucson, AZ: Neuropsychological Press, 1985.
55. Golden CJ, Hammeke TA, Purisch AD: Manual for the Luria-Nebraska Neuropsychological Battery. Los Angeles: Western Psychological Services, 1980.
56. Binder LM, Rattok J: Assessment of the postconcussive syndrome after mild head trauma. In Lezak M (ed): Assessment of the Behavioral Consequences of Head Trauma. New York: Alan R. Liss, 1989.

57. Newman PJ, Sweet JJ: The effects of clinical depression on the Luria-Nebraska Neuropsychological Battery. Int J Clin Neuropsych, 1986; 8:109–114.
58. Wells CE: Pseudodementia. Am J Psychiatry, 1979; 136:895–900.
59. Bender LM, Pankratz L: Neuropsychological evidence of a factitious memory complaint. J Clin Exp Neuropsych, 1987; 9:167–171.

— 7

Psychiatric Aspects of Minor Brain Injuries

David Rubinstein

Head injuries are classified commonly as major or minor. However, even a very minor head injury is not necessarily clinically insignificant. Head trauma is most frequently caused by automobile-related accidents. In fact, a survey conducted in San diego County revealed that 44% of brain injuries were secondary to motor vehicle accidents and 21% resulted from falls, 12% from assaults, 10% from sports, and 6% from firearms (1).

During our psychiatric practices we often find relatively subtle behavioral or affective changes in patients' personalities which appear to be etiologically enigmatic. Often the patient has suffered an overlooked trauma to the head, either recent or remote. For example, it is common to retrieve a history of a child whose head was hit after falling from a bicycle, or a wife who was beaten by her husband, or an alcoholic who failed to report head trauma while inebriated. In these cases, the patients fail to associate the trauma with the subsequent personality changes, possibly because they were fearful, ashamed, or amnestic.

"Minor" Head Trauma

Children and adults who suffer from mild brain (head) injuries complain of headaches, dizziness, fatigue, reduced concentration, poor memory, sleep-cycle disturbances, depression, and increased irritability. These complaints may last beyond the immediate visit to the emergency room, often for months to two years or more after the initial trauma. The pathophysiology of these symptoms has not been fully demonstrated, although strain injuries to the brain or upper brainstem have been etiologically implicated (2). Oppenheimer has demonstrated microscopic lesions in the brains of such patients (3).

It is likely that almost no head injury is minor or free from trauma to the underlying brain structures. Symptoms consequent to minor head trauma are essentially related to the cerebral concussion and to the psychological and neurological effects of the traumatic event; and they may result in conditions such as accident neurosis or a cluster of depressive manifestations (i.e., the post-traumatic stress disorder).

Minor head trauma presents an assortment of symptoms, which may be categorized into three groups: a) a post-traumatic concussion syndrome; b) a post-traumatic stress disorder; and c) a combination of both. We will examine the presenting manifestations of these separate diagnostic categories. The intensity and duration of symptoms are affected by a set of variables, including a) the psychological consequences of the impact; b) the emotional repercussions of body injury; c) premorbid personality features; d) compensation and litigation factors; e) the psychosocial and interpersonal effects of deficits. In order for the psychiatrist to provide appropriate therapy based on accurate diagnosis, it is essential to understand all of these organic and non-organic factors, and to sort out the role they play in each individual case.

Post-Traumatic Concussion Syndrome

Traditionally, concussions are defined as those head traumas with brief loss or alteration of consciousness lasting less than one hour and usually less than ten minutes, with rapid return to normal alertness and no evidence of neurologic dysfunction (4). Symptoms which appear in patients with brief loss of consciousness may clear up after a few hours following awakening. However, some may persist, and other symptoms may not appear for days or weeks following the accident.

A more flexible definition of cerebral concussion is articulated by Adams and Victor (5). These authors define it as a "usually reversible traumatic paralysis of nervous function; it may last for a variable period (seconds, minutes, hours or longer), and it is due to a change in the momentum of the head (either movement of the head is arrested by a blow, or movement of the head is arrested by a hard, unyielding surface)."

However, it has become increasingly clear that traditional criteria for the diagnosis of concussion need to be reviewed in the light of our clinical experiences. Often, concussion patients have had such a short period of alteration of consciousness that it will go almost or totally unnoticed at the time of arrival at the hospital. Steadman and Graham, for example, found that 73% of patients diagnosed with concussion were awake at the time of admission, and 85% of the admitted patients had a duration of unconsciousness of less than an hour (6). Furthermore, it is not unlikely that some injured patients report (erroneously) not having lost consciousness at all and not having suffered a direct trauma to their heads. Nevertheless, they may develop clinical manifestations of concussion immediately following the accident or during the follow-up period. Such clinical observations lead to a needed revision of traditionally held concepts, including a more precise inventory of post-concussion symptomatology, its physiopathology, and its prognostic implications.

A recent review of 103 consecutive patients in my practice with a history of having been involved in motor vehicle accidents revealed that 90 of them provided definite indications of having hit their heads at the time of impact, and 13 denied having hit their heads. Only 5 of the 90 patients indicated that the impact was either on the upper or lower mandibular regions. Strikingly, only 29 of the 90 patients affirmed they had briefly lost consciousness following the impact; 22 patients were uncertain about it; and 39 patients were certain about having maintained consciousness throughout the event. Even more striking was the fact that a mental status examination performed at the time of the first consultation revealed that 61 of the 90 patients demonstrated symptoms and signs of a post-traumatic concussion syndrome; only 27 of those patients had no hisotry of traditional criteria of concussion; and 2 were questionable. In addition, of the 13 patients who were certain about not having hit their heads, 3 revealed having lost consciousness briefly, and 2 of them still had manifestations of post-traumatic concussion syndrome.

The diagnosis of minor cerebral concussion was based on accepted neuropsychiatric criteria (5). In some cases, the patient was not unconscious at all, but only stunned or "saw stars." In others, the patient complained of amnesia for events immediately preceding and following the injury. However, in most cases there are definite symptoms of post-traumatic nervous instability, including headache, giddiness, fatigability, sleep-cycle disturbances, and nervousness which appear immediately following the impact of within a few days.

Obviously, the personality deficits developed from traumatic brain injuries will depend on the regions of the brain which have been most affected (7). The intensity and duration of these symptoms will vary with the degree of neural damage. *Frontopolar injuries* account for impaired judgment and insight, decreased problem-solving and reasoning ability, apathy, and diminished motivation. *Orbitofrontal dysfunction* is reflected by impulsivity, excitability, and impaired social judgment. Memory loss is frequently observed in *anterior temporal injuries*. Many patients demonstrate personality effects of diffuse subcortical damage such as motor incoordination, cognitive deficits, and decreased concentration. The force of the impact may also affect *brainstem* structures. In those cases we have observed acute loss of consciousness, long-lasting attention deficits, vestibular dysfunction, and various motor impairments, either cerebellar, pyramidal, or extrapyramidal.

Explanations of the physiopathological mechanisms leading to such manifestations have been gaining acceptance since publication of the work of Denny-Brown and Russell [8]. These authors pioneered the concept of a concussive paralysis of brain function, consequent to a change in the momentum of the head in either direction. Various causes of cerebral paralysis have been proposed since then. Trotter, for example, attributed the cerebral concussive paralysis to a brief period of cerebral ischemia inducing an immediate paralysis of cerebral function, with a tendency to rapid and spontaneous recovery [9]. However, Shatsky et al., by the use of high-speed cineangiography, demonstrated displacement of vessels but no deficits in blood flow associated with impact [10].

Acceleration-Deceleration of Brain in Concussion

A more rational and accepted explanation has been offered by Ommaya and Gennarelli [11]. These authors believe that the greatest damage is produced by acceleration-deceleration of the brain within the closed skull compartment. Mechanical forces operating during the acceleration-deceleration movements may cause direct and contrecoup cerebral injury; or they may produce horizontal or rotational movements of the brain. Horizontal movements of the brain, within the decelerating skull, contribute to coup or contrecoup lesions which are in line with the horizontal displacement of the skull, or with the point of impact on the skull. Gross, abrupt rotational brain movements tend to produce cortical or subcortical damage. Both types of brain movements, within a fixed skull, may cause lesions in the underlying brain tissues adjacent to the internal skull surface. For example, the orbital plate may cause damage to the frontal structures, orbitopolar or orbitofrontal; the sphenoid wing, to the anterior temporal lobe.

Microscopic examinations of autopsied brains have demonstrated widespread tissue disruption in the subcortical structures [12] owing to shearing forces affecting microscopic boundaries of moving and stationary brain structures. The degree of microscopic damage correlates with the intensity and degree of brain tissue movements. In minor head injuries, it may involve disrupted axons with micro-hemorrhages, with subsequent macrophage activity; in more severe injuries there are grossly visible hemorrhages with subcortical degeneration, and subsequent ventricular enlargement. These micro-scopic brain lesions have implications for behavioral sequelae.

Diagnosis of Minor Head Injuries

Our review of the clinical records of 103 consecutive patients pre-viously mentioned indicates that most of the habitual testing methods, such as the CT scan of the brain, EEG, and ordinary psychological evaluations, may be insufficient to reflect disruption of brain struc-tures and functioning. More sensitive evaluation methods are re-quired to demonstrate such deficits including careful mental status examination, comprehensive neuropsychological assessment, and computerized EEG studies with brain mapping. Only when the combined results of these methods are evaluated are we able to reach a clearer diagnosis of the patient's condition. The following cases, abstracted from our series of patients, are illustrative examples.

Case 1

A-67-year old male was involved in a motor vehicle accident. Twelve months later, at the time of his first consultation, he related that he had hit his head against the windshield but was uncertain whether he had lost consciousness. He was suffering from frequent headaches, sleep-cycle disturbances, sexual impotence, irritability, deficits in his recent memory functions and concentration, and marked depressive feelings since the accident. A mental status examination suggested strong evidence of a post-traumatic concussion syndrome. An EEG was normal. A neuropsychological assessment, however, revealed an impairment index of 0.9, suggestive of "severe cortical level of impairment of cognitive functioning with moderate impairment of non-verbal abstract reasoning and problem solving." A cognitive rehabilitation program associated with supportive psychotherapy, amitriptyline, and high doses of L-tryptophan and choline appeared to bring about the remission of all symptoms in a period of about six months.

Case 2

A 41-year-old female hit her head against the windshield at the time of impact in a motor vehicle accident. One month later, on examination, she had definite symptoms and signs of having suffered a concussion, although she was uncertain whether she had lost consciousness. An initial EEG was reported as abnormal with paroxysmal synchronous slowing during drowsiness and sleep. A second EEG, performed three months later, was normal. However, at that time a neuropsychological evaluation revealed an impairment index of 0.6 and was reported as "mild organic dysfunction with post-traumatic syndrome characterized by depression associated with acute cortical level impairment."

Case 3

A 28-year-old male presented one month following a motor vehicle accident in which he reported having hit his head against the windshield with no loss of consciousness. Mental status examination revealed marked symptoms of a cerebral concussion. An EEG was normal. A neuropsychological assessment reported "mild dysfunction in the posterior left hemisphere, along with much confounding of peripheral physical difficulties and probable sensory and motor deficits associated with brainstem injury."

Case 4

A 22-year-old male was examined two months after having suffered what appeared to be a minor head injury sustained when he hit his head against the windshield in a front-end collision. He was uncertain whether he had lost consciousness; if he had, it was for a period of a few seconds. He had definite recent memory deficits, poor concentration, poor attention span, and slow cognitive processes. A neuro-ophthalmological examination revealed a scotoma in the upper right quadrant of the right visual field. Two EEGs with nasopharyngeal leads and sleep deprivation, six months apart, were reported as normal. A neuropsychological evaluation demonstrated "mild organic dysfunction; this pattern of results is associated with non-progressive cortical level impairment which affected the anterior portion of right cerebral hemisphere and posterior portion of left cerebral hemisphere."

Post-Traumatic Stress Disorder

Symptoms found in patients following motor vehicle accidents are not limited to post-concussion syndrome. Frequently, we find typical manifestations of a post-traumatic stress disorder, as described in the diagnostic criteria of the *Diagnostic and Statistical Manual of Mental Disorders*, 3rd Edition (DMS-III-R) (13).

In our experience the majority of patients respond to the stress with symptoms characteristic of an increased arousal syndrome. These include sleep-cycle disturbances, trouble concentrating, irritability and outbursts of anger over trivial issues, and hypervigilance. These symptoms start almost immediately following the accident and last for a variable period of weeks, months, and occasionally up to two years.

Sleep-cycle disturbance, one of the most frequent symptoms, may consist of difficulty in initiating or in maintaining the sleep cycle. Often the patient has recurrent interrupted sleep toward the end of each REM period. This disturbance may be due to repetitive nightmares representing the scene of the accident or equivalent violent incident, or sleep may be interrupted for reasons the patient is unaware of.

Another symptom frequently reported is difficulty concentrating. The patient notices that he/she is unable to perform intellectual tasks with customary proficiency subsequent to the accident. It may take longer to read the page of a book, or he/she may have difficulties in the sequential subtraction of 7 from 100. Immediate memory functions are affected, so the patient has difficulty in reciting backwards a series of unrelated words or numbers. The patient may also complain of recent memory deficits; he/she may become forgetful of familiar facts and data he/she previously managed with ease.

A third common complaint is irritability, with propensity to explode in angry outbursts triggered by the most trivial issues. This has a deleterious effect on interpersonal relations, especially family relationships. Several of this author's patients have seen their marriages terminated because of their uncontrolled anger. They become insensitive to their spouses and children, feel alienated, and distance themselves from their immediate relatives and friends. Intimate relationships suffer; patients often complain of reduced libidinal drives with partial or total diminution of sexual activities.

Lack of energy, easy fatigability, a tendency to inertia, and loss of initiative are forerunners of a depressive syndrome. The patient may experience feelings of guilt, depressed mood, recurrent thoughts of doom, and eating disturbances. These symptoms may last for months following the accident and may require antidepressant treatment. Less frequently the patient may develop an episode of mania indistinguishable from other manic episodes. If affective changes do reach such alarming proportions, one must suspect a constitutional predisposition and inquire about premorbid pathologic personality features.

The most frequent symptom found among our patients was the persistent re-experiencing of the accident, as flashbacks or recurrent dreams, and physiologic reactivity on exposure to the circumstances associated to the accident. For example, whenever the patient drives a motor vehicle, or is driven, he experiences uncontrollable phobic symptoms associated with neurovegetative distress signals. After being involved in a collision with a truck, one of my patients insisted on sitting in the backseat of the family automobile driven by her husband; for months both avoided driving on a highway where trucks were frequent vehicles.

It could be argued that some symptoms result directly from the acute or chronic pain syndrome associated with the physical trauma experienced by the patient. Other symptoms, such as the anticipatory anxiety of re-experiencing the same traumatic event, the increased arousal manifestations with their physiological disturbances, and the avoidance behavior, are characteristic of a typical post-traumatic stress disorder. Zung developed a self-rating pain and distress scale to rate the intensity of the subjective complaints in these patients [14]. This scale assists the patient in reporting the degree, prevalence, and subjective perception of various symptomatic manifestations: somatosensory pain, mood changes, efficiency, sleep disturbances, psychomotor alterations, and alerrtness. A mean score of 35.6 or less would be considered normal; any score above this figure, to a maximum of 80, would be considered abnormal. Only 5 of our 103 patients scored within the normal range. All the rest scored somewhere between 38 and 76, with a mean of 51.2. The majority had high abnormal scores in mood, sleep cycles, and psychomotor items.

Combined Effects

When the patient suffers simultaneously from pain due to physical injuries, a post-concussion syndrome, and a post-traumatic stress disorder, all these symptoms are magnified and appear to follow a protracted course with complicated clinical manifestations. For example, memory deficits and concentration difficulties caused mostly by a concussion are enhanced by the associated stress disorder and its depressive component, the chronic pain being suffered, and by the analgesic treatment being prescribed.

During the diagnostic evaluation of such patients, it is crucial to assess and distinguish to what extent which syndrome is contributing to the symptom in question. Otherwise, a concussion syndrome may be overlooked and its cognitive deficits may be attributed erroneously to depression. We have found neuropsychological testing and computerized electroencephalography to be of inestimable value in such differential diagnoses.

Case 5

A 61-year-old male came for consultation following a motor vehicle accident during which he lost consciousness for a few seconds following impact. He could not recall with certainty if he had hit his head. When he arrived at the emergency room, he was alert and responsive, with no evidence of neurologic deficits. At the initial consultation, three months later, he appeared depressed and irritable. He complained of having lost interest in sexual relations with his wife and in all habitual activities, including his favorite sports activities. He also related frequently interrupted sleep cycles associated with "jerking of his legs," and problems with stammering. A clinical examination demonstrated that he was suffering from verbal apraxia, a depressive syndrome related to post-traumatic stress disorder, and restless leg syndrome, confirmed by a sleep study. Although a regular EEG was reported as normal, a neuropsychological assessment indicated that he was suffering from mild organic impairment affecting both cerebral hemispheres. The depressive symptomatology was affecting memory functions and cognition. Treatment approaches included the utilization of clonazepam 1 mg at bedtime, speech therapy, alprozolam 0.5 mg three times a day, amitriptyline 25 mg twice daily, and supportive psychotherapy. Total resolution of all symptoms was achieved after six months of treatment.

Psychodynamic Considerations

From a psychodynamic viewpoint we speculate that post-traumatic stress symptomatology is due to an abrupt breakdown of ego functions with mobilization of primitive defensive operations. Repression of the traumatic event may account for some deficits in recalling the events (post-traumatic amnesia) and for some dissociative phenomena (post-traumatic hysteria and conversion reactions) immediately following the accident. Denial may be reflected in compensatory euphoria and even hypomanic reactions. Identification with the aggressor explains frequent feelings of guilt and depressive symptoms.

Primary process phenomena may appear, such as "magical thinking," projection mechanisms, anticipatory anxiety, irritability, phobias related to moving vehicles, and poor impulse control. With deficient ego functions, more primary id and primitive superego phenomena tend to appear. The patient loses interest in object relations while blaming himself for deteriorating relationships. Increased narcissism tends to appear, with pervasive demands for sympathy, attention, and emotional nurturance to replenish an impoverished self-esteem.

For example, a 28-year-old black female was convinced that she had a "jinx" imposed by an envious sister-in-law; this explained to her the reason for her trauma. She became fearful of leaving her home to avoid the risk of being traumatized again by the same "curse." She felt depressed and blamed herself for the accident since she had provoked the sister-in-law's envy. Another 36-year-old female developed a manic episode following an automobile accident with denial of the accident and its emotional and physical consequences. The remission of manic symptoms with lithium therapy helped her to deal with the effect this trauma had on her daily functioning, including the loss of her job and an irreversible marital separation.

Variables Affecting Symptomatology

Psychiatric literature abounds with factors affecting clinical manifestations in these cases (15). We should briefly examine some of the outstanding ones.

Psychological Repercussions of Injury and Premorbid Personality Factors

The psychological effects of having been involved in a sudden, unexpected traumatic event are obvious. The person immediately feels anxious, scared, and shocked. A panic reaction ensues, with a variable length of recuperation from hours to days or weeks.

More important are long-term repercussions, especially if the individual has suffered intellectual or physical deficits. An active, high-striving person may develop marked depression when confined to a bed or a wheelchair or when faced with the inability to move easily without excruciating back pain.

The patient's age may be a significant factor in the intensity and duration of symptoms. Older persons tend to experience their limitations more adversely and view these deficits as further encroaching on an already limited life-style. Their capacity to mobilize healthier psychological resources in the face of stress may be diminished. On the other extreme, young patients may unrealistically underestimate the changes they have undergone. They insist they are well, when, in reality, they have significant cognitive and emotional disturbances which they do not recognize.

Mobilization of dependency needs may arouse either ego-syntonic or ego-dystonic reactions, depending on premorbid personality structure and dynamics. A narcissistic individual with intense dependency needs may take advantage of injuries sustained and prolong or exaggerate symptomatology. Patients with cyclothymic personality may develop either an enhancement or premorbid depressive features or a hypomanic episode, to manipulate environmental sympathy toward their pains and deficits. An alcoholic may increase his addictive habits, thus magnifying intellectual deficits. Sociopathic individuals may exaggerate their symptoms for secondary gains and financial compensation for their alleged injuries and suffering. In general, persons with personality limitations and/or instability are prone to react more adversely and with increased or prolonged symptomatology.

Interpersonal and Familial Factors

The patient's social and family environment cannot be ignored. These play a major role in the perception and expression of deficits and distress. We have described the formation of interpersonal dyadic relationships whereby an individual plays the role of "being sick" while a partner in the relationship is the "caretaker" (16,17). This type of partnership insures the survival of the relationship which may have been otherwise at risk. Obviously, dyadic partnerships tend to prolong and exaggerate the patient's symptoms; this is required by the unwritten contract they both try to protect. Incidentally, it is rather frequent to find that when one of the partners is recuperating from the distress suffered in a previous accident, the other partner suffers a second accident and the roles get reversed.

Problems in the marital relationship may have antedated the accident. In an effort to rationalize those difficulties, however, the traumatic event and its consequences become the excuse on which all interpersonal stresses are blamed. The patient and his/her spouse now have a valid reason to maintain alienation and detachment by virtue of a silent agreement. If the patient is the main source of income, the disability may produce significant upheaval as a result of the economic predicament of the family. Critical situations may arise with the patient's role being skewed and the spouse being forced to find compensatory functions to maintain the family's stability. In those cases, family intervention techniques are imperative to avoid a deterioration of the relationship.

Socio-Cultural Influences

It is also evident that some socio-cultural groups tolerate pain and disability better than others, while some may even foster the expression of distress and disability. These groups may communicate emotional distress and personality problems through the expression of aches and pains. It is rather frequent to encounter patients from selected cultural backgrounds complaining of diffuse, vague, and ill-defined pains after a motor vehicle accident. Others complain of "something wrong with the head" or of neuro-vegetative symptoms which cannot be cleared up for years following an accident. Others believe that the trauma affected all internal organs, including the heart, the liver, the brain, and all musculo-skeletal structures. In reality, these symptoms are culturally prevalent and a common denominator in most of the individuals surrounding the patient. Similarly, some individuals, often from economically deprived backgrounds in the United States, are prone to claim disability under the sponsorship of existing social security provisions. For these individuals it is an acceptable expedient condoned and cultivated by the culture they belong to.

Compensation and Litigation Influences

It has been debated whether symptoms presented by patients following minor head (brain) injuries, especially those caused by motor vehicle accidents, are valid or mere exaggerations to obtain financial compensation. Questions have been raised in view of the fact that some patients discontinue their treatments once the litigation is settled. It has been estimated that the expectation of compensation may exaggerate or perpetuate symptoms in one-quarter to one-third of all patients when the accident is someone else's fault (18–20). Other authors have stated that the incidence of malingering has been overestimated and that exaggerated symptoms are encountered less often than had been previously reported (6,21,22).

A resolution of this dilemma has been offered by Miller, who coined the term "accident neurosis" (19). In this condition the symptoms are an exaggeration of a concussion or of depression and anxiety. Physical examinations produce dramatic magnifications of physical signs; mental evaluations provide the opportunity for patients to augment their distress.

Certain clinical features are common in accident neurosis: It has been stated that there is a higher incidence in men, in unskilled workers, and following industrial accidents (4). In our experience with motor vehicle accidents, there is a higher incidence in persons under the age of 50, about equal distribution in both genders, no correlation with occupational skills, and prevalence in middle and lower socioeconomic classes.

At any rate, the notion of accident neurosis is real and valid. It has a psychogenic mechanism and it follows a predictable clinical course. Psychodynamically it is determined by both conscious and unconscious mechanisms. Whether compensation is sought becomes a secondary issue. The great majority of our patients presented genuine symptomatology. Some of them were discharged asymptomatic long before any settlement was reached and returned to their habitual occupation. Others continued with residual symptomatology, both cognitive and emotional, during a prolonged follow-up after settlement of their claims. Dynamics operating in accident neurosis are governed by variables involving premorbid personality factors and structure, familial interpersonal relationships, impact of the accident and injuries on the individual's physical and psychological capacities, and socio-cultural values and ethics.

Treatment Approaches

Minderhoud et al. reported that in a series of patients who had suffered a post-concussion syndrome, the number and frequency of symptoms was markedly reduced by treatment which included information, explanation, and encouragement (23). Those patients that were told they had a cerebral concussion displayed temporary complaints that resulted in a longer period of confinement to bed and more disabilities, although better results with respect to post-traumatic sequelae than those patients not informed of their diagnosis.

Our therapeutic experience was based on attempting to establish the nature of the symptomatic manifestations, that is, whether the patient had suffered a concussion, a post-traumatic stress disorder, or a combination of both, and whether other variables, such as the ones previously discussed, influenced the frequency and intensity of symptoms.

Several concomitant therapeutic approaches were utilized, including supportive psychotherapy, behavioral modification techniques, and pharmacotherapy. In some cases, the addition of marital counseling, speech therapy, and cognitive rehabilitation programs were found to be extremely helpful.

Supportive psychotherapy consisted essentially of ventilation of feelings, explanations, clarifications, reassurance, directives, and encouragement. We found that explaining to the patient the nature of his/her symptoms and correlating them with the traumatic event was extremely helpful, since many patients fear that they are "losing their mind." Allowing the patient to ventilate feelings provided the reassurance needed to encourage him/her to resume pre-traumatic activities and to establish an efficient therapeutic contract with the therapist. The patient had to be directed in accordance with current capabilities to avoid unwarranted complaints and disabilities. Often, insight into the patient's dynamics may be an added feature in the psychotherapeutic approach, helping to enlighten him/her about correlations between symptoms and current or preexisting conflicts in his/her personality.

Marital counseling was found to be imperative in all cases in which the patient's symptoms had seriously altered the dynamics of interpersonal relations with the impending risk of a separation or divorce. The spouse's participation in therapy seemed to reduce the marital crisis and induced cooperation with rehabilitation programs.

The technique of progressive relaxation was useful to induce a reduction of anxiety and of muscular aches owing to sprain and strain. Patients should be trained in this technique by rehearsing it in the presence of the therapist, and instructed to perform it repeatedly in the course of successive days. When sufficient training in this technique is achieved, a desensitization technique is also utilized to alleviate the phobic manifestations associated with riding or driving a motor vehicle. The patient is asked repeatedly to recount the accident. Whenever signs of anxiety are aroused, the exercise is stopped and restarted after a few minutes. This exercise utilized over successive sessions seems to alleviate the phobic symptoms.

Symptomatic relief was also achieved by the use of psychotropics, especially benzodiazepines and antidepressants. We prefer to prescribe smaller than usual dosages of these medications, because patients who have suffered a concussion may be oversensitive to their side effects. Alprazolam, in varied dosages from 0.25 mg at bedtime to 0.5 mg three times daily, and amitriptyline at dosages from 25 mg to 75 mg daily were utilized. When the depressive syndrome was significant and unresponsive to amitriptyline, fluoxetine 20 mg daily was prescribed with better results. Those patients with manic symptomatology responded well to the use of lithium carbonate 300 mg two or three times daily, according to the intensity of symptoms. Sleep was often secured with the utilization of temazepam 15 to 30 mg at bedtime.

In conclusion, minor head (brain) traumas are to be taken seriously by the practitioner. The patient's symptoms should be evaluated carefully. The condition should not be underestimated because of the potential for secondary gain. Symptoms vary in intensity and duration and are influenced by a set of factors which include premorbid personality elements, the effect of injuries and of intellectual deficits on the patient's pre-traumatic performance and capabilities, and socio-cultural and familial values and dynamics. Prognosis varies according to these factors, the presenting syndromes, and the severity of injuries. The psychiatrist who takes the trouble to understand and integrate these factors into his/her diagnostic and therapeutic plans may provide invaluable assistance to patients who have suffered minor head injury.

References

1. Krause JF, Black MA, Hessol N, et al.: The incidence of acute brain injury and serious impairment in a defined population. Am J Epidemiol, 1984; 119:186.
2. Gennarelli TA: Mechanisms and pathophysiology of cerebral concussion. J Head Trauma Rehabil, 1986; 1:23–30.
3. Oppenheimer DR: Microscopic lesions in the brain following head injury. J Neurol Neurosurg Psychiatry, 1968; 31:299–306.
4. Alexander MP: Traumatic Brain Injury. In Benson DF, Blumer D (eds): Psychiatric Aspects of Neurologic Disease, Vol. II. New York: Grune & Stratton, 1982.
5. Adams RD, Victor M: Principles of Neurology. New York: McGraw-Hill, 1976.
6. Steadman JH, Graham JG: Head injuries: An analysis and follow-up study. Proc R Soc Med, 1970; 63:23–28.
7. Blumer D, Benson DR: Personality changes with frontal and temporal lobe lesions. In Blumer D, Benson DF (eds): Psychiatric Aspects of Neurologic Disease, Vol. I. New York: Grune & Stratton, 1975; pp 151–170.
8. Denny-Brown D, Russell WR: Experimental cerebral concussion. Brain, 1941; 64:93.
9. Trotter W: Injuries of the skull and brain. In Choyce's System of Surgery. London: Cassell, 1932; Vol III, p 358.
10. Shatsky SA, Evans DE, Miller F, Martins AN: High speed angiography of experimental head injury. J Neurosurg, 1974; 41:523.
11. Ommaya AK, Gennarelli TA: Cerebral concussion and traumatic unconsciousness. Brain, 1974; 97:633–654.
12. Brooks DN, Aughton ME, Bond MR, et al.: Cognitive sequelae in relationship to early indices of severity of brain damage after severe blunt head injury. J Neurol Neurosurg Psychiatry, 1980; 43:529–534.
13. Diagnostic and Statistical Manual of Mental Disorders (Third Edition, Revised), Washington, DC: Am Psychiatric Ass, 1987; pp 247–251.
14. Zung WWK: A self-rating pain and distress scale. Psychosomatics, 1983; 24:887–894.
15. Lishman WA: The psychiatric sequelae of head injury: a review. Psychol Med, 1973; 3:304–318.
16. Rubinstein D, Timmins JF: Depressive dyadic and triadic relationships. J Marr Fam Counsel, 1978; 4:13–23.
17. Rubinstein D, Timmins JF: Narcissistic dyadic relationships. Am J Psychoanal, 1979; 39:125–136.

18. Miller H: Accident neurosis. Br Med J, 1961; 1:919–925.
19. Miller H: Mental after-effects of head injury. Proc R Soc Med, 1966; 59:257–261.
20. Kelly R: The post-traumatic syndrome. Proc IV Pahlave Int Cong Pahlave Med J, 1972; 3:530.
21. Parker N: Accident litigants with neurotic symptoms. Med J Aust, 1977; 2:318–322.
22. Rimel RW, Giordani B, Barth JT, et al.: Disability caused by minor head injury. Neurosurgery, 1981; 9:221–223.
23. Minderhoud JM, Boelens MEM, Huizenga J, Saan RJ: Treatment of minor head injuries. Clin Neurol Neurosurg, 1980; 82:127–140.

— 8

Sleep Abnormalities Following Head Trauma

Karl Doghramji and Joyce Zinsenheim

Introduction

The hallmark symptoms of disturbed sleep are insomnia and excessive daytime somnolence (EDS). The first of these, insomnia, is one of the most commonly encountered complaints in clinical medicine. Thirty-five percent of the adult population experiences it during the course of a year and about 17% considers it to be a serious difficulty (1). Simply stated, insomnia is the sensation of unrefreshing or interrupted sleep. Insomnia can be acute, in which case it is usually related to a disruptive emotional experience, travel across time zones, or other isolated events. This type of insomnia is usually transient and self-limited. Chronic and unrelenting insomnia, that is, insomnia which lasts more that a few months, is more often related to serious conditions such as major depression, chronic psychophysiological insomnia, central sleep apnea syndrome, and the chronic use of drugs and alcohol. It is also more typically the sleep complaint of brain-injured patients. Insomnia may also be characterized by inability to fall asleep within a reasonable time period, in which case it may be related to a disorder of the biologic clock, such as delayed-sleep-phase syndrome or a conditioned fear of falling asleep referred to as chronic psychophysiological insomnia. Insomnia may also refer to a difficulty

The authors thank Troy L. Thompson II, M.D., for his helpful suggestions regarding this chapter.

in staying asleep or awakening too early in the morning, symptoms more consistent with major depression.

The second major manifestation of altered sleep, EDS, may also be acute or chronic. In the latter case, milder levels of EDS may cause the sufferer to fall asleep during periods of relative inactivity such as while reading or watching television. However, when severe, individuals may fall asleep during times of greater activity, such as speaking, writing, or even eating. They may also experience sleep attacks, involuntary sleep episodes which usually strike without warning. The occurrence of sleep attacks during vulnerable moments such as while driving often constitutes a medical emergency mandating rapid evaluation and treatment. Symptoms often associated with EDS include difficulty with concentration, lapses in attention, impairment in memory and judgment, depression, irritability, and lethargy. Chronic EDS is a hallmark of obstructive sleep apnea syndrome, narcolepsy, periodic leg movements in sleep, the use of central nervous suppressant drugs, among others.

Victims of head trauma are known to suffer from difficulties with sleep and wakefulness. These are, in fact, some of the most challenging patients with which clinicians are faced since their problems are often chronic, unremitting, and refractory to treatment. Thus, patients may be incapacitated for years following their injuries (2). As a group, these symptoms are also some of the most frequently reported by head trauma patients. Rutherford (3), in a questionnaire survey of 145 inpatients who had undergone minor head injury six weeks prior, found insomnia to be the third most common of 17 symptom categories, the first 2 being headache and anxiety. Insomnia was reported by 15% of the population. Levin (4), in a multi-center study of post-concussional victims, reported that sleep disturbances ranked fourth among the fifteen most commonly reported complaints, the first three being headaches, fatigability, and dizziness. Sleep difficulties were reported in up to 50% of individuals in one site, and 44% overall. The second most frequently voiced symptom, fatigability, was reported in 56% of sufferers. This ill-defined complaint is widely recognized as one of the most debilitating symptoms encountered by head trauma victims and has been the focus of extensive and often fruitless evaluations. Although its causes may be multifactorial, it is often due to EDS. The consolidation of the insomnia and EDS groups reported by Levin yields a clear majority of patients having complaints concerning sleep and wakefulness.

The potential implications of these findings are immense. An estimated 500,000 new cases of brain injury occur every year (5) and account for 2% of all deaths and 26% of injury-related deaths in the United States (6). Head injuries are also a major cause of morbidity and long-term functional impairment. Added together, the annual economic cost of motor vehicle injuries is a staggering $14.4 billion, second only to the cost of cancer (7). If the nature and causes of sleep complaints could be understood and effective treatment modalities instituted, the potential seems great for effecting positive changes in the level of morbidity and possible mortality.

Polysomnography

Although it is often of interest to investigate the subjective complaints of sleep-disordered patients, more accurate data are obtained by conducting laboratory-based studies. The most thorough of these is polysomnography, a standardized technique for the simultaneous monitoring of multiple physiologic parameters during sleep. The first group of parameters pertain to sleep stages whose proper characterization requires the simultaneous monitoring of the electroencephalogram (EEG), electrooculogram (EOG), and electromyogram (EMG) of skeletal muscle, usually the submentalis. A complete clinical polysomnogram adds airflow monitors at the nose and mouth. Respiratory effort is detected with strain gauges placed around the chest and abdomen or by inductance plethysmography. Oxygen saturation is monitored by noninvasive transcutaneous sensors. Other parameters include the electrocardiogram and EMG of the anterior tibialis muscles, the latter intended to detect periodic leg movements. Finally, patients' gross body movements are continuously monitored by audiovisual means.

The most commonly employed form of polysomnography, referred to as the nocturnal polysomnogram (NPSG) is conducted during the typical sleeping hours of the patient and identifies pathological processes during sleep. Another form is the multiple sleep latency test (MSLT), a daytime study which objectively quantifies the degree of daytime somnolence. While being monitored in a manner similar to a NPSG, patients are asked to lie in a quiet and dark room during the day and not to resist the tendency to fall asleep. This procedure is followed at two-hour intervals beginning at 10:00 am and ending at 6:00 pm, and each subtest lasts between 10 and 30 minutes. The speed of falling asleep, referred to as the sleep latency, is inversely related to the degree of somnolence. Noncomplaining adults have a mean sleep latency across naps of 10 to 20 minutes, the exact frequency being a function of age. A mean sleep latency less than 10 minutes indicates a significant degree of EDS, and one less than 5 minutes indicates a pathologic level of EDS. In the latter case, the affected individual is highly susceptible to sleep attacks. The MSLT is useful in research settings as a means of objectively quantifying the severity of daytime somnolence. In clinical settings it is utilized to provided objective confirmation of EDS prior to the institution of long-term treatment. It is also vital in establishing or ruling out the diagnosis of certain sleep disorders such as narcolepsy or delayed-sleep-phase syndrome, and in monitoring the course of treatment of disorders which feature EDS.

Additional specialized forms of polysomnography are available, including the maintenance of wakefulness test (MWT), nocturnal penile tumescence monitoring, and gastroesophageal pH monitoring, among others (8,9).

The Architecture of Human Sleep

During quiet wakefulness the predominant frequency noted in the EEG of most individuals is 8 to 12 Hz. Research over the past few decades into sleep patterns has revealed that sleep is normally entered through stage 1; once sleep begins the predominant EEG frequency is a slower 4 to 7 Hz. A parallel decrease in EMG amplitude is noted, indicating a lessening of muscle tone, and the EOG reveals rhythmic and slow, rolling eye movements. Stage 2 soon follows and is marked by the intrusion of EEG sleep spindles, bursts of 12- to 14-Hz, highly synchronized activity lasting at least 0.5 seconds, and K-complexes, slow negative deflections usually occurring singly and followed by a positive component. Individuals may experience random thoughts and thought fragments during stages 1 and 2, and become less and less aware of their surroundings. With the approach of stages 3 and 4 of sleep, collectively referred to as delta sleep, the EEG frequency becomes even slower as 2- to 3-Hz synchronized waves predominate and eye movements cease. Cognitive mental processes are at their lowest level. Delta sleep is necessary for the refreshing and alerting quality of sleep; individuals whose sleep is deprived of this state awaken feeling sleepy despite sufficient time spent asleep. Stages 1 through 4 are collectively referred to as non-REM sleep and constitute approximately 75% of total sleep time in adults. Non-REM is a relatively quiet state during which skeletal muscle tone is continuously reduced compared to wakefulness; and cardiac, respiratory, and other automatic activity is monotonously regular and slow compared to wakefulness.

In contrast, during REM sleep the EEG displays low-voltage, fast, desynchronized activity. Although rapid eye movements (REMs) are noted on EOG, most skeletal muscles exhibit atonia, which is mediated through central nervous system (CNS) inhibitory impulses that are actively generated and that descend to peripheral muscles. This, as well as the observations that brain oxygen utilization and temperature in animals are enhanced during this stage, and that most sleepers report mental activity in the form of dreams when awakened from REM, has led investigators to conclude that REM is a paradoxical state during which the mind is active yet the body is paralyzed.

An orderly progression from stages 1 through 4 occurs within 45 minutes of falling asleep. Within 90 minutes of falling asleep, the first REM period appears. The period between sleep onset (the time of falling asleep) and the first REM period is also referred to as the REM latency. There is a continuous repetition of the 90-minute cycle from one REM period to the next throughout the night.

Transection studies in animals have demonstrated that the pons is both necessary and sufficient for the generation of many of the manifestations of REM sleep. Through lesion studies the site of REM sleep generation has further been isolated to the lateral pontine tegmentum, more specifically the nucleus reticularis pontis oralis (RPO) and a small region immediately ventral to the locus coeruleus. However, when one considers other phenomena associated with REM sleep, such as dreaming, which involves cortical structures, it becomes evident that many other brain regions must be involved. Possibly these structures are recruited by a small group of executive neurons within the brainstem (10).

Brain mechanisms involved in slow-wave sleep appear to be diffusely distributed and seem to extend from the medulla through the brainstem and hypothalamus into the basal forebrain. Here, they seem to interact in a reciprocal manner with neurons maintaining activation and wakefulness. Although a large number of neurotransmitters and modulators have been investigated in relationship to sleep, no one substance has yet been identified as being both necessary and sufficient for the generation of sleep or wakefulness. It appears, therefore, that these two states are governed by the complex interaction of many systems (11).

Sleep and wakefulness, like most biological processes, follow a cyclical pattern which corresponds to the 24-hour day. Investigations over the past few decades have indentified the suprachiasmatic nucleus (SCN) of the hypothalamus as an important structure in the regulation of at least some circadian rhythms. Although the free-running intrinsic period of the SCN is usually not exactly 24 hours in length, entrainment to the 24-hour daily cycle is achieved through neurosensory impulses. One such system is the retinohypothalamic tract (RHT), which transmits photic inputs to the SCN from retinal photoreceptors. Nonphotic stimuli such as feeding schedules and social cues, are also known to mediate SCN entrainment (12).

Although there remain many areas of investigation in basic sleep mechanisms, research over the past few decades has clearly discounted the notion that sleep is simply a lapse in wakefulness. Rather, it is now known to be a highly organized functional state with neurophysiological, psychological, and behavioral correlates. It is the product of actively generated central processes which, through the recruitment of the coordinated activity of other CNS structures, alter the activity of almost every peripheral organ. Implied in these statements is that damage to this intricate mechanism by head trauma might be anticipated to result in alterations in sleep architecture and physiology consistent with the neuroanatomic sites of damage. One purpose of this chapter is to explore hypothesized and experimental findings linking these factors to the nature and severity of insomnia, EDS, and emotional and cognitive changes.

Descriptive Studies of Sleep and Wakefulness Following Head Trauma

Initial investigations into the sleep of patients suffering from prior head trauma were primarily concerned with the possible role of polysomnographic findings in the prediction of the outcome of coma. Thus, most initial studies involved severely disabled and comatose patients. One of the first such studies was that of Bergamaso and colleagues (13), who performed serial polysomnograms limited to sleep-staging parameters on 18 comatose head trauma subjects. Even though their study lacked control subjects, they noted that some patients showed "typical polysomnographic sleep patterns." In almost all there was a decrease in the frequency of spindles and K-complexes. However, the pattern more often noted was a "biphasic" one. The first component was characterized by slow EEG activity and the paucity of movements and muscular activity, and was noted mainly during the day. The second component was characterized by faster and lower amplitude EEG activity and sawtooth waves with rapid eye movements on EOG, and was recorded mainly in the second half of the night. This apparent REM-NREM cycle was absent in another subgroup of patients who displayed a monophasic pattern characterized mainly by slow waves. In yet another subgroup, no definite patterns could be identified. Of interest is that the patients who displayed greater preservation of sleep architecture and circadian organization seemed to have a better prognosis. A gradual increase in organization of the EEG was noted as clinical state improved. On the basis of these observations, the authors suggested that polysomnography can be used as a prognostic tool during the period of coma.

In a similar study, Lessard and co-workers (14) investigated eight trauma-related and two drug-induced coma victims and seven normal individuals. The findings were similar to those of the previously discussed study. Unlike the control subjects, post-trauma patients lacked the characteristic sleep stages and many displayed a paucity of sleep spindles and K-complexes. In some patients, a cyclic variation of sleep EEG, i.e., periods of alternation between greater and lesser delta activity, could be identified. Most of these patients subsequently recovered, whereas most of the patients without evidence of cyclic variation died.

Subsequent investigators turned their attention to the sleep-wake abnormalities following recovery from the acute phase of head trauma. An extensive body of subjective data was gathered by Parsons and Ver Beek (15) who administered questionnaires to 75 subjects 3 months after minor head injuries sustained from motor vehicle accidents. The frontal and occipital regions of the head were primarily involved, and most patients had experienced loss of consciousness for up to one hour. Compared to their retrospective account of sleep prior to the injury, subjects experienced a greater frequency of spontaneous and prolonged awakenings within each night and over the course of the week. They assessed sleep quality as being worse following the accident, and they reported spending greater time following their final morning awakening at a lowered level of functioning. No association was noted between impact site and sleep-related complaints, yet the length of time in coma correlated positively with length of time spent in bed in the morning and negatively related to the number and vividness of dreams.

Although these subjective data are of interest, when taken alone they do not offer insights regarding pathophysiology. Hypotheses along these lines must also take into consideration objective testing results. Previous studies have shown that there is often a significant discrepancy between patients' subjective assessments of the magnitude and nature of their sleep difficulties and objective findings obtained by polysomnography. This is true of insomniacs as well as patients reporting EDS (16).

In an uncontrolled study, Harada and colleagues (17) performed longitudinal polysomnograms on 105 patients with miscellaneous clinical diagnoses associated with damage to the brain. Although patients were, presumably, conscious at the time of polysomnography, most were known to have sustained severe injuries to the brain. Only five patients in their sample were victims of traumatic head injury. They noted various changes, including a decrease in total sleep time, variable absence of delta waves, disappearance of sleep spindles and vertex sharp waves, and a "simplification" of the EEG during sleep to the point that in some patients a distinction between sleep stages could not be made. A variable loss of REM sleep was also noted which seemed to be more profound as the severity of coma increased. Although these findings are intriguing, the diversity of pathophysiological entities represented in their group poses an obstacle to making generalizations concerning the sleep disturbances of head trauma patients. Indeed, a variety of studies have shown that pathological processes affecting the CNS often lead to changes similar to the ones described above (18–20).

Ron and colleagues (21) performed polysomnograms limited to sleep-staging parameters in nine drug-free victims of severe head trauma and in nine controls. Patients had undergone variable periods of coma. Polysomnograms were performed one to three months after injury for four to seven nights while patients were conscious. In contrast to the normal subjects, head trauma patients had an excess of alpha bursts and sleep spindles in stages 2 and 3, EMG "tremor" in stage 3, fewer than usual eye movements in REM, and variable loss of EMG atonia. As time from the injury increased, some of these abnormalities abated and then ceased. Many patients initially lacked the typical REM-NREM cycling, which gradually returned as clinical state improved. A decrease in stage 1, and increases in stages 4 and REM, also paralleled improvement in clinical state. However, only the improvement rate in the percentage of REM was related to improvement rate of cognition variables; the relationship was a positive one. On the basis of their data, the authors suggest that REM may be important in information processing and memory, and that improvement in REM implies better prognosis in terms of regaining cognitive function.

Prigatano and colleagues (22) added to our understanding by performing limited polysomnography 6 to 59 months following injury in ten patients and in ten age-matched controls over the course of a single night. All patients had a history of closed head injury; were conscious at the time of study; and with the exception of one patient, had been comatose for at least 24 hours. Findings included a decrease in the percentage of stage 1 and an increase in the number of awakenings in patients. However, REM sleep was not altered in quality or proportion, in contrast to the previously reported study, even though patients complained of decreased or absent dreaming. Also unlike the previous study, no relationship was noted between REM measures and indices of cognitive function. In a controlled study, George and co-workers (23) performed polysomnographic studies on 16 patients. All had recovered from coma, some one month and the rest six months previously. Findings in the group studied one month after recovery included an increase in the number of awakenings, increased total wake time, and a decreased percentage of REM sleep. These abnormalities were more pronounced in patients in whom the duration of coma was longer (15–40 days) and in whom the level of injury was lower in the brain (mesendiencephalic). In patients with a relatively short coma duration (5–12 days) and with a higher level of brain injury (diencephalic), these findings were less pronounced. In the group studied six months after recovery of consciousness, the polysomnographic patterns were similar to those of controls, regardless of the site of the lesion.

Hanley (24) reported on a study of head injury patients who, at the time of the recording, no longer needed acute attention. Although details regarding duration of coma, length of time from the injury to the study, and other parameters are not stated, in comparison to the sleep patterns of established norms these patients had a lack of EOG bursts during REM, mixing of EEG stages, increased sleep latency and number of awakenings and brief arousals, increased wake time after sleep onset, sparse to absent stage 2 spindles often associated with temporal area damage, and the intrusion of low-amplitude waves into delta sleep.

Having reviewed some of the most relevant the literature on insomnia in head trauma patients, we now turn our attention to somnolence. It has long been known that CNS lesions can be associated with EDS (25). Narcolepsy, the best-researched EDS entity, features persistent daytime sleepiness as one of its hallmark symptoms. It is a lifelong and incurable disorder, presumed to be due to neurotransmitter abnormalities in the brain (26), although the precise pathophysiology has yet to be identified.

Excessive daytime sleepiness is also often reported by victims of head trauma (27). It has been our clinical impression from evaluating more than 20 head trauma patients that this is as great a concern for them as is sleep fragmentation. EDS is also of concern to clinicians and the public health community since it is often associated with cognitive errors and impaired concentration, which can lead not only to job errors and decreased productivity but also to automobile accidents and other catastrophes (28). Unfortunately, however, studies into EDS have been fewer and methodologically even less rigorous than those studying nocturnal sleep. Guilleminault and colleagues (29), in an uncontrolled study, examined 20 head trauma patients referred with a chief complaint of EDS. Nine had a history of coma lasting greater than 24 hours and five had a history of transient loss of consciousness. Reasearchers performed nocturnal polysomnography, which included respiratory monitoring. Eight patients had evidence of obstructive sleep apnea syndrome, which is often associated with EDS. Of interest was their observation that apneas resolved over the subsequent 26 months in five of these patients, although no mention is made of any possible changes in weight, which can influence apnea severity. Although the protocol for measuring EDS was not uniform across subjects (methods included continuous 24–36-hour recordings, 1 to 2 daytime naps, and MSLTs), there was evidence of moderate to severe sleepiness in most of the non-apnea patients. The patients who had experienced the longer coma periods seemed to have more persistent EDS over time. Askenasy and co-workers (30) also reported noting disorders of excessive somnolence (DOES) in 20% of their patients, although they do not specify which disorders were included in this category nor do they identify the methods by which EDS was measured.

In one of the most methodologically sound studies performed in this area to date, Manseau and Broughton (31) examined sleep and wakefulness in 16 severely head-injured subjects and matched controls. Patients had experienced variable periods of coma (mean of 24 days) in the acute phase of injury. Some patients complained of sleepiness, while others complained of insomnia. Nocturnal polysomnography and standard MSLTs were performed an average of 6.3 years after the trauma while patients were unmedicated and conscious. Major sleep pathologies such as sleep apnea and nocturnal myoclonus were excluded by prior polysomnography.

Polysomnography revealed that both subjectively sleepy and alert head trauma groups had significant alterations in sleep continuity when compared with controls; total sleep time was reduced, sleep latency was prolonged, and stage 2 was reduced. These changes were more pronounced in the sleepy group, and stage 2 proportion was less in this group than in the alert group. The MSLTs of head-injured subjects displayed longer sleep latencies, indicating a decreased level of daytime somnolence. Interestingly, this trend was also noted in the subjectively sleepy patients. Objective and subjective measures of sleepiness were not related. Multiple sleep latency tests were positively correlated with nocturnal sleep latencies. Although reaction time to cognitive tasks was prolonged in both head trauma groups, it was the same for these two groups. Coma duration was positively correlated with mean MSLT and the latency to delta sleep during nocturnal polysomnography. The authors concluded that sleepy head-injured subjects actually displayed hyposomnia rather than hypersomnia, and that sleep in the alert group more closely resembled that of the control group.

Synthesis of These Data

As is evident from the above discussion, investigations into sleep in head trauma patients are by no means conclusive. An inherent difficulty in this line of research is the ethical impossibility of performing carefully controlled prospective studies with human subjects. However, some of the inconsistencies in findings may reflect methodological inconsistencies and pitfalls. For example, many studies are weakened by the lack of proper control groups and the utilization of diagnostically heterogeneous groups of patients. Even studies confined to head trauma patients group those with open and closed head injuries. Some studies attempt to define the neuro-anatomic correlates of their findings, yet diagnostic procedures are not uniform across patients. Medications and other ingested substances are known to have profound effects on sleep architecture yet these are rarely accounted for. The possibility of coexisting medical and psychiatric conditions and their potential role in sleep architectural alterations are rarely considered. Examples of the latter include post-traumatic stress disorder (32) and depression (33), disorders to which victims of accidents and cerebral concussion are highly susceptible. These have profound effects on sleep continuity and architecture, most notably stage REM (34,35). In most studies, polysomnographic montages are limited to sleep staging parameters, thus disallowing the exclusion of patients with intrinsic sleep disorders such as sleep apnea syndrome and periodic leg movements in sleep which also have profound effects on sleep architecture. Because of these limitations, the data available to date on sleep architectural abnormalities allow only tentative generalizations, as discussed below, which await confirmation by future research.

During the acute comatose phase following severe traumatic head injuries, slow waves seem to predominate on the EEG, and there is a variable loss of sleep spindles and K-complexes. The normal REM-NREM cycle is also lost in severe cases. A gradual restoration of sleep architectural integrity occurs, parallels improvement in clinical state, and can be utilized as a prognostic tool during coma.

Following the resolution of coma, patients complain of persistent awakenings following sleep onset, many of which are prolonged. Many stay in bed later than their usual morning awakening time for a period of time proportional to the severity of their prior coma. Objective testing has confirmed patients' complaints of unrefreshing sleep by revealing a decrease in the total sleep time, frequent spontaneous nocturnal awakenings, and an increase in the total wake time. However, sleep latency may or may not be prolonged. With the passage of time, bursts of alpha waves begin to intrude into the EEG, spindles surge in frequency and are especially evident in stages 2 and 3 of sleep, and there may be an EMG tremor in stage 3 sleep. With clinical improvement these abnormal intrusions wane and delta and REM sleep, if previously impaired, gradually approach a normal pattern.

Unfortunately, no consensus exists as to possible alterations in REM sleep. Some report a decrease in the proportion of this stage or a decrease in the frequency of eye movements, some note a variable loss of atonia, and others report no change. There is also no consensus regarding the relationship between improvement of cognitive variables and serial changes in REM across time. One study reports a decrease in stage 2 sleep which is more severe in somnolent than alert patients.

Although many patients complain of daytime sleepiness, often leading to diminished ability to function during the day, daytime testing has not demonstrated an increased tendency to fall asleep. In fact, patients seem to have difficulty in falling and staying asleep both at night and during the day. Additionally, there is a discrepancy between patients' own assessment of the degree of sleepiness and the actual severity as assessed by MSLT. The degree of difficulty in initiating sleep during daytime naps seems to be related to the length of time spent in coma.

Given the preliminary nature of this information, any hypotheses regarding the relationship between sleep disturbances following head trauma and the syndromatic manifestations of the condition must be even more tentatively stated. It could be argued, however, that at least some of the abnormal findings in sleep and wakefulness cannot be explained on the basis of experimental errors and contaminants alone. The disappearance of a clear distinction between sleep stages may be one such finding and implies that, at least in severe cases, there is a disruption of the basic processes generating sleep and its various elements. Diffuse damage must involve multiple structures ranging from the pons to higher brainstem and, possibly, forebrain levels. REM sleep and dreaming have been thought to be important for emotional and cognitive well-being by providing the framework for processing and restructuring daytime information and traumatic events (36,37). Could disruptions in REM sleep in this population be responsible for the noted alterations in mood and cognitive abilities? The findings of improvement in REM sleep in parallel with improvement in cognitive function certainly support this formulation. Delta sleep deprivation has been shown to lead to daytime physical discomfort (38) and increased sensitivity to pain (39), symptoms commonly found in head trauma victims. To what extent can delta sleep alterations explain these and complaints of debilitating "fatigue"? The finding of a disruption in the normal circadian distribution of sleep stages indicates the possibility of damage to the hypothalamic area, as well. Does impairment of function of circadian oscillators underlie the observed tendency of patients to spend excessive time in bed during the day and their inability to fall asleep at night?

The lack of spindles during the coma phase and the report of the persistence of decreased stage 2 sleep in patients with impairment in daytime alertness are curious findings. Sleep spindles, which are highly synchronized waves, are generated in the thalamus by cells which have intrinsic oscillatory properties. Their rhythmicity is synchronized by a primary pacemaker located in the reticular thalamic nucleus. This system coordinates a large number of oscillators such that they display the same frequency, and hence result in the synchronized activity seen on EEG. Sleep spindles are also associated with the blockade of synaptic transmission of afferent impulses through the thalamus to the cortex at sleep onset and are thus thought to be important in cortical deactivation during sleep. Delta waves seen during stages 3 and 4 of sleep may also represent similar inhibitory phenomena. In contrast, during REM and waking desynchronized activity predominates. This implies a readiness of the neurons to receive afferent information and to respond, that is, a state of activation. In REM the information is internally generated, possibly by pontine mechanisms, and transmitted to the cortex. During wakefulness, this information is external. The finding of an impairment in spindles and stage 2 may be due to injury and functional impairment of thalamic nuclei which may be particularly vulnerable to the effects of head trauma. This, in turn, may result in a failure of cortical deactivating mechanisms which are necessary for sleep onset and possibly maintenance. Neuronal systems may therefore be in a constant state of activation. This may explain the observation of sleep continuity impairment, decreased total sleep time, and increased time spent awake. It may also explain the inability of patients to fall asleep (hyposomnia) during the day in the face of fatigue and excessive somnolence. The inability of thalamic gate-keeper systems to curb the bombardment of the cortex with impulses may lead to impairments in focusing and selective attention. An obvious and exciting implication from the preceding discussion is that alterations in sleep architecture and circadian distribution of sleep and wakefulness are not only epiphenomenal, but also pathogenic. If confirmed, such a construct can have tremendous diagnostic and prognostic implications.

Inplications Regarding Evaluation and Management

Prior to the initiation of treatment, a thorough diagnostic inquiry should be conducted, including an office-based evaluation directed toward uncovering disorders intrinsic to sleep. Although this strategy is recommended in the case of any patient who presents with a complaint of persistent EDS or insomnia, it is of special importance in head trauma patients in light of the possibility that sleep-related breathing and other sleep disorders may result from head trauma. Clinical guidelines for the evaluation process have been set forth in greater detail elsewhere (40,41). Thorough medical and psychiatric assessments are imperative. Symptoms of the major sleep disorders should be systematically asked for. These include, among others, loud snoring, gaps in breathing, unusual postures during sleep, and weight gain (obstructive sleep apnea syndrome); involuntary leg twitches during sleep (nocturnal myoclonus); sudden awakenings from sleep associated with gasping (gastroesophageal reflux and nocturnal panic attacks); and hypnagogic hallucinations, cataplexy, and sleep paralysis (narcolepsy). A more thorough list of the major sleep disorders appears in Table 8.1. Patients are typically completely unaware of the nocturnal activities and abnormalities described above. Therefore, the patient's bed partner can be of invaluable assistance in obtaining this information. Given the probability of circadian rhythm alterations in this population, the history should also include a review of the patient's sleeping habits, with particular attention to bedtime, time spent awake in bed, arising time, and the timing and duration of naps. Daily sleep logs completed by the patient over two weeks prior to the evaluation can reveal these circadian patterns more accurately, and can clarify habits such as the timing of meals and medication inges-

Table 8.1. Sleep disorders most commonly encountered in clinical practice.

DIMS: Disorders of initiating and maintaining sleep (insomnias)
    Psychiatric disorders (affective and personality disorders, schizophrenia, and others)
    Psychophysiological insomnia
    Drug and alcohol dependency
    Periodic leg movements in sleep
    Central sleep apnea syndrome
    Miscellaneous medical conditions
DOES: Disorders of excessive somnolence
    Obstructive sleep apnea syndrome
    Narcolepsy
    Idiopathic CNS hypersomnia
    Psychiatric disorders
    Periodic leg movements in sleep
    Miscellaneous medical conditions
Disorders of the sleep—wake schedule
    Delayed sleep phase syndrome
    Irregular sleep—wake pattern
    Advanced sleep—phase syndrome
    Frequently changing sleep—wake schedule owing to shift work or travel across time zones ("jet lag")
    Non-24-hour sleep—wake syndrome
Parasomnia
    Epileptic seizures
    Gastroesophageal reflux
    Sleepwalking
    Sleep terror
    Sleep-related enuresis
    Dream anxiety attacks
    Head-banging
    Bruxism
    Cluster headaches
    REM behavior disorder

Adapted from 45.

tion. The results of previous procedures and evaluations should be obtained. A physical examination and laboratory tests may be considered as indicated. Finally, polysomnography should be conducted if there is any doubt regarding the diagnosis or to confirm any suspected disorders of sleep or daytime somnolence. Polysomnography is also appropriate when routine interventions such as psychotherapy, behavioral therapy, pharmacotherapy, and careful adherence to sleep hygiene (discussed below) have not led to a resolution of the presumed disorder. Once the specific disorder is identified, treatment can be instituted with confidence. In the special case of the comatose patient, polysomnography can be of prognostic assistance, as noted above. Serial polysomnograms are often helpful in confirming clinical improvement.

In many cases, no diagnostic abnormalities are detected even following polysomnography. In such situations the most appropriate strategy is the identification of contributory or perpetuating factors and their management. One category of factors is alterations in sleep hygiene. Patients often attempt to relieve the symptoms of unrelenting insomnia or EDS by exercising "common-sense" measures which actually have the effect of aggravating the situation even further. They may compensate for lost sleep by spending excessive time in bed during the day through delaying their awakening time or napping. These behaviours actually have the effect of further fragmenting nocturnal sleep. Instead, patients should be advised to adhere to a regular awakening time regardless of the amount of sleep and to avoid naps. Many also resort to caffeine intake during the day to promote alertness, and alcohol at bedtime to promote sleep. Both should be avoided, as alcohol may further aggravate sleep disruption and caffeine may have a similar effect if taken after noon. Similarly, the ingestion of amphetamines and smoking tobacco can have a negative effect on sleep integrity. Although a large meal and excessive fluids close to bedtime may disturb sleep continuity, a small meal may have a beneficial effect. Contrary to popular belief, exercise just prior to bedtime does not induce sleep in most individuals; instead, exercise performed regularly, at a moderate pace, and no later than a few hours prior to bedtime may help deepen sleep. These and other helpful suggestions are outlined in Table 8.2.

Another common contributory factor is chronic psychophysiologic insomnia. The post-trauma period is intensely stressful, and this, coupled with the difficulties of hospitalization, can lead to chronic insomnia mediated through tension and anxiety. In many individuals the emergence of negative conditioning factors such as conditioned arousal at bedtime further aggravate sleep disturbance. In this disorder, termed chronic psychophysiologic insomnia, patients develop anticipatory anxiety over the prospect of another night of sleepless-

Table 8.2. Sleep hygiene measures.

1. Sleep as much as needed to feel alert during the day, but not more. Curtailing the time in bed seems to solidify sleep; excessive time spent in bed seems to fragment sleep.
2. Establish a regular arousal time in the morning which you can adhere to every day, including weekends and vacations. Such regularity strengthens circadian cycling.
3. Exercise performed regularly and not too close to bedtime probably deepens sleep.
4. Excessive noise may disturb sleep; insulate your room against loud noises.
5. Excessive warmth disturbs sleep. Keep the room temperature at a comfortable level.
6. A light snack prior to bedtime may improve sleep, although a large meal and excessive fluids close to bedtime may have the opposite effect.
7. Caffeinated beverages disturb sleep, even though you may not be aware of their effect.
8. Alcoholic beverages, which may assist in falling asleep, can significantly fragment sleep.
9. If you feel angry and frustrated because you cannot fall asleep, don't try harder to fall asleep; instead, leave the bedroom and do something not very stimulating, like reading a boring book.
10. The chronic use of tobacco disturbs sleep.

Adapted from 8.

ness followed by another day of fatigue. Anxiety typically increases as bedtime approaches, and reaches maximum intensity following retiring. Patients often spend hours in bed awake focused on, and brooding over, their sleeplessness. Their frustration is compounded as their concern over sleeplessness becomes a self-fulfilling prophecy with which they are faced night after night. Relaxation training, especially with skeletal muscle biofeedback, and cognitive techniques can interrupt such self-perpetuating insomnia. Patients conditioned to wakefulness at bedtimes can be helped by behavioral techniques which reestablish a connection between being in bed and sleeping.

The sleep pattern of many patients is highly fragmented, owing to nocturnal awakenings and daytime naps. Sleep restriction therapy was recently introduced (42), which strives to maximize the refreshing quality of sleep by consolidating it into a finite block of time. Prior to treatment, patients complete sleep logs over two weeks. Upon reviewing these, the clinician prescribes times in bed equivalent to their mean daily total sleep time as determined from their sleep logs. They report regularly to the clinician with their estimated time spent asleep during the treatment period. For each day, the clinician calculates the subjective sleep efficiency, that is, the ratio of the total time spent asleep to the time spent in bed. He then further restricts bedtimes by 15 minutes when the sleep efficiency is below 85%, and lengthens them when the sleep efficiency exceeds 90%. Although this method has never been systematically studied in head trauma patients, in our own experience some patients have reported significant and lasting improvement after eight weeks of treatment.

Benzodiazepine hypnotic agents can also interrupt a psychophysiologic cycle and promote sleep continuity. However, since tolerance and habituation to such agents is a common cause of insomnia, a recent National Institutes of Health consensus conference report (43) recommended that they be utilized in small doses and only intermittently. The long half-life hypnotics also pose the danger of daytime carry-over effects, such as impairment in driving performance. Benzodiazepines having short to intermediate half-lives offer an advantage in this regard, yet they may also pose risks such as daytime anxiety and anterograde amnesia in higher doses (44). Additionally, brain-injured victims may be more vulnerable to the adverse effects, especially the CNS-depressant qualities, of hypnotic agents. Special precautions, such as dosage reduction, should be exercised for them as well as for patients with impaired hepatic function, sleep apnea syndrome, alcoholism or drug dependence, and for the pregnant and elderly.

Conclusions

Although research over the past few decades has uncovered some of the polysomnographic abnormalities in patients with a history of head trauma, much work has yet to be done. It is clear, however, that sleep and wakefulness are definitely impaired in many head-injured patients. Therefore, when faced with complaints of daytime fatigue and sleepiness or interrupted sleep, the first task of the clinician is to identify underlying abnormalities through a careful office-based evaluation followed by polysomnography when indicated.

References

1. Mellinger GD, Balter MB, Uhlenhuth EH: Insomnia and its treatment. Arch Gen Psychiatry, 1985; 42:225–232.
2. Webb M: Severe post-traumatic insomnia treated with L-5-hydroxytryptophan. Lancet, 1981; June 20:1365–1366.
3. Rutherford WH: Sequelae of concussion caused by minor head injuries. Lancet, 1977; January 1:1–4.
4. Levin HS: Neurobehavioral outcome of mild to moderate head injury. In Hoff J, Anderson T, Cole T (eds): Mild to Moderate Head Injury. Boston: Blackwell Scientific Publications, 1989; pp 153–179.
5. Frankowski RF, Annegers JF, Whitman S: Epidemiological and descriptive studies part 1: the descriptive epidemiology of head trauma in the United States. In Becker DP, Povlishock JT (eds): Central Nervous System Trauma Status Report. Bethesda: NINCDS, 1985.

6. Sosin DM, Sacks JJ, Smith SM: Head injury-associated deaths in the United States from 1979 to 1986. JAMA, 1989; 262:2251–2255.

7. Hartunian NS, Smart CN, Thompson MS: The incidence and economic cost of cancer, motor vehicle injuries, coronary heart disease and stroke: a comparative analysis. Am J Pub Health, 1980; 70:1249–1260.

8. Hauri P: The Sleep Disorders. Kalamazoo, MI: The Upjohn Company, 1982.

9. Guilleminault C: Sleeping and Waking Disorders: Indications and Techniques. Menol Park, CA: Addison-Wesley, 1982.

10. Siegel JM: Brainstem mechanisms generating REM sleep. In Kryger MH, Roth T, Dement WC (eds): Principles and Practice of Sleep Medicine. Philadelphia: Saunders, 1989; pp 104–120.

11. Jones BE: Basic mechanisms of sleep-wake states. In Kryger MH, Roth T, Dement WC (eds): Principles and Practice of Sleep Medicine. Philadelphia: Saunders, 1989; pp 121–138.

12. Moore-Ede MC, Czeisler CA, Richardson GS: Circadian timekeeping in health and disease. Part 1. Basic properties of circadian pacemakers. N Engl J Med, 1983; 309:469–476.

13. Bergamaso B, Bergamini L, Doriguzzi T, et al.: EEG sleep patterns as a prognostic criterion in post-traumatic coma. Electroencephalogr Clin Neurophysiol, 1968; 24:374–377.

14. Lessard CS, Sances A, Larson SJ: Period analysis of EEG signals during sleep and post-traumatic coma. Aerospace Med, 1974; June, 664–668.

15. Parsons LC, Ver Beek, D: Sleep-awake patterns following cerebral concussion. Nurs Res, 1982; 31:260–264.

16. Carscadon MA, Dement WC, Mitler MM, et al.: Self-reports versus sleep laboratory findings in 233 drug-free subjects with complaints of chronic insomnia. Am J Psychiatry, 1976; 133:1382–1388.

17. Harada M, Minami R, Hattori E, et al.: Sleep in brain-damaged patients. An all night sleep study of 105 cases. Kumamoto Med J, 1976: 29: 110–127.

18. Feinberg I, Koresko RL, Heller N: Sleep: electroencephalographic and eye movement patterns in patients with chronic brain syndrome. J Psychiatr Res, 1967; 5:107–144.

19. Appenzeller O, Fisher AP: Disturbances in rapid eye movments during sleep in patients with lesions of the nervous system. Electroencephalogr Clin Neurophysiol, 1968; 25:29–35.

20. Bricolo A: Neurosurgical exploration and neurological pathology as a means for investigating human sleep. In Lairy G, Salzarulo P (eds): The Experimental Study of Human Sleep: Methodological Problems. Amsterdam: Elsevier, 1975; pp 51–82.

21. Ron S, Algom D, Harey D, et al.: Time-related changes in the distribution of sleep stages in brain injured patients. Electroencephalogr Clin Neurophysiol, 1980; 48:432–441.

22. Prigatano GP, Stahl ML, Orr WC, et al.: Sleep and dreaming disturbances in closed head injury patients. J Neurol Neurosurg Psychiatry, 1982; 45:78–80.

23. George B, Landau-Ferey J, Benoit O, et al.: Night sleep disorders during recovery of severe head injuries. Neurochirurgie, 1981; 27:35–38.

24. Hanley J: The signiture of post-concussion syndrome in the sleep tracing. Polysomnographic (EEG) patterns in nocturnal sleep following head injury. Neupsychiatr Bull, 1983; 8:1–4.
25. Bonduelle M, Degos C: Symptomatic narcolepsies: a critical study. In Guilleminault C, Dement WC, Passouant P (eds): Narcolepsy. New York: Spectiru, 1976; pp 313–332.
26. Kilduff TS, Bowersox SS, Kaitin KI, et al.: Muscarinic cholinergic receptors and the canine model of narcolepsy. Sleep, 1986; 9:102–106.
27. Gill AW: Idiopathic and traumatic narcolepsy. Lancet, 1941; 1:474–476.
28. Mitler MM, Carskadon MA, Czeisler CA, et al.: Catastrophes, sleep, and public policy: consensus report. Sleep, 1988; 11:100–109.
29. Guilleminault C, Faull KF, Miles L, et al.: Posttraumatic excessive daytime sleepiness: a review of 20 patients. Neurology, 1983; 33:1584–1589.
30. Askenasy JJM, Rahmani L: Neuropsycho-social rehabilitation of head injury. Am J Phys Med, 1988; 66:315–327.
31. Manseau C, Broughton R: Severe head injury: long term effects on sleep, sleepiness and performance. Sleep Res, 1990; 19:335.
32. Askenasy JJ, Gruskiewicz J, Braun J, et al.: Repititive visual images in severe war head injuries. Resuscitation, 1986; 13:191–201.
33. Robinson RG, Szetela B: Mood change following left hemispheric brain injury. Ann Neurol, 1981; 9:447–453.
34. Ross RR, Ball WA, Sullivan KA, et al.: Sleep disturbance as the hallmark of posttraumatic stress disorder. Am J Psychiatry, 1989; 146:697–707.
35. Inman DJ, Silver S, Doghramji K: Sleep disturbance in post traumatic disorder: a comparison with non-PTSD insomnia. J Trauma Stress, 1990; 3:429–437.
36. Berger L: Function of dreams. J Abnorm Psychol, 1967; 72:1–28.
37. Cartwright RD: Rapid eye movement sleep charactersitics during and after mood-disturbing events. Arch Gen Psychiatry, 1983; 40:197–201.
38. Agnew HW, Webb WB, Williams RL: Comparison of stage four and 1-REM sleep deprivation. Percept Mot Skills, 1967; 24:851–858.
39. Moldofsky H, Scarisbrick P: Induction of neurasthenic musculoskeletal pain syndrome by selective sleep stage deprivation. Psychosom Med, 1975; 37:341–351.
40. Doghramji K: Sleep disorders: A selective update. Hosp Commun Psychiatry, 1989; 40:29–40.
41. Doghramji K: Etiology, pathogenesis, and management of sleep disorders. Compr Ther, 1990; 16:49–59.
42. Spielman AJ, Saskin P, Thorpy MJ: Treatment of chronic insomnia by restriction of time in bed. Sleep, 1987; 10:45–56.
43. Consensus conference: Drugs and insomnia: The use of medications to promote sleep. JAMA, 1984; 251:2410–2414.
44. Griffiths RR, Lamb RJ, Ator NA, et al.: Relative abuse liability of triazolam: experimental assessment in animals and humans. Neurosci Biobehav Rev, 1985; 9:133–151.

— 9

Post-Traumatic Headache Syndrome

Arnold Sadwin, Robert Rothrock, Steven Mandel,
Donna Sadwin, and Lori O'Leary

Post-traumatic headache is the most common of many symptoms that occur after a minor head injury. In our series of over 4,000 patients who have had cerebral concussions, over 95% presented with head pain as one of the most distressing, persistent problems.

Whether this is termed a post-traumatic headache, a post-concussion syndrome, post-brain trauma cephalgia, or post-accident headache, the fact remains that both the patient and the physician are uncomfortable until the diagnosis has been clarified and a treatment program initiated. Other terms that have become synonymous with this syndrome are traumatic neurasthenia, traumatic psychasthenia, post-head-trauma syndrome, and post-traumatic nervous instability (1–2).

Until recent years, patients with the array of symptoms that can follow a cerebral concussion (Table 9.1) were felt to be suffering from some type of neurotic problem requiring psychiatric intervention. More recently, with the help of neurosurgical research, psychological testing, and electrophysiologic studies, there has been some clarification of the pathology associated with "minor" head injuries. The word *minor* is a misnomer, since the problem may result in major medical and social disruption in the life of the injured individual and his/her family.

Ironically, these patients appear to be normal, and their complaints are subjective, rendering it difficult for their loved ones to be sympathetic for any prolonged period of time. This creates a secondary cause for additional emotional problems, complicating the treatment

Table 9.1. Symptoms often seen in the post-concussion syndrome.

 1. Headaches
 2. Tiredness
 3. Light-headedness
 4. Difficulty concentrating
 5. Dizziness
 6. Memory difficulties
 7. Trouble expressing thoughts and word finding
 8. Blurring of vision
 9. Double vision
10. Bothered by bright lights
11. Bothered by loud noises
12. Ringing in the ears
13. Hearing loss
14. Balance difficulties
15. Clumsiness
16. Staggering
17. Change in handwriting
18. Dropping things
19. Lack of ambition
20. Loss of interest in sex
21. Depression
22. Irritability
23. Fear or anxiety
    a. Anxiety associated with the accident such as driving a car
    b. Fear of leaving the house
    c. Other unusual fears
24. Sleep disturbance
    a. Trouble falling asleep
    b. Trouble staying asleep
    c. Early rising in the morning
    d. Need for too much sleep
25. Bad dreams, usually about accidents of life-threatening experiences
26. Appetite change
    a. Loss
    b. Gain
    c. Craving for "junk" food, usually sweets
27. Weight change
    a. Loss
    b. Gain
28. Seizures
    a. Partial complex
    b. Grand mal
    c. Episodes of disorientation

program and requiring intervention. The physician can give the patient and the family great relief by objectifying the findings with the use of the latest techniques to separate the neurologic from the psychiatric aspects of this syndrome. Patients are relieved to find out that it is not a psychiatric disorder per se and that, in fact, they have suffered from microscopic brain damage. This results in either unconsciousness or "dysconsciousness" (the author's [A.S.] term for this altered state). Since the syndrome is usually self-limiting, the patient should be encouraged to expect improvement.

Incidence

The literature states that there are up to 8,000,000 cases of head injury in the United States each year.

The incidence of post-traumatic headache following head injury varies considerably in the literature. Penfield and Norcross found it in 28% of cases lasting more than 6 months (3); Guttman in 50% (4); Friedman in 40–60% (5); Jacobson in 72% (7); and Rowbothan in 80% (7).

In another study, Russell reports post-traumatic headaches in 100% of cases in patients over the age of 50. In our experience with over 4,000 cases, 95% of patients have complaints of headache.

In our series, the symptom complex following head injury includes some or all of the listed complaints, occurring either for prolonged periods of time or occasionally during the course of recovery (see Table 9.1).

Pathophysiology

Brain injury may occur when there is a sudden acceleration/deceleration and cranial soft tissue strikes the bony skull. This is characterized by diffuse structural axonal cell changes and physiologic alteration in function. There can be temporary disruption of the reticular system with an altered state of consciousness (dysconsciousness) and diffuse neurologic disruption. There may be a rotational component, depending on how the patient's head was positioned at the time of the impact. Stretching, twisting, and shearing of neuronal fibers causes microscopic lesions in the cerebral white matter. Loss of nerve cells and disturbance of Nissl body pattern in large pyramidal cells of laboratory animals with induced head injuries have been reported. Olendorph found increased cerebral circulation times in patients suffering from post-traumatic headaches. (9,11–15).

Headache Profile

Post-traumatic headaches are usually diffuse and constant for the first few weeks, although they may be unrelenting for the first two to three months. Their location may be anywhere in the head, unilateral or bilateral, and they may be throbbing or steady, sharp or dull. The severity of the head injury seems to be inversely proportional to the severity of the head pain. Blows to the head that cause a skull fracture often result in fewer complaints than do "mild" head injuries without fracture.

Patients often complain of a knife-like focal discomfort that may emanate from the point of impact, especially if there has been a scalp laceration. Sometimes the pain is described as a tight band-like feeling around the head or a pushing-out or pressing-in sensation.

After the headaches begin to subside, patients can occasionally identify occurrences that may exacerbate the pain. These include fatigue, excitement, crowds, bright lights, noises, attempts to concentrate, exertion, alcohol consumption, exposure to cold, postural changes (especially in bending forward), or stress. Often the headaches occur toward the end of the day, but some awaken the patient at night or are present upon awakening in the morning.

The description of the headache is only occasionally helpful in localizing the injury or predicting long-term outcome.

Post-traumatic headache has been described by some clinicians as a cross between a migraine headache and a tension headache. Muscle tension is often associated with the onset of pain, especially when there has been a cervical sprain. Such patients often complain of pain starting in the back of the neck radiating into the occipital region and then spreading to the frontal areas. These patients often have tenderness of the posterior cervical muscles. However, the cause of most post-traumatic headaches remains unknown.

Patients who have had a previous history of migraine and who may have been free of symptoms for quite some time may once again develop migraine headaches. Head trauma may also be the precipitating cause for a migraine syndrome to emerge. Some patients have experienced a combination of the addition of post-concussion headaches superimposed on their usual migraine episodes. Other associated injuries can influence the occurrence of headaches. These include entrapment syndrome secondary to nerve irritation or neuroma formation of a scalp injury. A local injection of Lidocaine often interrupts this kind of headache cycle and helps clarify the diagnosis.

Post-traumatic temporomandibular joint (TMJ) injury or dysfunction is often implicated as the cause of chronic head pain. Palpation of the TMJ area should help the examiner decide whether the patient should be sent to an appropriate dental specialist. Palpation of the facial bones, especially those overlying the sinuses, is also a useful screening technique for conditions appropriately referred to an otolaryngologist.

Dysautonomic cephalgia sometimes results from trauma to the soft tissue structures in the anterior triangle of the neck and irritation of the underlying autonomic fibers in the carotid sheath (16,17). Prolonged pain and spasm in the area with significant episodic unilateral throbbing headaches in the temporal or frontal regions are associated with facial burning, numbness, photophobia, blurred vision, vomiting, and Horner's syndrome. These may recur frequently and can last from hours to days. The differential diagnosis for the less commonly caused post-traumatic headaches includes injury to the greater superficial petrosal nerve and the afferent branches of the sphenopalatine ganglion which could result in cluster headaches. Accumulation of blood in the subdural spaces, rupture of pain-sensitive blood vessels or meningial irritation, inflammation, hydrocephalus, or tumor development should also be kept in mind.

Psychological Considerations

Head trauma can cause psychiatric symptoms in a patient who otherwise is making a stable adjustment to life. A post-traumatic stress disorder with flashbacks, sleep disturbance and nightmares, anxiety, depression, and phobia often accompanies head trauma.

It is important to know who the patient was and what he/she was going through at the time of the injury. Patients who have had a history of psychosis may experience recurrence. Patients with abnormal pre-trauma personalities also appear predisposed to post-traumatic symptomatology. Those who have never had any significant emotional problems may suddenly be confronted with a severe loss of self-esteem resulting from the array of problems that occur in the post-concussion syndrome.

A primary emotional lability can be seen secondary to the brain trauma itself. This is manifested by unreasonable mood swings and considerable irritability, leading to a change in personality with disruption of interpersonal relationships. Secondary depression with anxiety and phobia may be the result of the post-traumatic stress disorder. The examining physician should determine, if possible, what the patient's life was like, how the accident took place, and how it changed his/her status, in an effort to try to separate the primary organic from the secondary reactive emotional changes.

Therefore, the impact of head injury may be physical, psychological, social, and economical.

Neuropsychological Deficits

Neuropsychological studies done on post-concussion patients over the past several years have demonstrated a number of cognitive behavioral deficits primarily involving information processing, intellectual functioning, concentration, short-term memory, reaction time, attention span, and judgment. Common complaints include insomnia, increased fatigability, decreased motivation, blurred vision, intolerance to alcohol (18), and loss of sexual interest; depression or mania may occasionally occur.

Often neither the patient's family nor employer understands why the patient continues to have so much difficulty recovering from such a "minor" injury. It seems the harder the patient tries, the more anxious and frustrated he/she becomes.

Although it can be expected that the majority of patients will recover from most of the symptoms following a traumatic head injury, many of them do not. With careful assessment, it has been found that increasing numbers of patients retain disturbing defects for many years. Denker, in a follow-up study of 100 patients with minor head injury, reported that headache, dizziness, and various neuro-psychological symptoms persisted in approximately 33% of the cases for greater than one year and in about 15% of all cases after three years (19).

Headaches, memory problems, difficulty concentrating, irritability, depression, sleep disturbance, and so forth have led many patients to believe that they are developing Alzheimer's disease. It is important to reassure the patient that this is not what is happening.

The patient, the family, the employers, the attorneys, and the insurance companies all need clarification of the diagnosis and reassurance whenever possible. Besides the physical examination, it is recommended that the following studies be carried out, initially and periodically if indicated, when there is no improvement:

1. Thorough neurologic and general physical examinations
2. Personality psychological testing
3. Neuropsychological testing
4. Neurophysiologic studies including plain EEG, evoked potentials, and quantitative electroencephalogram (Thatcher)
5. MRI and/or CT scans of the brain

The results of these studies should be reviewed with the patient and all others concerned.

Clarification does not mean that the patient is necessarily ready to return to work. Rimel et al. prospectively followed 424 patients who sustained minor head trauma (20). Follow-up at three months showed persistent cognitive deficits in 59%. More than one-third of the patients employed prior to their initial injury had not yet returned to work.

Persistent symptoms and impaired intellectual functioning may result in prolonged disability or ultimately necessitate a change of employment to reduce both intellectual demands and emotional stress. Intensive rehabilitative therapy is necessary and is more effective the sooner it is begun.

Effects in Children

Minor head injury is one of the most common childhood mishaps. It is difficult to assess an altered mental state in a child who may have just struck his/her head. Sometimes there is a peculiar high pitched screaming which is quite different from the usual crying after less complicated injuries. Typically the child regresses. Symptoms may include recurrence of bed-wetting, thumb-sucking, clinging behavior, shyness, and incorrigible and aggressive behavior. Troublesome sleep disturbance has been observed, with an increased need for sleep during the day and poor sleeping at night with increased nightmares.

Such problems in children are very disruptive at home and in school. Both teachers and parents need to be educated about this syndrome and special consideration should be given to head-injured children until they have recovered. Rehabilitation in a child is sometimes more rapid than in an adult, and is often helped by medication such as syrup of compazine (21).

Diagnostic Studies

Clinical judgment should dictate the necessity for skull x-rays for any patient with a minor head injury. Masters et al. recently conducted a study of 7,035 patients, investigating the need for skull radiographic examination following head trauma (22). X-ray examination alone was not recommended for asymptomatic patients or in patients experiencing one or more of the following symptoms: headaches, dizziness, scalp hematcoma, laceration, contusion, or abrasion. Preferably a CT scan should be done, especially if the patient is not showing signs of rapid return of full consciousness. If the reverse is true, neurosurgical consultation is mandated to rule out skull fracture, cerebral contusion, or developing hematoma. Many neurosurgeons recommend skull x-rays for any patient with minor head injury (22). However, there is considerable disagreement surrounding this view. Magnetic resonance imaging has proven superior to CT scan of the brain to demonstrate hematoma, white matter pathology, edema, and other space-occupying lesions, especially in the subacute and chronic phases of the post-head-trauma syndrome (23,24).

A plain EEG and evoked potentials are occasionally helpful. Usually the plain EEG is read as normal, although abnormalities may be seen despite the absence of positive neurologic findings on examination.

Abnormal sleep EEG patterns have been reported as long as five days after head injury (25). Evoked potentials can reveal abnormalities especially in the brainstem (26).

Presently, we are using Thatcher software in our quantitative electroencephalographic studies (QEEG). In over 800 cases there has been a 92% clinical correlation in diagnosing the presence of the post-concussion state (27). The test should be done within weeks of the head injury, if possible, but sometimes the abnormalities persist for weeks, months, and even years. In about 25% of the closed head-injured patients, the Thatcher abnormalities may be permanent (26).

Abnormal auditory brainstem evoked potentials (BERA or ABR) have been reported in patients experiencing dizziness, vertigo, and heading loss, indicating slowing of central auditory processing (28,29). Electronystagmography (ENG) has also been used to investigate and correlate abnormal findings (30). Auditory brainstem evoked potentials and ENG are discussed in greater depth in the chapter on neurotological evaluation.

Visual changes or field defects should be evaluated by visual evoked potentials. Slow reaction time and abnormalities of the visual pathways have been demonstrated in patients with minor head injuries (31).

Persistent neuropsychological deficits should be investigated carefully. As a general rule, cognitive testing is best performed by those involved in the field of neuropsychology. Cognitive evoked potentials are presently being performed on an experimental basis in patients found to have neuropsychological deficits following minor head injury. Early findings indicate a delay in the P300 response, a finding commonly noted in amnesic patients.

Management

Management of the post-traumatic headache syndrome requires a great deal of patience and understanding. The therapist has to explain to the patient how a concussion takes place and what the consequences are. The patient deserves relief from the anxiety of not knowing what has happened to him/her. Many patients fear that they may be losing their minds or developing Alzheimer's disease.

During the first interview, if enough care is taken to establish that there has been a dysconscious state at the time of the injury, one can safely state to the patient that he/she has suffered microscopic, organic brain injury. The examiner will often see relief on the patient's face when he/she is reassured that his/her problems are not entirely of psychiatric origin. This initial naming and framing of the cause of the problems is one of the most important early steps in management. Each of the usual symptoms found in the post-concussion syndrome should be discussed with the patient so that he/she may feel free to discuss problems which otherwise would be kept secret because of shame, guilt, or ignorance.

The effects of sequelae on interpersonal relationships and the patients' vocation must also be addressed in the management program until maximum improvement is achieved. Communication with family, friends, teachers, fellow workers, and employers is often necessary. The patient needs a friendly, understanding physician who gives him/her enough time and attention, or who will send the patient to the appropriate specialist to deal with the often lengthy process of recovery. Establishment of realistic goals should not be biased by pressure from others. School authorities, parents, spouses, peer groups, and insurance companies who are paying for medical rehabilitation should be given sufficient information. This should help alleviate undue pressure placed on the patient to return to his/her former status before he/she is physically and mentally capable of doing so. The patient should be encouraged to keep pushing forward wherever possible to help speed full rehabilitation.

The process of recovery is gradual and varies considerably with the individual patient's level of intelligence, social and intellectual achievement, and degree of injury. Recovery can be adversely affected by the pressure of guilt, financial hardship, and lack of understanding. All of these deserve attention. The therapist has to digest all of the information and share results in order to obtain maximum cooperation. Unfortunately, in some cases, insurance companies may respond as if they were being taken advantage of, causing patients to feel that no one really cares and that they are suspected of exaggerating their problems. Physicians have to sort out the facts and communicate them clearly to the patient, insurance company, and other appropriate parties; but they must always be guided only by the patients' best long-term medical interests.

Many patients are left with partial disability. Unfortunately, many employers do not have re-entry programs for recovering employees to return to work on a gradually increasing basis. It is unrealistic to expect complete recovery overnight. Partial employment is often very helpful in hastening full recovery. However, trial employment may result in the disclosure of residual disabling intellectual impairment.

Treatment

Treatment for the various components of the post-concussion syndrome is most clear when each is addressed individually.

Headaches

The treatment of early, typical, constant, severe post-concussion headaches in which neurosurgical problems have been ruled out is carried out with one to two weeks' use of narcotic-containing agents such as Fiorinal with codeine (Sandoz Pharmaceuticals, East Hanover, NJ) or acetaminophen with codeine. After the first few weeks, it is generally recommended that the narcotic be discontinued. When the headaches begin to subside somewhat, patients may benefit during the day from Fiorinal capsules (which some patients have found more effective than the tablets). Other products such as Esgic (Forest Pharmaceuticals, St. Louis, MO) can be used as well. Patients who cannot take aspirin should be given Fioricet (Sandoz Pharmaceuticals, East Hanover, NJ) or Midrin (Carnrick Laboratories, Cedar Knolls, NJ) usually every four to six hours. If the headaches become less frequent and less severe, plain aspirin or acetaminophen may suffice. Limit the amount of these medications to avoid rebound headaches.

When a migraine has been precipitated, an attempt to treat headaches with this same program often meets with only moderate success. In that event, patients may benefit from the usual anti-migraine treatment programs. These generally include the prophylactic use of Inderal (Wyeth-Ayerst Laboratories, Philadelphia, PA) and Elavil (Merck Sharp & Dohme, West Point, PA). Small doses are recommended at first because of the usual low tolerance exhibited by post-concussion patients. Sometimes ergot derivatives are given in oral, sublingual inhalation, or suppository form. In more intractable types of migraine headaches, consideration should be given to dihydroergotamine injections D.H.E. 45 (Sandoz Pharmaceuticals, East Hanover, NJ) or Sumatriptan (Glaxo, Inc., Research Triangle Park, NC). Headaches that are associated with nerve entrapment, such as occipital neuralgia, may respond to nerve blocks with novocaine-derivative drugs with or without steroids. This treatment may warrant neurological or neurotological consultation.

Pain owing to temporomandibular joint dysfunction should be evaluated and treated by a TMJ specialist, or a general dentist skilled in management of TMJ problems. Treatment often includes a diligent program of physical therapy and alignment correction with a prosthesis. Patients often complain that the bite plate is hard to get used to. Comfort and improvement can be accomplished if the patient and the dentist are persistent and communicate well with each other.

Acupuncture and biofeedback have been helpful in reducing the severity and, at times, the frequency of post-concussion headaches. Untreated, these headaches can go on for weeks, months, or years.

Tiredness

The fatigue which follows minor head injury rarely responds to any form of treatment except for the passage of time. If depression is also a factor, some patients may respond to the carefully supervised use of antidepressants such as Prozac (Dista Products Co., Indianapolis, IN). We have found the liquid form of Prozac to be beneficial in titrating more carefully the low dosage needed in selected cases. Any anti-depressants should be used cautiously, starting with the lowest possible dosage.

Dizziness

Vertiginous episodes occur often as a result of a labyrinthine concussion which accompanies some closed head injuries. An otolaryngological (preferably neurotological) evaluation is recommended. Some patients have responded to anti-vertiginous medication. However, the side effect of sleepiness is a problem since it is compounded by the chronic state of fatigue. This subject is discussed in a separate chapter.

Blurring of Vision

Here is another symptom which should subside rather quickly. However, an ophthalmologic evaluation is indicated. Very often patients who have had a head injury around the age of 40 may need reading glasses for the first time. Additionally, a severe blow to the head may in dislodge particles in the vitreous, causing floaters, which may be permanent. Affected patients will need reassurance, which can be given to them by an ophthalmologist, in addition to expert ophthalmological assessment and treatment.

Tinnitus

Ringing in the ears and hearing buzzing sounds, water rushing, or hissing noises frequently are transient; but sometimes tinnitus may be permanent and cause a great deal of dismay. Otologic assessment is required and is discussed elsewhere in this book.

Concentration

Problems in concentration requiring the patient to reread material over and over again require considerable patience and practice to overcome. Neuropsychologists who are now specializing in cognitive rehabilitation have done remarkable work in helping post-concussion patients relearn how to focus their attention. Special teaching methods that have been used for years in treating mentally handicapped children can be applied in the treatment of patients with post-concussion complaints of concentration difficulties. Referral to a specialized neuropsychologist is recommended highly.

Memory

Recent memory impairment is one of the major problems that face almost all patients who have had a significant closed head injury. They soon realize they cannot rely on their former ability to retain and recall. They are advised to use a small reminder book kept on their person to schedule all the things that have to be done. Then they have to be reminded to carry and use the book and to try not to misplace it. This also applies to the various objects that they frequently misplace, such as keys, watches, money, important papers, etc. These should all be placed in the same location habitually. An extra set of keys should be kept in strategically located magnetic boxes. Many patients have locked themselves out of their car or home repeatedly. Patients who cook are advised to turn on the timer whenever they use the stove and to carry a small timer with them when they leave the kitchen to help prevent burning food, an all too frequent occurrence. Recently head-injured individuals may forget what they leave a room to get. They must learn to retrace their steps. They also have to learn how to deal with their forgetfulness. For example, absent-mindedness can lead to arguments with family members when the injured person forgets what he/she has said or been told.

Patient's complaints of memory impairment fluctuate; there are good days and bad days. Memory is often worse when the patient is tired or depressed. Sometimes antidepressant medication, which improves mood and gives patients more energy, leads them to believe that their memory has also improved. However, thus far, there has been no medication which has proven effective in the treatment of impaired memory. A cognitive rehabilitation counselor can be very helpful in treating this distressing and persistent symptom.

Sleep Disturbance

Sleep disturbed patients do benefit from the careful use of hypnotics. It is best to rotate minimal doses of these medications so that habituation may be kept at a minimum. The patients are advised to try them for a few weeks, but not to use them steadily thereafter. Often they are prescribed to be taken every other night. Some patients use them only during weekdays. In any event, patients should be weaned from these medications as soon as possible. Some patients who have had a past history of drug abuse should not be exposed to medication of this type. They may be advised to buy a small radio with an earplug to listen to during the night, rather than toss and turn in anguish over not being able to sleep. This is more beneficial than watching television or reading. The eyes may at least be rested in the dark, and patients are likely to get some light sleep. Meditation or hypnosis may also be helpful in some cases.

Depression

Treatment of depression is mandatory. It is helpful for the patient to have a Beck test at frequent intervals. This is a simple, standardized test consisting of 21 questions with four possible answers. Because of its simplicity, it can be given at frequent intervals to obtain a rough idea of the patient's emotional status. If test results are above 25, one should consider the use of antidepressants. Additionally, supportive psychotherapy should be utilized, including an explanation to the patient about the post-concussion syndrome. The physician should be cautious about the potential side effects of antidepressant medications: they may actually increase the severity of post-concussion headaches, irritability, and insomnia. In our practice we have found that art psychotherapy and group therapy have been helpful in the treatment of the depression and other psychiatric problems found in the post-concussion syndrome.

Irritability

Almost all head-injured patients are quite irritable, though they may not admit it. In extreme cases, there may be organic temporal lobe dysfunction which requires further assessment and treatment with the appropriate medications, including anticonvulsants. Otherwise, the irritability can be treated by psychotherapy, especially when it is explained to all concerned that it is a common, temporary symptom after a head injury.

Disorientation

Patients who have noted brief episodes in which they are lost in familiar places usually experience a panic reaction which must be dealt with as soon as it is diagnosed as part of the post-concussion syndrome. The sooner these patients understand that the momentary loss of orientation is to be expected and eventually will go away, the sooner they may anticipate it and learn not to panic when it happens. Group therapy has been very helpful in enabling patients to share this experience and reduce the stress that it causes.

Apprehension in an Automobile

Patients usually "white knuckle" in a car even if the head injury did not result from an auto accident. They are being very careful to avoid another insult to the brain and are understandably apprehensive about anything that puts them at risk. Even their own driving frightens them. Behavior modification and deconditioning managed by a skilled psychotherapist can be very effective in reducing the duration of this annoying problem. Patients who go untreated and feel that the symptom is something they can overcome by themselves are often disappointed months and years later when they are still phobic.

Seizures

A small percentage of patients develop bona fide seizure activity. It is often difficult to obtain a positive electroencephalogram. A clinical trial of the usual anticonvulsants such as Dilantin (Parke-Davis, Morris Plains, NJ), Tegretol (Geigy Pharmaceutical, Ardsley, NY), or Depakote (Abbott Laboratories, North Chicago, IL) is strongly recommended. Once again, it must be kept in mind that after head trauma patients' tolerance for medication is less than one would expect for age and weight. Repeated EEGs including 24-hour monitoring or EEG telemetry are often necessary to assist in the diagnosis of a post-traumatic seizure disorder.

Rehabilitation

Vocational rehabilitation as a treatment modality deserves special consideration. Usually the head-injured patient has orthopedic problems as well. Physical rehabilitation is warranted above and beyond the usual hot packs, moist heat, massage, electric stimulation, TENS (transelectrical nerve stimulator) unit, and passive and active exercises. It should include additional modalities such as hydrotherapy and work hardening programs. Physical rehabilitation should not be carried out without cognitive and emotional rehabilitation. Patients have to learn how to deal with sequential events without becoming overwhelmed or confused. They often fear their first day back at work, when the ultimate test of their recovery is made. Many of them fail to pass the test and either stop work or change jobs. Some patients are permanently disabled in spite of all rehabilitative efforts.

Prognosis

All of the above problems should be managed in individual, couple, and/or family therapy. Supportive group psychotherapy, which encourages patients to share helpful information, and individual art psychotherapy, which improves self-esteem, have been immeasurably helpful in shortening the post-traumatic syndrome.

Most post-concussion patients recover, but some do not. We have found that the older the patient is, the longer it takes and the more guarded the prognosis. Sometimes intellectual impairment is permanent in spite of all therapeutic efforts. Psychological support is particularly indicated in those unfortunate patients who do not show adequate improvement. It is recommended highly that these patients become involved in a support group such as the one that we have been conducting in Philadelphia for the past eight years. New group therapy members are told that over 1,000 patients have gone through the program, yet as they look around there are usually no more than four to eight people in the group. They hear that most have "graduated" and gone on with their lives and are not in need of continued supportive therapy. Some of them come back as "alumni" to report on their improvement to new group members and to offer encouragement to persevere. Hearing this from a former head-injured patient is valuable to the current sufferers.

Litigation and compensation generally play little, if any, role in determining the outcome in patients with post-traumatic headache syndrome following closed head injury. Legal settlement does not bring about the sudden termination of symptoms. Likewise, several studies confirmed the pressence of persistent post-traumatic symptomatology in individuals where no litigation or compensation was pending (18–20,32–36).

Since most patients have significant recovery, the overall prognosis is good, especially if an aggressive treatment program is utilized. It should also be noted that those patients who are unfortunate enough to have multiple concussions seem to do worse after each subsequent episode.

References

1. Trotter MS: The evolution of the surgery of head injuries. Lancet, 1930; 1:169–171.
2. Adams RD, Victor M: Craniocerebral trauma. In: Principles of Neurology. 3rd ed. New York: McGraw-Hill, 1985; pp 657–658.
3. Penfield W, Norcross N: Subdural traction and posttraumatic headache. Study of pathology and therapeusis. Arch Neurol Psychiatry, 1936; 36: 75–94.
4. Guttman L: Post-contusional headache. Lancet, 1943; 1:10–12.
5. Friedman AP: The so called post-traumatic headache. In Walker AE, Caveness WF, Critchley M (eds): Late effects of Head Injury. Springfield, IL: Charles C Thomas, 1969.
6. Jacobson SA: Mechanisms of the sequelae of minor cranio-cervical trauma. In Walker AE, Caveness WF, Critchley M (eds): Late Effects of Head Injury. Springfield, IL: Charles C Thomas, 1969; pp 33–45.
7. Rowbothan OF: Complications and sequelae of injuries to the head. Med Pr, 1941; 205:379–384.
8. Russell WR: The after-effects of head injury. Trans Med Chir Soc Endb, 1933–34; 113:129–141.
9. Povlishock JR, Becker DP, Cheng CL, et al.: Axonal change in minor head injury. J Neuropath Exp Neurol, 1983; 42:225–242.
10. Strich SJ: Shearing of nerve fibers as a cause of brain damage due to minor head injury: A pathological study of twenty cases. Lancet, 1961; II:443–448.
11. Ommaya AK, Gennarelli TA: Cerebral concussion and traumatic unconsciousness. Brain, 1979; 97:633–654.
12. Oppenheimer DR: Microscopic lesions in the brain following head injury. J Neurol Neurosurg Psychiatry, 1968; 31:299–306.
13. Groat RA, Simmons JQ: Loss of nerve cells in experimental cerebral concussion. J Neuropathol Exp Neurol, 1950; 9:150–163.
14. Groat RA, Windle WR, Macoun HW: Functional and structural changes in monkey brain during and after concussion. J Neurosurg, 1945; 2: 26–35.
15. Olendorph WH, Ktano M: Radioisotope measurement of brain blood turnover time as a clinical index of brain circulation. J Nucl Med, 1967; 8:570–587.
16. Vigayan N, Dreyfus PM: Post-traumatic dysautonomic cephalgia. Arch Neurol, 1975; 32:649–652.
17. Vijayan N: A new post-traumatic headache syndrome: Clinical and therapeutic observations. Headache, 1977; 17:19–22.
18. Stuss DT, Hugenhultz H, Richard MT, et al.: Subtle neuropsychological deficits in patients with bood recovery after closed head injury. Neurosurgery, 1985; 17:41–47.
19. Denker PG: The postconcussion syndrome: prognosis and evaluation of organic factors. NY State J Med, 1944; 44:379–384.
20. Rimel RW, Giordani B, Barth JT, et al.: Disability caused by minor head injury. Neurosurgery 1981; 9:221–228.

21. Dillon H, Leopold RL: Children and the post-concussion syndrome. JAMA, 1961; 175(2):86–92.

22. Masters SJ, McClean PM, Acarese JS, et al.: Skull x-ray examination after head trauma: Recommendations by a multi-disciplinary panel and validation study. N Engl J Med, 1987; 316:84–91.

23. Han JS, Kaufman B, Alfidi RJ, et al.: Head trauma evaluation by magnetic resonance and computed tomography: a comparison. Radiology, 1984; 150:71–77.

24. Levin HS, Amparo E, Eisenberg HM, et al.: Magnetic resonance imaging and computerized tomography in relation to the neurobehavioral sequelae of mild and moderate head injuries. J Neuro Surg, 1987; 66:706–713.

25. Prigatano G, Stahl M, Orr W, et al.: Sleep and dreaming disturbances in closed head injury patients. J Neurol Neurosurg Psychiatry, 1982; 45:48–80.

26. Gerson I, Medical Director, University Services, Philadelphia, PA, Personal communication.

27. Thatcher RA, et al: EEG discriminant analysis of mild head trauma. EEG Clin Neurol, 1989; 73:94–106.

28. Noseworthy JH, Miller J, Murrary TJ, et al.: Auditory brainstem response in post-concussion syndrome. Arch Neurol, 1981; 38:275–278.

29. Schoenbauber R, Gentilini M, Orlando A: Prognostic value at auditory brain-stem responses for late post-concussion symptoms following minor head injury. J Neurosurg, 1988; 68:742–744.

30. Eviator L: Vestibular testing in basilar artery migraine. Ann Neurol, 1981; 9:126–130.

31. MacFlynn G, Montgomery EA, Fenton CW, et al.: Measurement of reaction time following minor head injury. J Neurol Neurosurg Psychiatry, 1984; 47:1326–1331.

32. Kelly R, Smith BN: Post-traumatic headache syndrome: Another myth discredited. J Roy Soc Med, 1981; 74:275–277.

33. McKinlay WM, Brooks DN, Bond MR: Post-concussional symptoms, financial compensation and outcome of severe blunt head injury. J Neurol Neurosurg Psychiatry, 1985; 46:1084–1091.

34. Gronwall D, Wrightson P: Delayed recovery of intellectual function after minor head injury. Lancet, 1974; 2:605–609.

35. McMillan TM, Gluexsman EE: The neuropsychology of moderate head injury. J Neurol Neurosurg Psychiatry, 1987; 50:393–397.

36. Elkind AH: Headache and head trauma. Clin J Pain, 1989; 5:77–87.

— 10

Neurotologic Evaluation and Treatment Following Minor Head Trauma

Robert Thayer Sataloff and Joseph R. Spiegel

Introduction

Otologic symptoms occur commonly following head injury. Dizziness, tinnitus, hearing loss, and even facial paralysis may occur following trauma, often in association with headache, memory loss, lethargy, irritability, and other neurologic complaints discussed elsewhere in this book. For many years, auditory and vestibular symptoms following trauma were considered psychogenic. However, organic causes for these complaints have been established and accepted for at least the last two decades [1,2]. Following severe head injury, the mechanisms are clear. They include localized middle or inner ear injury from direct trauma to the ear and temporal bone, labyrinthine concussion, injury to the seventh and eighth neurovascular bundles (ipsilateral or contra coup), and injury to the brainstem or higher pathways. In cases of severe head injury, isolated auditory and vestibular symptoms are unusual, but severe dizziness and ataxia, inability to discriminate or process speech signals, tinnitus, and other otologic problems occur frequently in association with other signs and symptoms of neurologic injury. Vestibular symptoms associated with mild head trauma and "inner ear concussion" are also well recognized [3]. When neurotologic symptoms occur following minor head trauma, they may be the most prominent post-traumatic complaints, or they may be subtle. Consequently, all patients with symptoms of hearing loss, tinnitus, dizziness, or facial nerve dysfunction following head trauma should undergo comprehensive neurotologic evaluation.

Neurotology is a subspecialty of otolaryngology. Although the field is nearly 30 years old, there are still few practitioners who have the experience or fellowship training beyond otolaryngology residency to qualify them as neurotologists. Otolaryngologists subspecializing in this area are specially trained in the diseases of the ear and ear-brain interface, and in skull base surgery for problems such as acoustic neuroma, glomus jugulare, intractable vertigo, total deafness, and traditionally "unresectable" neoplasms. They are distinct from otoneurologists, whose background is in neurology but who have special interest in disorders afflicting the hearing and balance system.

History

The neurotological examination begins with a comprehensive history. The history must include not only information about the ear and otologic complaints, but also a complete description of the injury, general medical history, and any other information that might help elucidate true causation.

The Head Injury

Teleologically, the ear is an extremely important structure. It is deeply embedded in the head, protected by the otic capsule, the hardest bone in the body. Hearing and balance were critical to the survival of animals and prehistoric humans. Consequently, they are well protected. In general, if the head injury is not severe enough to cause loss of consciousness, it is unlikely to cause significant, measurable hearing loss, although dips in 3,000- to 6,000-Hz range may occur. However, other otologic complaints such as difficulty processing sentences, tinnitus, and dizziness may occur with lesser injuries. The ear is more readily injured by temporal and parietal blows than by those directed at the frontal or occipital bone. Consequently, it is important to determine the exact nature of the injury, the point at which the head was struck, and estimate of the force of injury, whether there was rebound or whiplash injury, whether loss of consciousness occurred, and whether there had been any previous episodes of head trauma or otologic symptoms. Since hearing loss, dizziness, and tinnitus are often not noticed until a day or more following injury, the time of onset of symptoms seems less helpful than one might expect. However, time of onset is important to establish, especially if symptoms are noticed immediately at the time of the accident (in which case the trauma is the most likely cause), or many weeks after the accident (in which case a post-traumatic etiology is somewhat less likely).

Hearing Loss

There are a great many causes of hearing loss, including pathology localized to the ear, hereditary syndromes, systemic disease (diabetes, syphilis, etc.), noise, and other causes (4). Sometimes symptoms caused by such problems are reported or noted for the first time immediately following injury. In some cases, the underlying condition may even predispose the ear to post-traumatic dysfunction. In any situation in which both ears are subjected to similar trauma and only one ear develops signs or symptoms, the physician must search diligently to rule out underlying disease. In all patients, a thorough history may be most revealing. Inquiries should include at least the following questions:

1. In which ear do you think you have hearing loss?
2. How long have you had a hearing loss?
3. If you first noticed it in relation to your head injury, exactly when did you become aware of it?
4. Who noticed it: you, family members, or others?
5. Did your hearing decrease slowly, rapidly, or suddenly?
6. Is your hearing now stable?
7. Does your hearing fluctuate?
8. Do you have distortion of pitch?
9. Do you have distortion of loudness (bothered by loud noises)?
10. Can you use both ears on the telephone?
11. Do you have a feeling of fullness in your ears?
12. Are you aware of anything (foods, weather, sounds) that makes your hearing better or worse?
13. Does your hearing change with straining, bending, nose-blowing, or lifting?
14. Did you have ear problems as a child?
15. Have you ever had ear drainage?
16. Have you had recent or frequent ear infections?
17. Have you ever had ear surgery?
18. Have you ever had ear surgery recommended, but not performed?
19. Have you ever had a direct injury to your ear?
20. Have you ever had problems similar to your current complaints prior to your current injury?
21. Do you have ear pain?
22. Have you had recent dental work?
23. If you have dentures, when were they adjusted last?

24. Do you tend to grind your teeth?
25. Does anyone in your family have a hearing loss?
26. Has anyone in your family undergone surgery for hearing?
27. Do you have parents, brothers, or sisters with syphilis?
28. Have you ever had a venereal disease?
29. Have you ever worked at a job noisy enough to require you to speak loudly in order to be heard?
30. Do your ears ring, or do you have temporary hearing loss when you leave your noisy work environment?
31. Do you have any noisy recreational activities, such as rifle shooting, listening to rock and roll music, snowmobiling, motorcycling, wood-working, etc?
32. Do you wear ear protectors when exposed to loud noise?
33. Do you frequently scuba dive?
34. Do you fly private aircraft or skydive?
35. Do you have ear noises or dizziness?

In combination with questions about tinnitus, vertigo, and general health, these questions usually supply the information necessary to establish a diagnosis once a physical examination and appropriate testing have been completed.

Tinnitus

Tinnitus is a term used to describe perceived sounds that originate within a person, rather than in the outside world. Although nearly everyone experiences mild tinnitus momentarily and intermittently, continuous tinnitus is abnormal, but not unusual. The National Center for Health Statistics reported that about 32% of all adults in the United States acknowledge having had tinnitus at some time [5]. Approximately 6.4% characterize the tinnitus as debilitating or severe. The prevalence of tinnitus increases with age up until approximately 70 years and declines thereafter [6]. This symptom is more common in people with otologic problems, although tinnitus also can occur in otologically normal patients. Nodar reported that approximately 13% of schoolchildren with normal audiograms report having tinnitus at least occasionally [7]. Sataloff studied 267 normal elderly patients with no history of noise exposure or otologic disease and found 24% with tinnitus [8]. As expected, the incidence is higher among patients who consult an otologist for any reason. Fowler questioned 2,000 consecutive patients, 85% of whom reported tinnitus [9]. Heller found that 75% of patients complaining of hearing loss reported tinnitus, and Graham found that approximately 50% of deaf children also complained of tinnitus [10,11]. According to Glasgold and Altman, nearly 80% of patients with otosclerosis have tinnitus

(12), and House and Brackmann reported that 83% of 500 consecutive patients with acoustic neuromas had tinnitus (13).

Among the common misconceptions about tinnitus is that it is idiopathic and incurable. Neither of these assumptions is always correct. Awareness of conditions that cause tinnitus, however, has not been as helpful to tinnitus research as might be expected. Recognizing causal relationships has not shed much light on the actual mechanisms by which internal sounds are created.

Tinnitus is a difficult problem for the physician and patient in all cases. Tinnitus may be either subjective (audible only to the patient) or objective (audible to the examiner, as well). Subjective tinnitus is more common by far with current methods of tinnitus detection. Consequently, it is usually difficult to document its presence and quantify its severity, although a few tests are currently available to help with this problem. Although the character of tinnitus is rarely diagnostic, certain qualities are suggestive of specific problems. A seashell-like tinnitus is often associated with endolymphatic hydrops, swelling of the inner ear membranes associated with Meniere's syndrome, syphilitic labyrinthitis, trauma, and other conditions. Unilateral ringing tinnitus may be caused by trauma, but it is also suggestive of acoustic neuroma. Pulsatile tinnitus may be caused by arterial venus malformations or glomus jugulare tumors, although more benign problems are more common. The history of a tinnitus problem should include the following questions:

1. Are your noises localized?
2. If so, are they in your right ear, left ear, both ears or head?
3. How long have you had head noises?
4. Was there a particular incident (cold, explosion, head injury) that seems to have started your tinnitus?
5. What was the time relationship between the incident and onset of your tinnitus?
6. Has your tinnitus changed since it first appeared?
7. Is it constantly present?
8. Is it episodic?
9. Are you completely free of tinnitus between attacks?
10. Recently, have attacks occurred more frequently, less frequently, or without change?
11. How frequently do you have attacks?
12. Are your noises more apt to occur at a particular time of the day or night?
13. Is there an activity that brings on the noises or makes them worse?
14. Are the noises worse when you are under stress?
15. Are there any foods or substances to which you are exposed that

aggravate the noises (alcohol, cigarettes, coffee, chocolate, salt, etc.)?

16. Are the noises worse during any one season?
17. Is there anything you can do to decrease the noises or make them go away?
18. Are there any activities or sounds that make the tinnitus less disturbing?
19. Can you characterize the noise (ringing, whistling, buzzing, seashell, heartbeat, hissing, bells, voices)?
20. To which of the followng would you compare the loudness of your noise:
    a. A soft whisper
    b. An electirc fan
    c. A diesel truck motor
    d. A jet taking off
21. Is the loudness fairly constant?
22. If it varies, does it vary slightly or widely?
23. Does the noise sound the same in both ears?
24. What medications or treatments have you tried?
25. How would you rate the severity of your tinnitus:
    a. Mild (aware of it when you think about it)
    b. Moderate (aware of it frequently, but able to ignore it most of the time; occasionally interferes with falling asleep)
    c. Severe (aware of it all the time, very disturbing)
    d. Very severe (aware of it all the time, interferes with daily activities, communication and sleep)
26. Do you think other people should be able to hear the noises?
27. Do the noises sound as if they are coming from inside or outside your head?
28. Are your head noises ever voices?
29. Do you have a feeling of fullness in your ears?
30. If so, does it fluctuate with the tinnitus?
31. Has anyone else in your family had tinnitus?
32. Do you have hearing loss or dizziness?

In some cases, the answers to these questions, combined with other information obtained through history, physical examination, and testing, permit identification of a specific cause of tinnitus. For example, ringing tinnitus associated with fluctuating ear fullness and hearing loss during straining can be caused by a perilymph fistula. This is a fairly common injury following trauma. Seashell-like tinnitus associated with ear fullness and fluctuating hearing loss unassociated with straining or forceful nose-blowing suggests endolymphatic hydrops. These symptoms may develop many weeks after a traumatic episode, in contrast with fistula symptoms, which are more likely to be recognized shortly after a head injury. Both types of tinnitus may be amenable to treatment.

Dizziness

Vertigo, like deafness and tinnitus, is a subjective experience and is a symptom, not a disease. Its cause must be sought carefully in each case. The terms *dizziness* or *vertigo* are used by patients to describe a variety of sensations, many of which are not related to the vestibular system. It is convenient to think of the balance system as a complex conglomerate of senses that each send the brain information about one's position in space. Components of the balance system include the vestibular labyrinth, the eyes, neck muscles, proprioceptive nerve endings, cerebellum, and other structures. If all sources provide information in agreement, one has no equilibrium problem. However, if most of the sources tell the brain that the body is standing still, for example, but one component says that the body is turning left, the brain becomes confused and we experience dizziness. It is the physician's responsibility to analyze systematically each component of the balance system to determine which component or components are providing incorrect information, and whether correct information is being provided and analyzed in an aberrant fashion by the brain. Typically, labyrinthine dysfunction is associated with a sense of motion. It may be true spinning, a sensation of being on a ship or of falling, or simply a vague sense of imbalance when moving. In many cases, it is episodic. Fainting, light-headedness, body weakness, spots before the eyes, general light-headedness, tightness in the head, and loss of consciousness are generally not of vestibular origin. However, such descriptions are of only limited diagnostic help. Even some severe peripheral (vestibular or eighth nerve) lesions may produce only mild unsteadiness or no dizziness at all, such as seen in many patients with acoustic neuroma. Similarly, lesions outside the vestibular system may produce true rotary vertigo, as seen with trauma or microvascular occlusion in the brainstem, and with cervical vertigo.

Dizziness is a relatively uncommon problem in healthy individuals. In contrast to a 24% incidence of tinnitus, Sataloff et al. found only a 5% incidence of dizziness in their study of 267 normal senior citizens (8). Causes of dizziness are almost as numerous as causes of hearing loss, and some of them are medically serious (multiple sclerosis, acoustic neuroma, diabetes, cardiac arrythmia, etc.). Consequently, any patient with an equilibrium complaint needs a thorough examination. Although dizziness may be caused by head trauma, the fact that it is reported for the first time following an injury is insufficient to establish causation without investigating other possible causes. In taking history from a patient with equilibrium complaints, at least the following questions should be asked:

1. When did you first develop dizziness?
2. What is it like (light-headedness, blacking out, tendency to fall, objects spinning, you spinning, loss of balance, nausea or vomiting)?
3. If you or your environment is spinning, is the direction of motion to the right or left?
4. Is your dizziness constant or episodic?
5. If episodic, how long do the attacks last?
6. How often do you have attacks?
7. Have they been more or less frequent recently?
8. Have they been more or less severe recently?
9. Under which circumstance did your dizziness first occur?
10. Exactly what were you doing at the time?
11. If you first noted dizziness after your head injury, how many hours, days, or weeks elapsed between the injury and your first balance symptoms?
12. Did you have any other symptoms at the same time, such as neck pain, shoulder pain, jaw pain, ear fullness, hearing loss, or ear noises?
13. Did you have a cold, the flu, or "cold sores" within the month or two prior to the onset of your dizziness?
14. Are you completely free of dizziness between attacks?
15. Do you get dizzy rolling over in bed?
16. If so, to the right, to the left, or both?
17. Do you get dizzy with position change?
18. If so, does your dizziness occur only in certain positions?
19. Do you get dizzy from bending, lifting, straining, or forceful nose-blowing?
20. Do you have trouble walking in the dark?
21. Do you know of a cause for your dizziness?
22. Is there anything that will stop the dizziness or make it better?
23. Is there anything that will bring on an attack or make your dizziness worse (fatigue, exertion, hunger, certain foods, menstruation, etc.)?
24. Do you have any warning that an attack is about to start?
25. Once an attack has begun, does head movement make it worse?
26. Do you have significant problems with motion sickness?
27. Do you get headaches in relation to attacks of dizziness?
28. Do you get migraine headaches?
29. Are there other members of your family with migraine headaches?
30. Does your hearing change when you are dizzy?

31. Do you have fullness or stuffiness in your ears?
32. If yes, does it change when you have an attack of dizziness?
33. Have you had previous head injuries?
34. Have you ever injured your neck?
35. Do you have spine disease like arthritis (especially in the neck)?
36. Have you had any injuries to either ear?
37. Have you ever had surgery on either ear?
38. What drugs have been used to treat your dizziness?
39. Have they helped?
40. Do you have hearing loss or tinnitus?

It is important to pursue a systematic inquiry in all cases of disequilibrium not only because the condition is caused by serious problems in some cases, but also because many patients with balance disorders can be helped. Many people believe incorrectly that sensorineural hearing loss, tinnitus, and dizziness are incurable; but many conditions that cause any or all of these symptoms may be treated successfully. Ruling out causes not related to injury is also essential in accurately establishing a diagnosis of post-traumatic dizziness. When post-traumatc dizziness can be identified, it is equally important to separate peripheral causes (which are almost always treatable), from central causes such as brainstem contusion (in which the prognosis is often worse).

The Facial Nerve

Although facial paralysis will not be covered extensively in this chapter, certain principles are worthy of emphasis. Facial paralysis is not "Bell's palsy" until all other diagnoses have been excluded. There is a dangerous tendency to ascribe this idiopathic diagnosis to all cases of facial paralysis, spontaneous or post-traumatic. The facial nerve runs from the facial nucleus in the brainstem, bending around the abducens nucleus; courses from the brainstem across a short expanse of posterior fossa; enters the internal auditory canal in its anterior/superior compartment; becomes covered with bone in its labyrinthine segment as it leaves the internal auditory canal; courses anteriorly; bends at the geniculate ganglion; courses horizontally and vertically through the mastoid; exits through the stylomastoid foramen; and innervates muscles of facial expression. It also carries special sensory fibers for taste, preganglionic parasympathetic fibers to the lacrimal and submandibular glands, and sensory fibers to the skin of the posterior/superior aspect of the external auditory canal. Any portion of the nerve may be involved by disease or injured. Diseases causing facial paralysis include not only viruses (especially herpes) and Bell's palsy but also facial neuromas, acoustic neuromas, cancers of the ear and parotid gland, multiple sclerosis, and other serious conditions. Trauma to the face or temporal bone may also cause edema and paresis or paralysis of the nerve. In rare cases, relatively minor head injury has been associated with facial paralysis, presumably caused by shearing action as the nerve enters the internal auditory canal. Very rarely, facial spasm may also occur following head trauma. Like other neurotologic problems, facial paralysis requires extensive evaluation before a valid diagnosis can be rendered.

General Medical History

In addition to the questions above directed specifically to otologic problems, the neurotologist must obtain a complete general medical history. Many systemic conditions are associated with otologic symptoms such as hearing loss, tinnitus, and dizziness. Such conditions include diabetes, hypoglycemia, thyroid dysfunction, cardiac arrythmia, hypertension, hypotension, renal disease, collagen vascular disease, previous meningitis, multiple sclerosis, herpes infection, previous syphilis infection (even from decades ago), glaucoma, seizure disorders, and many other conditions. Psychiatric conditions are also relevant because many of the medications used to treat them and other systemic diseases may cause otologic symptoms as side effects; so can a variety of antibiotics and toxic chemicals, such as lead and mercury. Previous radiation treatment to the head and neck may result in microvascular changes that cause hearing loss, tinnitus, or dizziness. Even excess consumption of alcohol or caffeine may produce symptoms that could be confused with other etiologies such as trauma.

Physical Examination

Physical examination of the patient with neurotological complaints begins with a general assessment as the patient enters the physician's office. While physical examination outside the head and neck is deferred to other specialists, initial observations of skin color and turgor, gait, affect, and other characteristics frequently provide valuable information. Neurotological examination starts with the ears. In addition to complete otoscopic examination, a pneumatic otoscope is used to move each eardrum firmly back and forth to determine whether this maneuver causes dizziness and nystagmus. If there is a hole in the eardrum, this is called a fistula test. If the eardrum is intact, it is called Hennebert's test. Although technically conjugate deviation of the eyes is required for the test to be positive, in general practice a clear subjective response of dizziness is considered a positive test, especially if nystagmus is present. A positive Hennebert's test may occur with endolymphatic hydrops or a fistula. Hitzelberger's sign is sought by testing sensation of the lateral posterior/superior aspect of the external auditory canal. This is the area that receives sensory supply from the facial nerve. Lesions putting pressure on the nerve such as acoustic neuromas or anterior/ inferior cerebellar auditory vascular loops often cause a sensory deficit in this area, or positive Hitzelberger's sign. The eyes are examined for extraocular muscle function and spontaneous nystagmus. This examination is aided by Frenzel glasses, which prevent visual fixation. It is important to note that the examiner's eye is an order of magnitude more sensitive in detecting nystagmus than an electronystagmograph; so direct observation of the eyes should not be omitted. Other cranial nerves should also be examined. The olfactory nerve may be tested by asking the patient to inhale vapors from a collection of different scents. The optic nerve is tested at least by visual confrontation, if not by referral to an ophthalmologist. Trigeminal nerve sensation is tested by assessing sensation in all three divisions on both sides. The trigeminal nerve also supplies motor fibers to muscles of mastication which can be evaluated by assessing jaw movement and lateral muscle strength. In addition to Hitzelberger's sign, the facial nerve is assessed through observations of facial movement and tone. Tear flow, stapedius muscle reflex, salivary flow, and taste can also be tested. The glossopharyngeal nerve is evaluated by testing the gag reflex in the posterior third of the tongue and sensation along the posterior portion of the palate, uvula, and tonsil. Abnormal vocal cord motion is often the most obvious sign of tenth nerve dysfunction. The eleventh cranial nerve weakness is diagnosed in the presence of sternocleidomastoid or trapezius muscle weakness, and twelfth nerve dysfunction causes unilateral tongue paralysis. Examination of the nose and oral cavity is performed routinely and does not differ from examination of any other otolaryngologic patient, except that special attention is paid to nasal obstruction when taste and smell disorders have been identified, and to clear rhinorrhea, which may indicate a cerebrospinal fluid leak following head injury. Examination of the larynx should include special attention to symmetry of vocal fold motion, and to any signs of direct laryngeal trauma which may occur in association with minor head injury, especially if an automobile driver strikes the steering wheel. In addition, hoarseness or any other voice change should be noted and investigated. Examination of the neck includes palpation not only of the anterior neck, but also of the posterior aspect. Muscle spasms and tenderness of the cervical vertebrae are often associated with limitation of motion, especially in patients who have dizziness associated with changes in head and neck position. Attention should be paid to the regions of C1 and C2, especially in patients with post-traumatic dizziness. Neck examination should also include auscultation of the carotid arteries and palpation of the superficial temporal arteries. If there is any question of vascular insufficiency, ultrasound of the carotid and vertebral arteries or arteriography should be considered. In addition, Romberg testing, gait assessment, cerebellar function testing, and other neurologic evaluation should be carried out as described elsewhere in this book.

When systemic diseases are suspected as the cause of neurotologic symptoms, referrals should be made to an internist, cardiologist, endocrinologist, neurologist, ophthalmologist, or other specialist for complete assessment. An appropriately high index of suspicion will lead the neurotologist to make such referrals frequently.

Testing

Neurotologic evaluation is never complete without indicated testing. This usually includes a hearing test, assessment of the balance system, radiologic studies, and selected blood tests.

Auditory Testing

For any patient with otologic complaints, an audiogram is mandatory. However, routine hearing tests have many limitations and shortcomings. Frequently, additional special tests are required. They cannot be discussed in great detail in this short chapter, and the reader is advised to consult other literature for more details (4).

Routine Audiogram

An audiogram is a written record of an individual's hearing level measured by objective response to pure tone stimuli at 250, 500, 1,000, 2,000, 3,000, 4,000, 6,000, and 8,000 Hz. These tones are generated electronically by the audiometer. This frequency range includes most of the speech spectrum (frequencies below 3,000 Hz). The test requires patient cooperation and voluntary response. It tests only the ability to hear extremely soft tones, and gives no information about the patient's ability to handle more complex signals or understand words. In addition, it samples hearing thresholds across a very broad range. For example, it gives no information about the condition of hair cells and nerve endings that respond to frequencies between 6,000 and 8,000 Hz or those that respond to higher frequencies. This information can be obtained through other specialized tests.

With 0 dB representing average normal hearing, a 60 dB threshold can also be called a 60 dB "hearing level." Though both terms describe the same condition, the term *hearing level* is preferred. An audiogram should be performed on calibrated equipment in a sound-proof test room. Air conduction tests the ability of the ear to receive and conduct sound waves entering the external auditory canal. Normally, these waves cause the ear drum to vibrate, and the vibrations are transmitted through the ossicular chain to the oval window. When air conduction is impaired as a result of damage to the outer or middle ear but the sensorineural mechanism of the inner ear is intact, there will be a difference between air conduction and bone conduction. Such a mechanical hearing loss may be caused by many conditions, such as fluid in the ear, ossicular fixation, ossicular disruption from trauma, and chronic disease. Bone conduction measures the patient's ability to hear sound vibrations transmitted directly to the cochlea through the bones of the skull, bypassing the outer and middle ear. Bone conduction is not impaired in simple conductive hearing loss. Thus, conductive hearing loss can be distinguished from sensorineural hearing loss by audiometric testing. Essentially, the audiogram is similar to traditional tuning-fork testing, except that it is better controlled and quantified. Routine audiograms also include speech reception threshold (SRT), which tests the softest intensity at which a patient can correctly identify 50% of spondee words (two-syllable words of equal stress per syllable) read through the audiometer earphones. The discrimination score utilizes a different list of one-syllable phonetically balanced words read at a comfortable listening level approximately 30 dB above SRT. The discrimination score is the percentage identified correctly and should be between 90% and 100%. Patients with sensorineural losses may have decreased discrimination, and in certain conditions (such as acoustic neuroma) discrimination may be dramatically decreased even when pure tone thresholds are fairly normal.

Correct procedure must be observed carefully when calibrating, performing, and interpreting audiograms. There are many potential pitfalls, and errors can be made easily. It is often advisable to supplement routine audiometry with special tests. In most cases, it is possible to distinguish between sensory (inner ear) and neural (nerve) hearing loss. Head trauma may produce damage in either site. Typically, head trauma damages the outer hair cells, initially in the region between 3,000 and 6,000 Hz, producing a sensorineural hearing loss. However, neural and central injury may also be present (cases 1 and 2). Hearing abnormalities have been reported in as many as 20%

of patients who have sustained minor head injury (14). Clinically, this percentage seems somewhat high if pure-tone audiometry is the sole criterion; but it is probably in the right range when both pure-tone and brainstem response audiometry are used to screen patients for hearing loss.

Tests for Recruitment

The phenomenon of recruitment is a disproportionate increase in the sensation of loudness of a sound when its intensity is raised. The principle value of detecting recruiment is that it helps to trace the site of the lesion in the auditory pathway to the hair cells of the cochlea. The patient often provides clues to the presence of cochlear damage when he or she is questioned about his or her hearing difficulty. He or she may say that loud noises are very bothersome in his or her bad ear or that the sound seems to be tinny and harsh and very unclear. He or she may volunteer that music sounds distorted or flat. These complaints should not be confused with the annoyance voiced by a neurotic patient who hears well but is bothered by such noises as the shouting of children. A well-defined sensorineural hearing loss is a prerequisite before recuriment can be used as a basis for localizing an auditory deficit to the cochlea.

Tuning Fork

Recruitment can be detected in some cases with the aid of a 512-Hz tuning fork if a hearing loss affects the speech frequencies, as often occurs in endolymphatic hydrops. The test is done by comparing the growth of loudness in the good ear with that in the bad ear. The fork is struck once gently and held up to each of the patient's ears, and he or she is asked in which ear the tone sounds louder. Naturally, he or she will say the tone is louder in the ear that has normal hearing. Then, the intensity of the tone is increased by striking the fork once again quite hard (but not too hard, or the tone will be distorted). The patient then is asked again to indicate in which ear the tone now sounds louder, with the fork held first near the good ear and then quickly moved about the same distance from the bad ear. If complete or hyper-recruitment is present, the patient will now exclaim in surprise that the tone is as loud or louder in his or her bad ear. This means that there has been a larger growth in the sensation of loudness in his or her bad ear, in spite of a hearing loss.

Alternate Binaural Loudness Balance Test

Testing for recruitment with a tuning fork is a rather rough technique, but it may help in diagnosing recruitment. More precise tests have been devised to test for recruitment, but most of these are suitable for use only when one ear is impaired and the other is normal. The technique in common use is called the alternate binaural loudness balance test, which matches the loudness of a given tone in each ear.

This is done with an audiometer and involves presenting a tone of a certain intensity to the good ear and then alternately applying it to the bad ear at various intensities; the patient is asked to report when the tone is equally loud in both ears. Initially, a brief tone 15 dB above threshold is applied to the good ear. Then the tone is presented briefly to the bad ear 15 dB above its threshold, and the patient is asked whether the tone was louder or softer than that heard in the good ear. According to his or her response, necessary adjustments are made to the intensity going to the bad ear until a loudness balance is obtained with the good ear. Then, the intensity to the good ear is increased by another 15 dB, and another balance is obtained with the bad ear. Loudness balancing is continued in 15-dB steps until sufficient information is obtained about the growth of loudness in the bad ear. This technique requires that the same frequency be balanced in the two ears and the tone be presented alternately to the good ear, which serves as the reference. Also, the difference in threshold between the two ears should be at least 20 dB for this test to be valid.

If the difference in loudness level between the two ears is unchanged at high intensities, recruitment is absent. If the loudness difference gradually decreases at higher intensities, recruitment is present. If the loudness difference completely disappears between the two ears at higher intensities, the condition is called complete recruitment and is indicative of damage to the inner ear. There may be hyper-recruitment, in which the tone in the bad ear sounds even louder than the tone in the good ear at some point above threshold. Recruitment may occur at varying speeds. If it continues regularly with each increase in intensity, it is called continuous recruitment, and this is indicative of inner ear damage. Recruitment that is found only at or near threshold levels is not characteristic of inner ear damage but occurs often in sensorineural hearing impairment.

Detection of Small Changes in Intensity

Another method of demonstrating recruitment involves the patient's ability to detect small changes in intensity. A recruiting ear detects smaller changes in loudness than normal ears or those with conductive hearing loss. At levels near threshold, a normal ear is likely to require a change of about 2 dB to recognize a difference in loudness, but in an ear that recruits, only a 0.5 dB increase may be necessary to detect the loudness change.

As the intensity of the tone then increases in normal ears, the change necessary for detecting the difference in loudness becomes smaller, whereas the recruiting ear requires about the same change as it did near threshold level.

Short Increment Sensitivity Index Test

Another test for localizing the site of damage to the cochlea is the short increment sensitivity index (SISI) test. It measures the patient's ability to hear small, short changes of sound intensity. The test is done monaurally by fixing the level of a steady tone at 20 dB above the patient's threshold at each frequency to be tested and superimposing on this steady tone 1 dB increments of about 200 msec duration, interspersing the increments at 5 second intervals. The patient is to respond each time he hears any "jumps in loudness." If he or she hears five of the 1-dB increments, his or her sensitivity index is 25%. A score of between 60% and 100% at frequencies about 1,000 Hz is positive for cochlear disorders, whereas a score below 20% is considered to be negative. Scores between 20% and 60% are inconclusive.

A revision of the test called the high-intensity SISI uses a similar technique, but with very loud tones rather than near threshold tones. In high-intensity SISI testing, patients with cochlear hearing loss and those with normal hearing will exhibit a high percentage of response to the short increment increases. However, patients with retrocochlear disease, such as an acoustic neuroma, will continue to have low percentage scores. Thus, both the classical SISI and the high-intensity tests help to differentiate not only between cochlear and noncochlear but also cochlear and retrocochlear pathology.

Other Tests

There are more tests using speech discrimination and Bekesy audiometry that also help to determine the presence of cochlear damage; these are supplementary to the basic tests described. They are especially helpful when both ears have a hearing loss, because a "control" ear is not essential to the test procedure. Stapedius reflex testing also is useful in these cases.

Testing for Diplacusis—Distortion of Pitch

Another simple and fairly reliable office test can be done with a tuning fork to help to localize the site of auditory damage in the cochlea. This test explores not distortion of loudness (recruitment) but distortion of pitch, which is called diplacusis. Distortion is the hallmark of hair cell damage.

A 512-Hz tuning fork is struck and held near the normal ear and then near the opposite ear. If the damage is localized in the cochlea, the patient may report that the same tuning fork has a different sound when it is heard in the bad ear. Usually, he or she will say that the pitch is higher and not as clear but rather fuzzy. It is important to clarify to the patient when this test is performed that he or she is being asked to evaluate pitch, not intensity; otherwise, inaccurate results may be obtained.

Hearing Tests Using Speech to Detect Central Hearing Loss

Special tests using modified speech are becoming very useful in deciding whether a hearing loss is caused by damage in the central nervous system. Lesions in the cortex do not result in any reduction in pure-tone thresholds, but brainstem lesions may cause some high frequency hearing loss. Routine speech audiometry is almost always normal in cortical lesions. Sometimes it is impaired in brainstem lesions but with a characteristic pattern. Since neither pure-tone nor routine speech tests help to localize damage in the central nervous system, more complex tests have been developed to help to provide this information.

A chief function of the cortex is to convert neural impulses into meaningful information. Words and sentences acquire their significance at the cortical level. Because quality, space, and time are factors governing the cortical identification of a verbal pattern, the tests are designed so that they explore the synthesizing ability of the cortex when one or more of these factors is purposely changed. Such tests are helpful in people such as the individual described in case 1.

Binaural Test of Auditory Fusion

One such test of central auditory dysfunction is the binaural test of auditory fusion. Speech signals are transmitted through two different narrow-band filters. Each band by itself is too narrow to allow recognition of test words. Subjects who have normal hearing show excellent integration of test words when they receive the signals from one filter in one ear and the other filter in the other ear. Poorer scores are made by patients with brain lesions and are indications of a functional failure within the cortex.

Sound Localization Tests

Sound localization tests are being used in the diagnosis of central lesions. Deviation of the localization band to one side points to a cerebral lesion on the contralateral side or to a brainstem lesion on the ipsilateral side.

Other Tests

Distorted voice, interrupted voice, and accelerated voice tests likewise are used in detecting central lesions. In the distorted voice test, phonetically balanced (PB) words are administered about 50 dB above threshold through a low-pass filter that is able to reduce the discrimination to about 70% or 80% in normal subjects. Patients with temporal lobe tumors present an average discrimination score that is poorer in the ear contralateral to the tumor.

The interrupted voice test presents PB words at about 50 dB above threshold, interrupting them periodically 10 times/sec. Subjects with normal hearing obtain about 80% discrimination; those with temporal lobe tumors have reduced discrimination in the ear contralateral to the tumor.

In the accelerated voice test, when the number of words per minute is increased from about 150 words to about 350 words, the discrimination approaches 100% in subjects who have normal hearing, but the threshold for maximal response is raised by 10 to 15 dB. In patients with tumors of the temporal lobe, there is a normal threshold shift, but the discrimination never attains 100% in the contralateral ear. In cortical lesions the impairment always seems to be in the ear contralateral to the neoplasm and moderate in extent. Brainstem lesions exhibit ipsilateral or bilateral impairments.

Ipsilateral and contralateral stapedius reflex tests also provide useful information.

Testing for Functional Hearing Loss

Whenever a patient claims to have a hearing loss that does not seem to be based on organic damage to the auditory pathway, or whenever the test responses and the general behavior of the patient appears to be questionable, a variety of tests can be performed to help determine whether the loss is functional rather than organic.

Suggestive Clues

The most suggestive findings are inconsistencies in the hearing tests. For instance, a patient has a hearing threshold level of 70 dB in one test and a 40-dB threshold when the test is repeated several minutes later; or the audiogram of a patient shows a 60-dB average hearing loss bilaterally, but the patient inadvertently replies to soft speech behind his or her back; or he or she has an SRT of 20 dB in contrast to a 60-dB pure-tone average; or the patient gives poor or no responses in bone conduction tests, indicating severe sensorineural involvement, but has suspiciously good discrimination ability for the apparent degree and type of loss. However, care must be exercised. Certain organic conditions, such as Meniere's disease, multiple sclerosis, and severe tinnitus, may also cause inconsistent responses.

Also, the patient's behavior may not be consistent with the degree of loss claimed, especially in cases of bilateral functional hearing loss. Usually, a patient with severe bilateral deafness is very attentive to the speaker's face and mouth in order to benefit from lip-reading. A functionally deaf person may not show this attentiveness. He or she also may have unusually good voice control, which is not consistent with the degree of loss. Occasionally, a functionally deaf person will assume a moronic attitude or repeat part of a test word correctly and labor excessively over the last half of the word. These and other subtle clues should alert the examiner to the possibility of the presence of a purely functional hearing loss or a functional overlay on an organic hearing loss (case 3).

Lombard, or Voice Reflex, Test

When a patient claims deafness in one ear, but it is suspected of being functional, several simple tests are available to determine the validity of the loss. The patient is given a newspaper or a magazine article to read aloud without stopping. While he or she is reading, the tester presents noise to the good ear. This may be done by rubbing a piece of typing paper such as onion-skin paper over the patient's good ear. If the patient's voice does not get significantly louder, it is highly suggestive that he or she can hear in his or her supposedly "bad" ear. Because hearing is partly a feedback mechanism that informs the speaker how loud he or she is speaking, a person with normal hearing will speak more loudly in a very noisy area so that he or she can hear himself or herself and be heard above the noise. If the patient does not raise his voice when noise is applied to one ear, it means that he or she is hearing himself or herself speak in the other ear, and consequently that ear does not have the marked hearing loss indicated on the pure-tone or speech audiogram. Instead of rubbing paper against the patient's ears as the source of noise, a Barany noise apparatus or the noise from an audiometer noise generator is extremely effective in this test, because the level of the noise can be controlled. This type of test is called the Lombard, or voice reflex, test, and although it does not help to establish thresholds, it does give the examiner some idea of whether the loss is exaggerated.

Stenger Test

The Stenger test depends on a given pure tone presented to both ears simultaneously. The tone will be perceived in the ear where it is louder. If the sound in one ear is made louder, then the listener will hear it in that ear and he or she will not realize that a weaker sound exists in the other ear.

A tone is presented to the good ear about 10 dB above threshold and, at the same time, 10 dB below the admitted threshold in the bad ear. If the patient responds, the test is a negative Stenger because he or she heard the tone in the good ear without realizing there was a weaker tone in his or her bad ear. If the patient does not respond, it is a positive Stenger because he or she heard the sound in his or her assumed bad ear without realizing there was a tone of weaker intensity presented to his or her good ear.

This test can be done with speech as well as pure tones. There must be a difference of at least 30 dB between thresholds of the good and bad ear for the test to be effective. Also, a two-channel audiometer is needed to administer the test.

The Stenger test also enables the examiner to obtain an approximation of the patient's true thresholds in the bad ear (15). This is done by presenting the pure tone 10 dB above threshold in the good ear and presenting a pure tone at 0 Hz in the bad ear. The tone in the bad ear is increased in 5-dB steps until the patient stops responding. (Remember, he or she is hearing the tone in his or her good ear at first.) The Stenger pure tone threshold of the bad ear is approximately 15 dB above his or her true threshold.

Repetition of Audiogram Without Masking

Still another test to indicate whether a patient really has a total unilateral hearing loss or may be malingering is to repeat the audiogram, but this time without masking the good ear. Since a pure tone presented to the test ear can be heard also in the non-test ear when the loudness of the tone is 50 to 55 dB above the threshold of the non-test ear, at least some shadow curve should be present in the absence of masking. If the patient does not respond when the intensity levels reach this point, then the chances are that he or she has a functional deafness in the test ear. If the patient does report hearing the tone, he or she should be questioned carefully about its location. Again, total lack of response is an indication of the dilemma that the functional patient faces when he or she feels that his or her claim is threatened with exposure.

Delayed Talk-Back Test

The monitoring effect of an ear can also be disrupted if a person listens to himself or herself speak through earphones while the return voice is delayed in time. A delay of 0.1 to 0.2 seconds causes symptoms similar to stuttering. If this occurs when the feedback level is lower than the admitted threshold, functional loss is present. In the delayed talk-back test (also called the delayed auditory feedback test), which is done through a modified tape recorder, it is possible to detect significant hearing losses but not the minor exaggerations that occur occasionally in medico-legal situations. This is so because delayed feedback affects the rhythm and the rate of the patient's speech at levels averaging 20 to 40 dB above threshold.

Psychogalvanic Skin Response Test

A great deal of testing has been done with the psychogalvanic skin response test, which is close to being an objective test of hearing, though it still has many shortcomings. This test is done with special equipment and is based on the conditioned-response mechanism. The patient is conditioned so that each time he or she hears a tone, it is followed about a second later by a definite electric shock in his or her arm, to which is strapped an electrode. Through electrodes placed on the patient's fingers or palms, it is possible to measure the change in skin resistance or the so-called electrodermal response excited by the electric shock in the patient's leg. Each time that the patient receives a shock, the skin resistance is altered and can be read on a meter or recorded on a moving graph. After the patient is conditioned well, the electric shock is stopped, and only the sound is given. In a well-conditioned patient, about a second after the sound is applied, he or she will "expect" the shock again and show a typical change in his electrodermal responses. It can be concluded, then, that each time the patient gives a positive reading on the recording equipment after a sound is given, he or she hears the sound. By lowering the intensity of the stimulus, a threshold level can be obtained. At certain intervals, it is necessary to reinforce the conditioned response mechanism by reapplying the electric shock.

This is an excellent technique, based to some extent on the traditional lie detector method, but many complicating factors make it far from a completely reliable method of measuring a hearing threshold level objectively and reliably. It is excellent, however, if it is used in conjunction with a battery of other tests, in helping to establish the organic or the nonorganic basis of any hearing threshold.

Use of Excellent Audiometric Technique

One of the most effective methods of obviating false audiograms for intentional functional hearing loss is to use excellent audiometric technique. Malingering and inaccurate responses are discouraged by a tester who uses excellent technique. Malingering normal hearing also is possible. If a patient is given a sound and is asked repeatedly, "Do you hear it?" he or she will be tempted to say yes, even if he or she does not hear it, whenever some advantage of remuneration is at stake, such as obtaining employment.

Testing for Auditory Tone Decay

Just as marked recruitment usually is indicative of damage in the inner ear, abnormal tone decay (abnormal auditory fatigue) usually is a sign of pressure on or damage to the auditory nerve fibers. This phenomenon may be of particular importance in that it can be an early sign of an acoustic neuroma or some other neoplasm invading the posterior fossa.

Administration of Test

The test for abnormal tone decay is very simple to perform and should be done routinely in every case of unilateral sensorineural hearing loss, especially when no recruitment is found. The test is based on the fact that whereas a person with normal hearing can continue to hear a steady threshold tone for at least one minute, the patient who has a tumor pressing on his or her auditory nerve is unable to keep hearing a threshold tone for this length of time. The test is performed monaurally with an audiometer. A frequency that shows reduced threshold is selected, and the patient is instructed to raise a finger as long as he or she can hear the tone. The tone then is presented at threshold or 5 dB above threshold, and a stopwatch is started with the presentation of the tone. Each time the patient lowers his or her finger, the intensity is increased 5 dB, and the time is noted for that period of hearing. The tone interrupter switch never is released from the "on" position during any of the intensity changes. The test is one minute in duration.

Findings

A person with normal tone decay usually will continue to hold up his or her finger during the entire 60 seconds. Occasionally, he or she may require a 5- or 10-dB increase during the first part of the test, but he or she then maintains the tone for the remainder of the time. A patient who has abnormal tone decay may lower his or her finger after only about 10 seconds, and when the tone is raised 5 dB, he or she may lower his or her finger again after another 10 seconds and continue to indicate that the tone fades out repeatedly, until after 60 seconds there may be an increase of 25 dB or more above the original threshold. Some patients may even fail to hear the tone at the maximum intensity of the audiometer after one minute, whereas originally they may have heard the threshold tone at 25 dB. Masking may be required. This finding of abnormal tone decay is highly suggestive of pressure on the auditory nerve fibers. A tuning fork can also be used to detect abnormal tone decay by testing for threshold, then fatiguing the ear and retesting for threshold.

Diagnostic Self-Recording Audiometry: Bekesy Audiometry

Another method of measuring abnormal tone decay is with a Bekesy audiometer. This is a type of self-recording audiometer that is being used with increased frequency for threshold and special testing. Physicians should be acquainted with its operating principles and the information that it can supply.

Procedure and Mechanism

This method of establishing pure-tone thresholds permits the patient to trace his or her own audiogram as the tone or tones are presented to him or her automatically. Each ear is tested separately. The patient holds a hand switch and has on a set of earphones through which he or she hears the tone. As soon as he or she hears the tone, he or she presses the switch—which causes the sound to decrease in loudness—and holds it down until the tone is gone. This procedure continues until the full range of frequencies has been tested.

The switch controls the attenuator of the audiometer that decreases or increases the intensity of the tone. A pen geared to the attenuator makes a continuous record on an audiogram blank of the patient's intensity adjustments. The audiogram is placed on a table that moves in relation to the frequency being presented. Several methods of frequency selection are available. The audiometer can be set up to produce the frequency range continuously from 100 to 10,000 Hz, or it can be arranged to test hearing in a two-octave range, or if desired, to test threshold for a single frequency for several minutes.

The test signal can be continuous, or pulsed at a rate of about $2\frac{1}{2}$ times/sec. Operation of the patient's hand switch attenuates the signal at a rate of about 2.5 to 5 dB/sec according to the speed selection made by the examiner. Thus, a test routinely performed with Bekesy self-recording audiometry can determine thresholds with both pulsed and continuous tone presentations. If the pulsed tone is used first, a pen with a specific colored ink is placed in the penholder, and the thresholds are recorded. When the pulsed-tone testing is completed, a pen with a different color is placed in the penholder, the frequency is reset to the original point, and the switching is changed to provide a continuous tone. The patient traces another audiogram, as he or she did for the pulsed tones. It is important that the patient not see the equipment in operation, because awareness of the movements of the pen and the action of the hand switch may affect his or her responses and result in an invalid audiogram.

Value

With proper instruction to the patient, Bekesy audiometry not only provides an accurate picture of thresholds but also supplies other valuable information. By comparing the thresholds for the pulsed and the continuous tone, the physician can get a reasonably good indication of the site of the lesion within the auditory system.

Types of Bekesy Audiograms

In normal or conductively impaired ears, the pulsed and the continuous tracings overlap for the entire frequency range tested. This is a type I audiogram. In the type II audiogram, the pulsed and the continuous tones overlap in the low frequencies, but between 500 and 1,000 Hz the continuous frequency tracing drops about 15 dB below the pulsed tracing and then remains parallel with the high frequencies. Type II audiograms occur in cases of cochlear involvement. Sometimes the pen excursions narrow down to about 5 dB in the higher frequencies. Cases of cochlear involvement sometimes also show type I tracings.

In the type III audiogram, the continuous tracing drops suddenly away from the pulsed tracing and usually continues down to the intensity limits of the audiometer. Eighth nerve disorders usually show type III audiograms. Another type of audiogram found in eighth nerve disorders is the type IV tracing, in which the continuous tone tracing stays well below the pulsed tracing at all frequencies.

Interpretation of Bekesy Audiograms

There is some feeling that the amplitude of the Bekesy audiogram provides considerable information about the presence of the absence of recruitment. For example, tracings of very small amplitude might lead one to believe that the patient can detect changes in intensity much smaller than the average subject and that he or she therefore has recruitment. Unfortunately, this is not the case. It is more likely that tracings of small amplitude are suggestive of abnormal tone decay rather than of recruitment. A great deal of the interpretation depends on the on and off period of the tone presented.

Nondiagnostic Self-Recording Audiometry and Computerized Audiometry

Nondiagnostic computerized audiometry measures pure-tone thresholds only. Computerized audiometry has special applications, especially in industry and selected research settings. Neither will be discussed in detail in this chapter.

Impedance Audiometry

Impedance audiometry supplements otoscopic and audiometric findings and provides additional capabilities to hearing evaluation. Impedance audiometry is an objective method for evaluating the integrity and function of the auditory mechanism. It includes four separate types of measurement and has the potential for a much wider role as research in its use continues. The procedures most often used are (a) tympanometry, (b) static compliance, (c) stapedius reflex thresholds, and (d) acoustic decay test.

Tympanometry

The eardrum and connecting ossicles form a mechanism that should transfer vibrating energy efficiently. Tympanometry measures the mobility of this system. It is analogous to pneumatic otoscopy. If the system becomes stiffer and more resistant because some condition impedes its free movement, we are able to measure the abnormal impedance (or its reciprocal "compliance"). The compliance or impedance of the middle ear system is measured by its response to variations in air pressure on the eardrum. The entrance of the ear canal is sealed with a probe tip containing three holes: one for supply of air pressure, one for a low-frequency probe tone (usually of 220 Hz), and a third opening connected to a pick-up microphone. As controlled degrees of positive and negative air pressure are introduced into the sealed ear canal, the resulting movement (or reduced movement) of the mechanism is plotted or automatically graphed on a chart called a tympanogram.

Static Compliance

This is a single numerical value representing the acoustic compliance of the middle ear at rest. It is compared to the known compliance of normal and abnormal ears. However, the normative data are influenced by age and sex, and there is some overlap of compliance values obtained in various conditions—normal and abnormal. These factors create some question as to the diagnostic usefulness of static compliance measurements. In general, low compliance is indicative of a stiff middle ear system, and high compliance is indicative of a flaccid middle ear system. The probe tone and pickup microphone are used to measure static compliance. The sound pressure level (SPL) of the tone will increase as the cavity size is decreased, or the SPL of the probe tone will decreased as cavity size is increased, just as a singer will sound louder in a small hall than in a large one. The changes in SPL of the tone are received by the pickup microphone and read in cubic centimeters of equivalent volume. The benefits of volume measurements include delineating space-occupying lesions in the middle ear or mastoid (the volume would be less than normal), identifying perforated tympanic membranes (the volume would be greater than normal), and evaluating the patency of the tubes placed in the tympanic membrane for ventilation purposes (the volume would be greater than normal).

Acoustic Reflex Thresholds

This test determines the level in dB at which the stapedius muscle contracts. Normally, the reflex for pure tones is elicited at about 90 dB above the hearing threshold. For broad-band noise, it occurs at about 70 dB above threshold. The contraction occurs bilaterally, even when only one ear is stimulated. In patients with cochlear damage and associated recruitment, the reflex may occur at sensation levels less than 60 dB above the auditory pure tone threshold (Metz recruitment). In bilateral conductive losses and in some unilateral losses, the acoustic reflex may be absent bilaterally. In a unilateral cochlear loss not exceeding 80 dB, acoustic reflexes may appear unilaterally when the stimulation earphone is on the "dead ear" side. These factors then can be diagnostically important, especially when masking is impractical.

Acoustic Reflex Decay Test

In the normal ear, contraction of the middle ear muscles to a sound 10 dB above the acoustic reflex threshold can be maintained for at least 45 seconds without detectable decay or adaptation. In the presence of an acoustic neuroma or other retrocochlear lesion, however, the middle ear muscle contraction may show fatigue or decay in less than ten seconds. In some cases, it may be entirely absent.

Other impedance tests include the ipsilateral reflex test for the differential diagnosis of brainstem lesions; facial nerve test for localizing the site of a lesion in facial paralysis; eustachian tube tests for determining eustachian tube function; fistula test in which the air pressure will cause dizziness and deviation of the eyes if a fistula into the inner ear exists; and test for presence of a glomus tumor in which meter variations in synchrony with the pulse beat can be observed.

Impedance audiometry is especially useful in difficult to test patients such as very young children, the mentally retarded, the physically disabled, and the malingerer. Like all other tests, it is not 100% accurate and must be interpreted with expertise.

Continuous Frequency Testing

As mentioned previously, routine audiograms sample only a few frequencies. Several audiometers are now available that will test frequencies between those traditionally measured. Such testing is valuable in many cases. For example, a patient who complains of tinnitus following an injury and has a normal routine audiogram may show a drop at an unusual frequency in the effected ear, such as 5,325 Hz. Such a finding helps substantiate and explain the tinnitus.

Tinnitus Matching

Several devices are available to help quantify tinnitus, and some newer audiometers include tinnitus matching capabilities. These tests allow reasonably good quantification of tinnitus pitch and loudness. Interestingly, even very loud tinnitus is rarely more than 5 to 10 dB above threshold.

High-Frequency Audiometry

It is often useful to test frequencies above 8,000 Hz. Audiometers can be obtained that permit audiograms up to 20,000 Hz. Testing to 12,000 or 14,000 Hz provides the desired information in most cases, and testing at frequencies above 14,000 presents special difficulties. High-frequency testing is especially valuable for differentiating presbycusis from occupational hearing loss, detecting early effects of ototoxic drugs, and potentially in selected trauma cases.

Electrocochleography

This method of assessing difficult-to-test patients involves placing an electrode in the ear and measuring directly the ear's electrical response to a sound stimulus. Most commonly, the electrode is placed through the eardrum into the promontory, although noninvasive canal electrodes are now available and work well. In children, this may require a short-acting general anesthetic. This evoked potential test has proven clinical value in several areas, particularly—

1. Confirming wave I in the brainstem response. This is especially useful if the ABR expresses an equivocal result.
2. Confirming endolymphatic hydrops in Meniere's patients. This is helpful, for example, with patients who cannot tolerate an electronystagmogram evaluation.

Evoked Response Audiometry

Accurate hearing testing in infants, mentally retarded patients, neurologically disabled patients, and others who cannot or will not volunteer accurate responses is a special problem. A few objective tests (those requiring no patient cooperation) are now available. Impedance audiometry is objective, but it is difficult to determine hearing thresholds from it in some cases.

Evoked response audiometry is similar to electroencephalography or brain wave testing. Painless electrodes are attached to the patient. A darkened, "soundproof" room is used. A computer is required to isolate the auditory response from the rest of the electrical activity from the brain. Pure-tone or broad-band stimuli can be used. There are two types of evoked response audiometry.

Cortical Evoked Response Audiometry

This method focuses on electrical activity at the cerebral cortex level. It allows measurement not only of auditory signals, but also of other brain wave variations that are associated with the perception of sound. Therefore, it may prove a valuable tool in evaluating not only thresholds, but also whether or not a sound actually reaches a level of perception in the brain.

Brainstem Evoked Response Audiometry (BERA)

This technique is somewhat newer, but it has become very popular clinically. Testing can be done with pure tones or broad-band noise, and threshold levels can be determined. The test can be used on infants and has even been advocated for routine screening in newborn nurseries. It also can be performed under general anesthesia, and it remains useful even in the presence of deep coma. Brainstem evoked response audiometry measures electrical peaks occurring in the brainstem along the auditory pathway. The sites of origin of the waves are still controversial, but probable locations are commonly accepted as follows: Wave I is produced at the auditory level; wave II, at the cochlear nucleus; wave III, at the superior olive; wave IV, probably at the level of the lateral lemniscus in the pons; wave V, at the inferior colliculus; wave VI, probably at the thalamus; and wave VII, possibly at the cortical level. Absence of distortion of peaks or delay between peaks can help localize lesions in the auditory pathway. For example, difference in latency between a patient's ears currently appears to be the most sensitive test for detecting acoustic neuromas. However, BERA can have other localizing value. Absence of wave II with a normal wave I might suggest a brainstem vascular accident with a normal peripheral hearing mechanism. Separation between waves IV and V suggests demyelinating disease, such as multiple sclerosis, causing conduction delay. Abnormal brainstem evoked auditory responses have been reported following minor head trauma (14,16). The most prominent abnormality appears to be reversible conduction delay apparent at high stimulus repetition rate (clicks of greater than 50 per second). Brainstem auditory evoked response testing should be performed early, and these abnormalities may disappear within two months following injury in some patients. In some cases, other abnormalities may be seen even at lower stimulus repetition rates, including differences in absolute wave V latency, and interwave latencies of waves III to V. The brainstem auditory evoked response findings following minor hearing injury are most consistent with ischemia and synaptic dysfunction rather axonal damage.

Vestibular Testing

The balance system is extremely complicated, and ideal tests have not been developed. Research is currently under way to develop tests that will assess accurately the entire, composite functioning of the balance system and test each component in isolation. At present, the most commonly performed test is electronystagmography. Posturography is just coming into use, and vestibular evoked potential testing is under investigation. A brief review of vestibular physiology is helpful in understanding balance tests. The semicircular canals are arranged in three planes at right angles to each other (x, y, z axes), and work in pairs. The cupulae of the semicircular canals are stimulated by movement of endolymphatic fluid, and each canal causes the nystagmus in its own plain. That is, the horizontal canal produces horizontal nystagmus; the superior canal causes rotary nystagmus; and the posterior canal produces vertical nystagmus. Caloric testing stimulates primarily the horizontal semicircular canal and gives little or no information about function of the superior and posterior semicircular canals in most cases. The position of gaze and plane of the head are of great importance in vestibular testing, especially when the semicircular canals are stimulated by rotation, rather than water irrigation. For rotary testing, it is useful to remember that ampullopedal flow (toward the cupulae) produces greater stimulation than ampullofugal flow (away from the cupulae) in the horizontal semicircular canal, but the opposite is true for the superior and posterior canals. Therefore, the response to rotation represents the combined effect of stimulating the sensory system of one semicircular canal while suppressing that of its counterpart on the other side of the body. Rotational excitation and selective head position may be used to give information about the semicircular canals that is difficult or impossible to obtain from caloric stimulation. The clinical value of this additional information is controversial, and rotational testing is not common in the United States (although it is used more frequently in Britain).

Electronystagmography

Electronystagmography (ENG) is a technique for recording eye movements that detects spontaneous and induced nystagmus. It allows measurement of eye movements with eyes opened or closed and permits quantification of the fast and slow phases, time of onset and duration, as well as other parameters. Although some centers use only horizontal leads, the use of both horizontal and vertical electrodes is preferable. Electronystagmography must be done under controlled conditions with proper preparation, which includes avoidance of drugs (especially those active in the central nervous system). Even a small drug effect may cause alterations in the electronystagmographic tracing. The test is performed in several phases. These include calibration (which assesses cerebellar function), gaze nystagmus, sinusoidal tracking, optokinetic nystagmus, spontaneous nystagmus, Dix Hallpike testing, position testing, and caloric testing. The test may give useful information about peripheral and central abnormalities in the vestibular system (case 4). Interpretation is complex. However, a table summarizing electronystagmographic findings and their meaning is available (4). Electronystagmography is especially helpful when a unilateral reduced vestibular response is identified in conjunction with other signs of dysfunction in the same ear. In such cases, it provides strong support for a peripheral (eighth nerve or end organ) cause of balance dysfunction.

Dynamic Posturography

For approximately 15 to 20 years, platforms have been used to try to assess more complex integrated functioning of the balance system. Until recently, most were static posture platforms with pressure sensors used to measure body sway while patients tried to maintain various challenging positions such as Romberg and Tandem Romberg maneuvers. Movement was measured with eyes closed and opened. The tests had many drawbacks, including inability to separate proprioceptive function and to eliminate visual distortion. In 1971, Nashner introduced a system of dynamic posturography which has been developed into a test system which is now available commercially (17).

Dynamic posturography uses a computer controlled moveable platform with a sway-referenced surrounding visual environment. In other words, both the platform and visual surround move, tracking the anterior-posterior sway of the patient. The visual surround and platform may operate together or independently. They are capable of creating visual distortion or totally eliminating visual cues. The platform can perform a variety of complex motions, and the patient's body sway is detected through pressure-sensitized strain gauges in each quadrant of the platform. The typical test protocol assesses sensory organization through six test procedures and movement coordination through a variety of sudden platform movements. Balance strategies are assessed using both the sensory organization and movement coordination test batteries. Dynamic posturography provides a great deal of information about total balance function that cannot be obtained from tests such as ENG alone.

Evoked Vestibular Response

Evoked vestibular response testing is analogous to brainstem auditory evoked testing. However, vestibular evoked potentials are still not being used clinically. Current research indicates that this test is likely to be valuable in the near future, and clinical trials to assess its efficacy are already underway.

Metabolic Tests

Metabolic tests must be selected on the basis of clinical need in each individual case, of course. However, certain conditions have such profound importance in neurotologic symptoms that they are sought with nearly routine frequency.

Luetic labyrinthitis is a highly specific syphilis infection of the inner ear. Most commonly, it occurs when infection has been congenital or has occurred many years or decades in the past. Treponemes become sequestered in the perilymph, changing life-cycle characteristics and dividing only every 90 days (as opposed to every 33 hours in normal *Treponema pallidum* infections). Luetic labyrinthitis can cause hearing loss, tinnitus, and vertigo. Untreated, it may eventually cause total deafness. It is one of the causes of treatable sensorineural hearing loss and frequently responds well to steroids and prolonged antibiotic use. Routine serologic testing (RPR—Rapid Plasma Roagin and VDRL—Venercal Disease Research Laboratory Test) is normal. In order to detect luetic labyrinthitis, an FTA (fluorescent treponemal antibody-absorbed test) absorption test or MHA-TP (microhemagglutination assay for Treponemal pallidum antibody) must be obtained.

Diabetes and especially reactive hypoglycemia may produce symptoms of dizziness. In some cases, hypoglycemia may provoke symptoms similar to endolymphatic hydrops. A five-hour glucose tolerance test is often necessary in dizzy patients to rule out this condition.

Even mild hyperthyroidism may produce fluctuatiing hearing loss, tinnitus, and disequilibrium in some patients. It is frequently necessary to obtain triiodothyronine, thyroxine, and thyroid-stimulating hormone serum levels to establish this diagnosis.

Diabetes mellitus and collagen vascular disease produce vascular changes which compromise perfusion and may cause otologic symptoms. In addition to routine screening for diabetes, tests for collagen vascular disease, including rheumatoid factor, anti-nuclear antibody, and sedimentation rate, may be indicated.

Autoimmune inner ear pathology has been well documented. When suspected, a variety of tests of immune function are required.

In at least a small number of patients, allergies may cause otologic symptoms. In the authors' experience, this association is less common than some literature would suggest. However, in the appropriate clinical setting, allergy evaluation and treatment may be required for otologic symptoms, including dizziness, tinnitus, and hearing loss.

Hyperlipoproteinemia has been associated with sensorineural hearing loss, as well. When sensorineural hearing loss of unknown etiology is under investigation, measurement of cholesterol and triglyceride levels should be included.

A great may other tests may be appropriate, depending upon clinical presentation. Many viruses, Lyme disease, sickle cell disease, and numerous other problems may cause neurotologic symptoms that are difficult to differentiate from symptoms caused by trauma without appropriate studies.

Radiologic Tests

Neurotologic diagnosis has been revolutionized by modern radiologic technology. In virtually all patients with otologic symptoms, radiologic investigation is mandatory, especially in patients who have suffered head trauma.

Magnetic Resonance Imaging

Magnetic resonance imaging (MRI) is the mainstay of radiologic evaluation of the neurotologic patient. Magnetic resonance imaging of the brain is discussed in the chapter by Dr Gonzales in this book. In the neurotologic patient, it is essential to rule out demyelinating disease, neoplasms, subdural hematomas, and other conditions that may be responsible for the patient's neurotologic complaints. High-resolution gadolinium-enhanced MRI of the internal auditory canal is required to rule out acoustic neuroma. Very high quality studies are necessary, and they should be performed on a magnet of at least 1.5 Tesla strength.

Computed Tomography

Computerized tomography (CT scan) has been performed much less frequently in the last few years because of improvements in MRI. However, CT testing may still be extremely valuable. Magnetic resonance imaging does not show bony detail. A high-resolution CT of the ears may show even hairline fractures or other abnormalities in the bone of great clinical importance that may be invisible on MRI. One should not hesitate to order both studies, especially in patients who have suffered trauma.

Air-Contrast CT

Air-contrast CT involves infusion of 3 to 5 cc of air through a lumbar puncture. The procedure should be performed with a small needle and is done routinely on an outpatient basis. Air is allowed to rise into the cerebellar pontine angle, and the internal auditory canal and neurovascular bundle can be visualized well. This test was standard for detection of small acoustic neuromas before MRI was developed. Now it is performed much less commonly, but it still has use. It shows the region much more clearly than MRI and often allows detection of abnormalities such as anterior/inferior cerebellar artery loop compression of the eighth cranial nerve, a condition that cannot be seen routinely on MRI.

Ultrasound

When there is a question regarding the adequacy of carotid or vertebral blood flow, ultrasound provides a noninvasive, painless, expeditious method for assessing blood flow. If the results are equivocal, if significant vascular compromise is identified, or if there is very strong clinical suspicion of vascular occlusion despite an unimpressive ultrasound, arteriography may be required. While this test is more definitive, it may be associated with serious complications, and is ordered only when truly necessary.

Facial Nerve Testing

Facial nerve testing is done routinely when a motor abnormality is observed (case 2). However, tests may also be helpful in the absence of obvious motor abnormalities, especially if a pressure lesion is suspected, such as acoustic neuroma or vascular compression.

Simple Topognostic Tests

The validity and reliability of topognostic facial nerve testing have not been proven. Nevertheless, they often provide helpful information regarding the site of a facial nerve lesion. A modified Schirmer tear test helps determine whether the lesion is proximately distal to the greater superficial petrosal nerve and auricular ganglion. The stapedius reflex decay test establishes this relationship to the stapedius muscle. Testing of taste on the anterior two-thirds of the tongue, or testing salivary flow from the submandibular glands, locates the lesions in relation to the chorda tympani nerve. Peripheral branches of the facial nerve can be tested with a facial nerve stimulator. Although minimal nerve excitability testing is performed most commonly, maximal nerve excitability may provide more information. It usually requires 1 or 2 mA of current above the nerve threshold. Assessment of all of these tests is subjective.

Electromyography

Standard facial electromyography records muscle action potentials produced by voluntary efforts to move muscles. Responses are recorded using needle electrodes inserted into the muscle, and the signal is monitored on an oscilloscope visually and acoustically. Muscle function and degeneration can be detected.

Electroneuronography

Electroneuronography is similar to electromyography except that it uses surface electrodes and evoked rather than volitional stimuli. A stimulating electrode is placed over the main trunk of the facial nerve at the stylomastoid foramen, and a recording electrode is placed over the muscle to be tested. This technique allows measurement of latency and conduction velocity, although latency has proven a more useful measure. Recording of threshold is possible to read; however, supramaximal stimuli are generally used. Several parameters can be measured and have proven useful clinically.

Treatment

Discussion of the treatment of hearing loss, tinnitus, dizziness, and facial paralysis has filled many books, and complete discussion is certainly beyond the limitations of this chapter. However, a few points are worthy of emphasis.

Sensorineural hearing loss, tinnitus, and vertigo are not uniformly incurable, as is popularly assumed. In many cases, underlying causal or contributing factors can be identified and treated with consequent amelioration of otologic symptoms. Such conditions include luetic labyrinthitis, diabetes, hypoglycemia, hyperthyroidism, among others. When treatable causes cannot be identified, most patients can still be helped to some degree.

Hearing Loss

Conductive hearing loss can generally be overcome with amplification (hearing aids) or cured surgically. It rarely results from minor head trauma unless the blow is directly to the ear. If hearing loss occurs following trauma, it is usually sensorineural. Often, partial or complete spontaneous resolution of the hearing loss occurs. If the diagnosis is made within the first week or two, therapy with corticosteroids may be helpful as with other nerve injuries, although its efficacy is unproven. Vasodilator medication is also used widely, but its value is also not established scientifically. If hearing loss is permanent and affects the speech frequencies enough to be troublesome to the patient, it is almost always possible to prescribe appropriate hearing aids to compensate for the loss.

Tinnitus

Unless a correctable structural or metabolic cause is found, tinnitus is usually not curable. Most patients adjust well to their tinnitus, but some are extremely disturbed by it. An enormous number of medications have been used to treat tinnitus, generally without success. Tinnitus maskers are recommended by some physicians, but their value is also limited for the vast majority of tinnitus sufferers.

Maskers are devices similar to hearing aids. They introduce a noise into the ear that the patient is able to control. Some patients find this helpful, but most do not. External masking with a radio or fan is helpful to many people, especially at night if the tinnitus interferes with their ability to fall asleep. Many patients find tinnitus less disturbing if they wear a hearing aid. Consequently, in a patient with tinnitus and even a mild hearing loss, it may be worthwhile to try amplification sooner than one ordinarily would in a patient not troubled by tinnitus.

A few patients are truly distraught and disabled by tinnitus. In some patients, tinnitus persists even in a totally deaf ear. Such patients may be candidates for eighth nerve section, a neurotologic procedure in which the nerve is cut, separating the ear from the brain. However, this procedure is only successful 50% to 70% of the time. If the tinnitus is believed to be associated with a vascular loop compressing the eighth nerve, microvascular decompression can be performed through the posterior fossa. This procedure may be helpful, but the tinnitus must be extremely disturbing in order to justify an operation of this sort. In selected cases, patients can learn to tolerate their tinnitus. Stress management, hypnosis, and biofeedback may be helpful in some patients.

Dizziness

Dizziness of central etiology following minor head trauma is discussed elsewhere. In general, when dizziness is caused by cerebral, cerebellar, or brainstem contusion, it is associated with other neurologic problems and is difficult to treat. The outlook for dizziness caused by vestibular injury is better.

Many medications are helpful in controlling peripheral vertigo. Meclizine is among the most common. It causes drowsiness in many people, but it is often effective in controlling vertigo. Scopolamine, administered through a transdermal patch, is also effective in controlling dizziness from a labyrinthine injury, such as post-traumatic inner ear concussion. However, its side effects limit its use in many patients who are bothered especially by mouth dryness and dilation of the pupils causing blurred vision. Diazepam is also effective in suppressing vertigo, but long-term use of this potentially habit-forming drug should be avoided when possible. Prochlorperazine also helps many patients, sometimes producing good clinical improvement with low doses of 5 to 10 mg once in the evening. In post-traumatic hydrops, diuretic therapy with hydrochlorothiazide decreases vertigo, stabilizes hearing, and decreases fullness and fluctuation in many patients.

Patients with positional vertigo present special problems. It is helpful to distinguish benign positional paroxysmal vertigo (BPPV) from cervical vertigo. Benign positional paroxysmal vertigo occurs when the patient's head is turned in a certain position. Typically, vertigo is induced when the patient rolls to one side in bed. During electronystagmography, BPPV shows a short delay before onset on nystagmus, and the severity of nystagmus decreases with repeat testing. Benign positional paroxysmal vertigo is generally not helped by medications such as meclizine and diazepam. Vestibular exercises which provoke vertigo and develop compensatory pathways and suppression are preferable. Cervical vertigo is usually accompanied by limitation of neck motion and tenderness. Turning the neck into certain positions causes dizziness, and symptoms can sometimes even be provoked by pressure over certain tender points in the neck or over the greater occipital nerve. Many treatments have been suggested for cervical vertigo. However, cervical manipulation and physical therapy generally produce the best results.

If dizziness is caused by a perilymph fistula, and if the patient seeks medical attention promptly, a short period of bed rest is the first line of treatment. If the symptoms persist after five days of bed rest, or if they have been present for a long period of time before the diagnosis is made, surgical repair is warranted. This is accomplished with local anesthesia through the external auditory canal. The perilymph leak in the oval window or round window (or both) is repaired. Because of the hydrodynamics of the ear, the incidence of recurrent fistula formation is high, and the risks of permanent sensorineural hearing loss, tinnitus, and disequilibrium are substantial.

If medical treatments for peripheral vertigo fail, several surgical approaches are available. For endolymphatic hydrops, endolymphatic sac decompression provides relief of dizziness in approximately 70% of people. Despite the 30% failure rate, it is appropriate in selected cases. Vestibular nerve section is a more definitive procedure. This may be performed by entering the posterior fossa through the mastoid or just behind the sigmoid sinus. The eighth nerve is divided, preserving cochlear fibers and sectioning the vestibular division of the eighth nerve. The experience of the authors parallels that of other authors reporting success rates above 90% with this procedure. If there is no usable hearing, the entire eighth nerve can be divided. Interestingly, this procedure does not appear to improve the success rate substantially. Failures are probably due to disequilibrium produced by a lesion more central in the vestibular pathway, or located elsewhere in the vestibular system altogether. Despite all efforts, it is not possible to identify such conditions in all patients prior to surgery.

Occasionally, it is impossible to determine which ear is responsible for dizziness, especially if there are signs of abnormality bilaterally. In such cases, bilateral medical labyrinthectomy is possible. This procedure takes advantage of the ototoxicity of streptomycin. Patients must be selected carefully (18), and the procedure must be carefully controlled (19). When bilateral labyrinthectomy is complete, patients generally adapt well so long as they have visual cues. However, they are not able to function in total darkness.

Physical Therapy

Although the value of physical therapy in patients with balance disorders has become apparent only recently, it should not be underestimated. It is useful in patients who have failed conventional treatment and in those who have persistent minor equilibrium problems after partially successful treatment. Physical therapy for balance disorders is quite specialized (20). The physical therapy team must have special interest and expertise in balance disorders, special equipment for balance rehabilitation, and willingness to devote substantial energy and resources to balance rehabilitation. Most physical therapy departments do not have experience and expertise in this area, and their results with patients with balance disorders are not encouraging. However, when an appropriately trained team is involved, it can be exceedingly helpful. Such therapy is useful not only in patients with vestibular disorders. In patients with post-traumatic central disequilibrium, it is often the only help available.

Conclusions

Neurotologic symptoms occur commonly in people who have suffered head injuries. In some cases, they are causally related to the trauma. In others, other conditions cause or contribute to the patient's symptoms. In all cases, systematic, comprehensive evaluation should be carried out. In most cases, help in some form is available.

Case Reports

Case 1

A 29-year-old female was involved in a motor vehicle accident while traveling at about 55 miles per hour. She was a passenger and was not wearing a seat belt. Hers' was the fifth car in a multi-car accident.

When her vehicle struck the car in front of her, she was thrown forward and hit the windshield with her forehead, breaking the windshield glass. She did not lose consciousness and was not hospitalized. She noted immediate head, neck, and back pain. Four days later she developed nausea, a sensation of motion sickness, rotary vertigo, and slightly slurred speech. Her dizziness was severe enough to cause her to fall into walls and furniture on several occasions. She also noted high-pitched, ringing tinnitus in the right ear and hearing loss. In addition, she complained of memory deficits. Over the next several months, her headaches and memory loss persisted. She had short retrograde amnesia and significant antegrade memory deficits. Her hearing deteriorated gradually bilaterally; and although she had mild hearing fluctuation, it remained consistently diminished beginning four months following her injury. Her disequilibrium improved but did not resolve completely. Her symptoms were unaffected by forceful nose-blowing, bending, or straining. She had no other medical problems.

Otoscopic examination, Hitzelberger's sign, and Hennebert's sign were normal. She had no diplacusis. The rest of her otolaryngologic examination was normal except for marked neck tenderness and limitation of motion. Initial audiogram revealed low-normal hearing thresholds (Fig. 10.1A) four days after injury. Four months after injury, her thresholds had deteriorated substantially (Fig. 10.1B).

DATE	RIGHT EAR AIR CONDUCTION							LEFT EAR AIR CONDUCTION					
	250	500	1000	2000	4000	8000		250	500	1000	2000	4000	8000
A	20	20	15	20	20	30		20	20	20	20	15	30

	RIGHT EAR BONE CONDUCTION							LEFT EAR BONE CONDUCTION					
A-	15	20	20	15	20			25	20	20	20	25	

DATE	RIGHT EAR AIR CONDUCTION							LEFT EAR AIR CONDUCTION					
	250	500	1000	2000	4000	8000		250	500	1000	2000	4000	8000
B	30	35	25	20	35	40		40	50	55	60	45	55

	RIGHT EAR BONE CONDUCTION							LEFT EAR BONE CONDUCTION					
B-	45	55	60	55	60			40	50	65	65	60	

Fig. 10.1. Audiogram of case 1 four days (**A**) and approximately four months (**B**) after injury.

Electronystagmogram one week after injury showed right beating spontaneous nystagmus, abnormal Dix-Hallpike tests, and 100% reduced vestibular response on the left. Three days later left caloric response was still reduced, but better. Three-and-a-half months later, spontaneous nystagmus had disappeared, positional nystagmus was improved, and vestibular response was diminished bilaterally. Auditory evoked response audiogram within a week of the accident showed conduction delays suggestive of retrocochlear pathology on the right consistent with brainstem contusion. The latencies were improved $3\frac{1}{2}$ months later, although there was still a suggestion of right retrocochlear injury. Computed tomography and gadolinium-enhanced MRI of the brain and internal auditory canals were normal. Repeat studies $3\frac{1}{2}$ months later were also normal. Central auditory testing was markedly abnormal, and brainstem thresholds were within normal limits. Complete metabolic evaluation, including FTA, thyroid function studies, and other tests was also normal. Medications were not successful at improving hearing thresholds.

Comment: This is an unusual case of progressive sensorineural hearing loss caused by minor head trauma. The peripheral mechanism was clearly injured as indicated by the initial ENG; but the hearing loss is central.

Case 2

A 32-year-old male was injured at work when he was thrown against the wall, striking the right side of his head. He was stunned for a few seconds and had short-term retrograde amnesia. He also had headache and minor memory deficits following the injury. One day after the accident, he noted complete right peripheral facial paralysis. Neurotologic examination was normal except for facial paralysis and a positive Hitzelberger's sign on the right. Audiogram revealed a small 4,000-Hz dip on the right (Fig. 10.2) with an even smaller dip on the left. Computed tomography and MRI were normal. Electroneuronography three months after the injury still revealed 100% electrical degeneration on the right. The patient had declined facial nerve decompression. Partial recovery of voluntary facial motion occurred over the next several months.

Facial paralysis is common after penetrating trauma, fractures, or surgery. It is seen less frequently after minor head trauma and is felt to be due to edema within the facial nerve canal, particularly in the labyrinthine segment where the nerve leaves the internal auditory canal to enter the middle ear, because this is the most narrow segment. The slight 4,000-Hz audiometric dip is typical following inner ear concussion.

DATE	RIGHT EAR AIR CONDUCTION							LEFT EAR AIR CONDUCTION					
	250	500	1000	2000	4000	8000		250	500	1000	2000	4000	8000
	20	15	15	15	30	15		5	10	5	5	20	10

RIGHT EAR BONE CONDUCTION						LEFT EAR BONE CONDUCTION					

Fig. 10.2. Audiogram of case 2 obtained approximately one month following injury. Discrimination scores were 100%.

Case 3

A 37-year-old man was walking through a store when a box weighing approximately two pounds fell less than three feet from an upper shelf, striking him in the top of the head. He claimed to have been knocked unconscious, although there were no witnesses to the event. He also reported memory loss, difficulty concentrating, hearing loss in his left ear, and dizziness. Initial audiogram showed a severe left hearing loss with 0% discrimination (Fig. 10.3). During discrimination testing, he repeated "guess" words similar to those presented to him, but never got one correct. The Stenger test was positive and suggested normal hearing. In addition, while instructions were being given through the earphone in his right ear at low intensity, they were suddenly switched to his left ear. He continued to respond for two sentences before he realized that his left ear was being used. Brainstem evoked response thresholds were also normal. Electronystagmogram was normal, but there were numerous eyeblinks and voluntary muscle contraction artifacts.

DATE	RIGHT EAR AIR CONDUCTION							LEFT EAR AIR CONDUCTION					
	250	500	1000	2000	4000	8000		250	500	1000	2000	4000	8000
A	10	10	5	10	10	10		75	65	70	80	65	70
B	10	10	5	10	10	10		15	10	15	10	15	20

RIGHT EAR BONE CONDUCTION						LEFT EAR BONE CONDUCTION					

Fig. 10.3. Audiogram of case 3 showing reported thresholds and threshold estimates with the Stenger test.

DATE	RIGHT EAR AIR CONDUCTION							LEFT EAR AIR CONDUCTION					
	250	500	1000	2000	4000	8000		250	500	1000	2000	4000	8000
A	5	0	0	0	0	5		5	0	0	0	5	20
B	5	10	5	-5	-5	5		0	5	0	-5	5	10

RIGHT EAR BONE CONDUCTION							LEFT EAR BONE CONDUCTION				

Fig. 10.4. Audiogram of case 4.

Case 4

A 43-year-old male worked as a computer repairman and did not have a history of significant noise exposure. He had no problems until he slipped on ice while descending a flight of stairs and fell backwards, snapping his neck and striking his occiput on the top step. He then slid down the remaining eight stairs. Although he did not lose consciousness, he was "dazed." Immediately, he noted headache, neck pain, and dizziness, which he described as a motion sensation, as if he were "on a boat." In addition, he complained of bilateral "cricket-like" tinnitus. He developed memory and concentration deficits that have persisted for more than eight years. Examination revealed strongly positive Hennebert's sign in each ear, marked neck tenderness and limitation of motion, and normal cerebellar testing. Audiogram showed a bilateral high frequency dip typically seen following significant trauma (Fig. 10.4). Brainstem evoked response audiogram showed conduction delays with increased click rate, suggestive of a brainstem injury. Electronystagmogram revealed no reduced vestibular response but spontaneous nystagmus and positional nystagmus. Maneuvers with rapid neck twisting produced slightly greater nystagmus than gentle positioning. These findings are common following trauma to the inner ear and neck. Electronystagmogram also revealed abnormal saccadic pursuit and pendular tracking, suggestive of central injury. This patient's trauma resulted in injuries to three components of his balance system: brainstem, inner ears, and neck.

References

1. Pearson BW, Barker, HO: Head injury—Same otoneurological sequelae. Arch Otolaryngol, 1973; 97:81–84.
2. Rubin W: Whiplash and vestibular involvement. Arch Otolaryngol, 1973; 97:85–87.

3. Tuohimaa P: Vestibular disturbances after acute mild head trauma. Acta Otolaryngol (Stockh.), 1979 (Suppl 359); 87:1–67.
4. Sataloff RT, Sataloff J: Occupational Hearing Loss. New York: Marcel Dekker, 1987.
5. National Center for Health Statistics: Hearing status and ear examinations: Findings among adults, United States, 1960–1962. Vital and Health Statistics, Series 11, No. 32, U.S. Dept. of HEW, Washington, DC, November 1968.
6. Reed GF: An audiometric study of two hundred cases of subjective tinnitus. Arch Otolaryngol, 1960; 71:94–104.
7. Nodar RH: Tinnitus aurium in school-age children: A survey. J Aud Res, 1972; 12:133–135.
8. Sataloff J, Sataloff RT, Lueneburg W: Tinnitus and vertigo in healthy senior citizens with a history of noise exposure. Am J Otolaryngol, 1987; 8(2):87–89.
9. Fowler EP: Tinnitus aurium: Its significance in certain diseases of the ear. NY State J Med, 1912; 12:702–704.
10. Heller ME, Bergman M: Tinnitus aurium in normally hearing persons. Ann Otolaryngol Rhinol Laryngol, 1953; 62:73–83.
11. Graham JM: Tinnitus in children with hearing loss. CIBA Foundation Symposium 85, Tinnitus, London, England, 1981, pp 172–181.
12. Glasgold A, Altmann F: The effect of stapes surgery on tinnitus in otosclerosis. Laryngoscope, 1966; 76:1624–1532.
13. House JW, Brackmann DE: Tinnitus: Surgical treatment. CIBA Foundation Symposium 85, Tinnitus, London, England, 1981, pp 204–212.
14. Podoshin L, Ben-David Y, Fradis M, Pratt H, et al.: Brainstem auditory evoked potential with increased stimulus rate in minor head trauma. J Laryongol Otolaryngol, 1990; 104(3):191–194.
15. Rintelmann W (ed): Hearing Assessment. Baltimore, MD: University Park Press, 1979; 404–406.
16. Al-Hady MR, Shehata O, El-Mously M, Sallam FS: Audiologgical findings following head trauma. J Laryngol Otolaryngol, 1990; 104(12):927–936.
17. Nashner, LN: A model describing vestibular detection of body sway motion. Acta Otolaryngol Scand, 1971; 72:429–436.
18. Sataloff RT, Hughes M, Small A: Vestibular "masking": A diagnostic technique. Laryngoscope, 1987; 97(7):885–886.
19. Graham MD, Sataloff RT, Kemink JL: Titration streptomycin therapy for bilateral Meniere's disease: A preliminary report. Otolaryngol Head Neck Surg, 1984; 92(4):440–447.
20. Whitney SL, Furman JMR, Hirsch BE, Kamerer DB: Physical therapy for patients with balance disorders. Clin Management, 1991; 11(1):42–48.

— 11

Temporomandibular Joint Disorders

Anthony Farole

Disorders of the temporomandibular joint (TMJ) sometimes result from minor head trauma. The TMJ has been referred to as the "great impostor" because disorders that affect this area can mimic so many other pain syndromes and pathological processes of the head and neck area (Table 11.1). It is important, therefore, that the clinician learn about the signs and symptoms of TMJ disease so that disorders of this area can be correctly included or excluded in a differential diagnosis when appropriate. The purpose of this chapter is to outline the most current concepts regarding multidisciplinary understanding of TMJ disorders. This will be useful information for the specialist and non-specialist. Diagnosis, therapy, and current suggested research are included.

Temporomandibular joint dysfunction is no more a single disease or entity than heart disease; the disorder should be considered a major category under which the various subtypes can be listed. Figure 11.1 is a categorization that will be referred to in this chapter when discussing the various subtypes. Before this discussion, however, a brief description of the pertinent anatomy of this joint is relevant.

The TMJ is a synovial joint between the temporal bone and the mandible. It has both upper and lower compartments or joint spaces that result from and are separated by the intervening articular disc (Fig. 11.2). The superiormost portion of the mandible, which forms the lower portion of the joint articulation, is the mandibular *condyle*. It is capped with fibrocartilage, as is the *glenoid fossa*, the superiormost articulating surface of the temporal bone. The articular *disc* or

Table 11.1. Facial pain.

Atypical facial pain
Muscle-bone-joint
  Myofascial pain dysfunction (MPD)
  Temporomandibular joint disease (TMJ)
  Eagle's syndrome
  Inflammation: Gradenigo & Tolosa Hunt syndromes
  Tumor
  Trauma
Mouth
  Teeth, tongue, and mucous membrane diseases
  Parotid gland and duct diseases
  Burning tongue—mouth
Eyes/ears/nose/throat
  Diseases (e.g., glaucoma)
  Stresses (e.g., noise)
  Infection (e.g., sinusitis)
  Tumor (e.g., nasopharyngeal malignancy)
  Trauma
Vascular Diseases
  Headache
    Cluster
    Migraine (lower half)
  Carotid artery disease
    Post-surgery
    Aneurysm
    Carotidynia
    Raeder's syndrome
  Inflammation
    Giant cell (temporal) arteritis
    Wegener's granulomatosis
    Sinus thrombophelbitis
Cranial nerve disease
  Cranial neuralgias
    Trigeminal
    Glossopharyngeal
    Geniculate
  Herpes zoster
  Post-traumatic neuroma
Central nervous system (CNS) pain
  Peripheral origin
    (Deafferentation syndrome)
    Post-herpetic neuralgia
    Post-traumatic neuralgia
    Phantom tooth, nose
  CNS origin
    Lesions of the brainstem trigeminal system
    Thalamic syndrome
Referred pain
  Angina pectoris
  Cervical spine or muscle lesions
  Intracranial diseases

Reprinted with permission from Solomon S: Facial Pain-Differential Diagnosis and Treatment. Clin J Pain, 1986; 2:11–18.

Internal Derangements
 Disc displacement
  With disc reduction
  Without disc reduction
  Disc deformity
  Disc or disc attachment tear
  Intracapsular adhesions

Myofascial pain dysfunction (MPD)
  No organic disease
  Diagnostic imaging negative

Osteoarthrosis
  Cartilage and/or bone changes of condyle/glenoid fossa can present with
  or without osteoarthritis

Any of the three major categories can occur alone or give rise to one or both
of the other two categories:

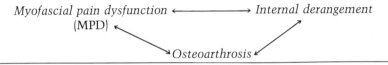

Fig. 11.1. Dysfunctions of the temporomandibular joint.

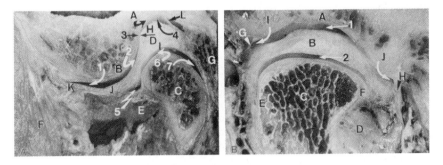

Fig. 11.2. Gross anatomy of the TMJ. Reprinted with permission from
Murakami K.I. Arthroscopic Anatomy of the Temporomandibular Joint. In:
Oral and Maxillofacial Surgery Clinics of North America. Disorders of the
TMJ I: Diagnosis and Arthroscopy. Philadelphia: W.B. Saunders Company
1989: p. 69–77.

meniscus also consists of fibrocartilage. Most other joints of the human body are lined by hyaline cartilage. The sternoclavicular joint is also lined by fibrocartilage, and it is thought that the functional and embryological development of these joints may account for the difference in cartilage type. There is a greater amount of type I collagen in fibrocartilage compared to hyaline cartilage, which is richer in type II collagen (1). A synovial membrane lines the joint and is found in both upper and lower joint compartments. The synovium is greatest in quantity in the anterior and posterior pouches, lateral and medial gutters. It is thinnest in the areas subject to close direct articulation or contact like the glenoid fossa and *articular eminence*—that portion of the articulating surface of the upper joint space anterior to the glenoid fossa which slopes downward and forms a convex articulating surface.

The functional movements of the mandible require complex interactions of the disc, condyle, and glenoid fossa-articular eminence areas (Fig. 11.2). In addition to hinge movement, this diarthroidial (two "hinges") joint permits *translation* or gliding of the condyle on the disc surface and excursive movements to each side. Further, the right and left side TMJs must synchronize movements. The right and left sides function in tandem in straight opening and closing of the jaw. One side may need to pivot while the contralateral side is translating (sliding) forward, as occurs during right- and left-sided jaw movements. Two other functional anatomic structures deserve mention because of the vital role they play in normal and dysfunctional joints. The first is the *posterior attachment* of the disc to the posterior aspect of the glenoid fossa. This posterior attachment is also known as the bilaminar zone because of the two layers of connective tissue, one elastic and one non-elastic (Fig. 11.3). These layers sandwich adipose tissue, also referred to as the retrodiscal fat pad. It is the posterior attachment of the disc that is subject to stretching, tearing, and loss of elasticity that may contribute to disc displacement and that can contribute to *internal derangements* (Fig. 11.4). The last functional unit important in the understanding the TMJ is the attachment of the lateral pterygoid muscle. This muscle has two heads—an upper, smaller head that serves as the anterior attachment to the disc and a lower, larger head that attaches by tendinous insertion into the neck of the mandibular condyle (Fig. 11.5). The two muscle heads run forward and medial to reach their attachment to the pterygoid plate of the sphenoid bone. Spasm of this muscle can lead to dysfunctional movements or asynchrony of the glenoid fossa, disc, condyle relationship. Electromyographic studies have demonstrated that the two heads of the lateral pterygoid muscle often function reciprocally—that is, during one phase of mouth opening the superior head is contracting while the inferior head is relaxed (2–4).

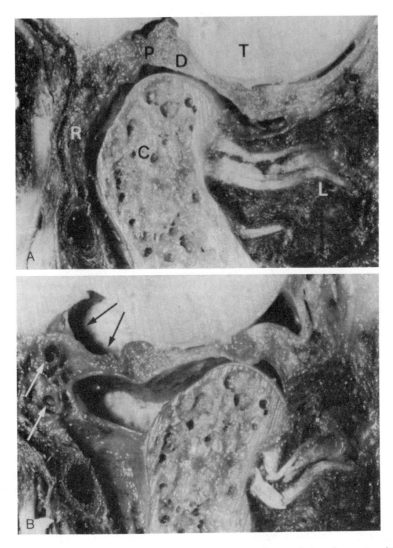

Fig. 11.3. Sagittal sections of the right TMJ during closing (**A**) and opening (**B**) of the mandible. Reprinted with permission of Temporomandibular Joint Laboratory, UCLA Dental Research Institute, Los Angeles, California.

As a synovial joint, the TMJ can share many of the pathological processes that afflic other joints of the body. These include any of the arthritic conditions, such as osteoarthritis, rheumatoid arthritis, gout, and other afflictions like osteomyelitis (although rare), intracapsular and extracapsular fractures, hematomas, adhesions, synovitis

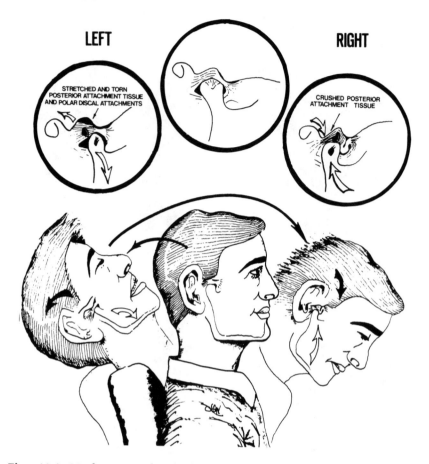

Fig. 11.4. Mechanism of whiplash-related internal disc derangement. Reprinted with permission from Weinberg S., Lapointe H. Cervical Extension-Flexion Injury (Whiplash) and Internal Derangement of the Temporomandibular Joint. Journal of Oral and Maxillofacial Surgery 1987; 45:2 653–656.

and other inflammatory conditions, and primary and metastatic tumors (5).

It is beyond the intent and scope of this chapter to cover all TMJ disorders. The discussion will be limited to the differential diagnosis of the two most common afflictions of the TMJ that we see most frequently. These are *internal derangements* and *myofascial pain* and *dysfunction* (MPD). It must also be understood that these two processes can and often do occur simultaneously. Therapeutically, it is important to distinguish which of the two categories is present. An internal derangement of the TMJ is one in which there is asynchrony of the anatomical subunits of the condyle, glenoid fossa, articular disc, and its attachments (generally within the capsule of the joint).

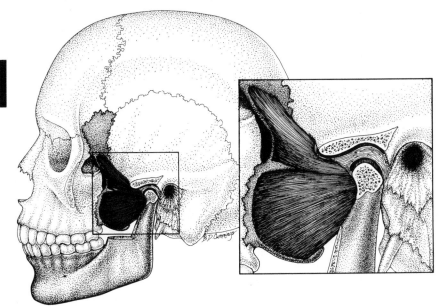

PART 1

Fig. 11.5. Attachments of the lateral pterygoid muscle. Reprinted with permission from Travell J.G., Simons D.S. Myofascial Pain and Dysfunction The Trigger Point Manual. Baltimore/London: Williams & Wilkins, 1983: p. 260–272

These derangements are also termed intracapsular and can often show demonstrable abnormalities on diagnostic tests like plain radiographs, magnetic resonance imaging (MRI), or computed tomograhy (CT) (Fig. 11.6). Myofascial pain and dysfunction, on the other hand, may not have any associated radiographic abnormalities. In Laskin's classic definition of MPD (6), as it relates to masticatory dysfunction, one of the criteria for diagnosis of MPD was absence of radiographic abnormalities. These two major categories will be discussed in greater detail later.

Diagnosis of TMJ disorders is made by a systematic evaluation of the masticatory system and should include a history, physical examination, and appropriate radiographs when indicated. Special imaging of the TMJ is best left to the consulting specialist.

History

The patient with a TMJ disorder may present with complaints of unilateral or bilateral jaw pain. The location of pain is important both in distinguishing TMJ disease from other disorders and in the categorization of either internal derangement or MPD. Point tenderness

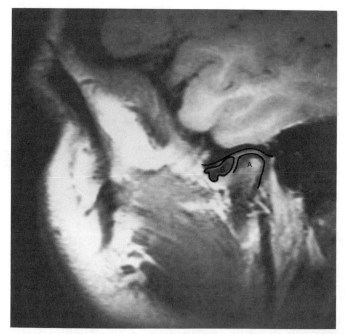

A

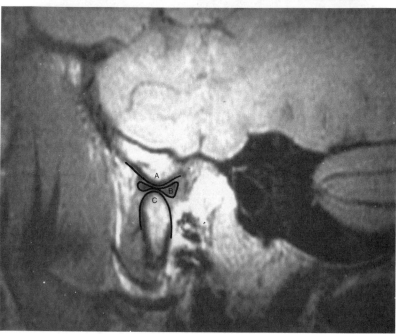

B

Fig. 11.6. **A**: Photograph of TMJ MRI illustrating displaced disc, B, and condyle, A. **B**: Photograph of TMJ MRI in open position with reduced disc, B. Articular eminence, A, and condyle in open position, C, are seen. **C**: Computed tomography scan of TMJ, depicting severe degenerative changes to condyle and joint fossa associated with a failed synthetic disc replacement.

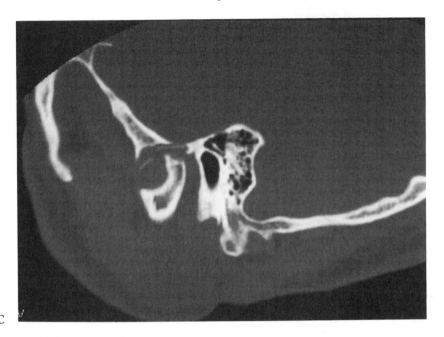

C

Fig. 11.6 *Continued*

over the joint capsule itself—either spontaneous or provoked by palpation—is suggestive of an intracapsular problem. Diffuse discomfort in the jaw musculature, as in the temporal or massetter area, especially if it is bilateral, is indicative of MPD. It must be realized, however, that these two problems can and do coexist, so that both direct and referred pain can be present. The timing of pain is also important. Early-morning or awakening jaw pain or stiffness is common after nocturnal bruxism, clenching, or myoclonus owing to other reasons. Mastication difficulties can be due to both MPD and internal derangement. Pain upon jaw motion versus rest is an important clue to rule in or out a TMJ disorder. Unless there exists significant inflammatory arthritis, head or jaw pain is unlikely to be due to TMJ disease during resting of the mandible.

Joint noise is often present with TMJ disorders. Patients often describe the noise as popping, cracking, clicking, grating, grinding, or other adjectives. Clicking or popping with jaw movements is often associated with a displaced disc. When questioned, the patient may report a reciprocal or closing click. This sound is often softer that the opening snap. Both sounds can be associated with the articular disc "reducing" into a normal position during opening and displacing into an abnormal position during jaw closure (Fig. 11.7). Isolated jaw clicking without symptoms of pain, inability to open or close fully, or locking need not be treated. Clicking does indicate an anatomical

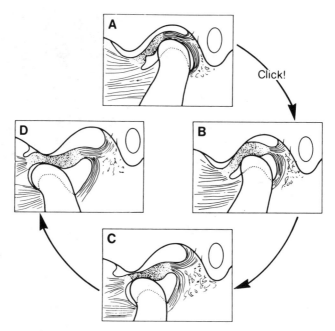

Fig. 11.7. Mechanism of early click due to slight anterior displacement of the articular disc. Reprinted with permission from Travell J.G., Simons D.S. "Introduction to Masticatory Muscles" *Myofascial Pain and Dysfunction: The Trigger Point Manual.* Baltimore/London: Quintessence Publishing 1983: p. 165–182.

abnormal positioning of the disc/condyle relationship but is not necessarily a predictor of future functional disability. Joint sounds such as crepitus or grating are generally present when degeneration of the articular cartilage is present. This can be present with any of the arthritides and in advanced disc disease if the disc or its attachments are torn or completely detached or displaced (non-reducing). The resulting grating sound is produced by frictional forces between the unprotected mandibular condyle onto the glenoid fossa during jaw movement. A history of clicking, followed by a period of no clicking, followed by crepitus is associated with progressive internal derangement. It represents the disc initially clicking, but reducible, then not reducible (totally displaced), then complete perforation or detachment resulting in crepitus and advanced osteoarthritis.

The most common motion problem associated with TMJ disorders is hypomobility or a perceived decrease in mouth opening. This can be associated with either MPD or internal derangement. As such it either represents a mechanical problem or is secondary to reflex myospasm restricting movement. However, hypermobility associated with synovitis or capsular pain can also be present. Those patients will demonstrate a normal or supernormal ability to open their mouth. They may also give a history of episodic subluxation or dislocation of the mandible. The patient may be able to reduce the dislocations or they may report visits to a health professional or emergency room to be manually reduced. Although rare, these disorders can be associated with hyperflexibility states such as Marfan's syndrome or Ehlers-Danlos syndrome (7).

Other symptoms that may be reported by patients presenting with TMJ disorders include headaches, which may be vascular or muscular; tinnitus; muffled hearing; tooth pain or sore teeth; earaches; of neck and shoulder pain. These symptoms are not unique to TMJ disorders. Therefore, appropriate workup and referral to a neurologist, otolaryngologist, general dentist, rheumatologist, or a related specialist should be considered. It is important to be aware that multiple sclerosis, myasthenia gravis, tic doloreaux, connective tissue disorders like lupus erythematosis and scleroderma, primary and metastic tumors of the head and neck, otitis, electrolyte imbalances, tetanus, calcium imbalances, migraine, and cervical disc disease, among others, can all mimic TMJ disorders and cause a misdiagnosis. Psychosomatic pain, neurosis, psychosis, and psychiatric disturbances can lead to somatization of patient's problems to the jaw area (8,9). Patients with anxiety and stress sometimes will apply their tension to the jaw area in the form of clenching the jaws or daytime or nighttime grinding (bruxism). This can directly injure joint structures or trigger jaw muscle spasm by repetitive microtrauma (8). Behavior therapists, psychologists, and psychiatrists can all play a role in the overall management of these problems. Referral is indicated when appropriate.

The physical examination follows the comprehensive history. It begins by general observation of the patient for symmetry, or abnormal posturing of the head, neck, or jaw. By observing the patient's general demeanor, an appreciation for the presence or absence of stress, anxiety, or depression can be gained. The muscles of mastication are examined and palpated. Hypertrophy or atrophy and tenderness during rest and function are signs and symptoms to be charted. The muscles examined should include the temporalis, masseter, lateral and medial pterygoids, digastric, suprahyoids, sternocleidomastoid, trapezius, and posterior neck muscles. Range of motion is measured in millimeters from the edges of the upper and lower incisors if present. Normal mouth-opening range is 45 mm, 10 mm to each side—measured from the midline of the dentition and about 10 mm of protrusive or forward movement of the mandible.

The presence of pain during any of these movements is noted, as is clicking or other joint sounds. The area immediately over the TMJ is just anterior to the tragus of the ear. This is palpated for tenderness. The patient is asked to open and close to allow palpation of joint movement, evaluation of symmetry or restrictive movement, and detection for tenderness during moton. Bidigital palpation with the index fingers in the ear canals also allows for sensitive appreciation of joint dynamics. The dental occlusion is noted for discrepancies related to abnormal bite patterns. The etiology of TMJ problems may be related to dentoskeletal malocclusions such as overbite, underbite, open bite patterns, asymmetries, and others. Obvious dental decay or abscesses are noted, as tooth pain can easily be referred to the TMJ area and could be the only source of the patient's TMJ problem.

After the physical examination is complete, a diagnosis or differential diagnosis is formulated. If indicated, further diagnostic testing or referral is made. The next section will review diagnostic TMJ imaging and the potential role it plays in therapeutic decision making.

TMJ Imaging

No single diagnostic image will provide total information about TMJ anatomy, pathology, and joint dynamics. The specific image requested will vary from one clinician to another depending on availability, area

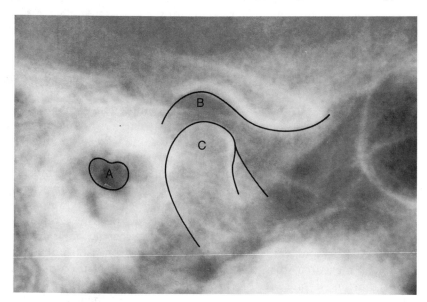

Fig. 11.8. TMJ "spot film." Auditory canal (A), joint space (B), and condyle of mandible (C) are shown.

of interest, and quality of image in the clinician's locale. Plain bone radiography in the form of a panoramic radiograph, TMJ spot film, or tomography can give useful information regarding shape, presence of degenerative changes, and screening to rule out adjacent abnormalities like tumor (Fig. 11.8). Normal and abnormal joint space and range of motion can be appreciated if both open and closed views are obtained. Computed tomography may be useful, especially in known deformity cases where three-dimensional reconstructions may offer useful information regarding potential reconstruction decisions. However, for soft tissue detail of disc position, CT has no useful role (10). Arthrography is a useful test to determine disc position and, when performed under fluoroscopy, can allow assessment of joint dynamics. Perforations and adhesions can also be detected by arthrography. It should be noted that the articular disc is indirectly viewed by this technique and it is minimally invasive. Done by experienced personnel, arthrography very rarely involves complications. On occasion arthrography has proven therapeutic. The mechanism is presumably by lysis of articular adhesions, allowing freedom of disc movement. There is no question that the application of MRI imaging to the TMJ has provided the most useful and informative diagnostic image to date. Many believe it to be the "gold standard" in assessing disc position and disc morphology. It offers the advantage of direct imaging of the articular

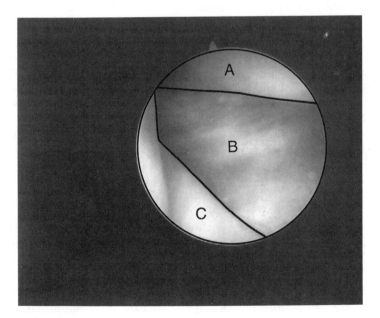

Fig. 11.9. Arthroscopic view of right TMJ. Anterior slope of articular eminence (a), medial capsule with pterygoid shadown (b), and articular disc (c) are seen.

disc, allowing assessment of both shape and position. It is, also, noninvasive and emits no ionizing radiation. Although true dynamic imaging is not possible at this time, cine-MRI can create a motion video approximating true dynamic viewing. TMJ arthroscopy, a surgical procedure usually performed under general anesthesia, adds another diagnostic ability. It provides a dimension of viewing not possible using any of the methods discussed, namely, direct intra-capsular viewing (Fig. 11.9). The fibrocartilage of the glenoid fossa, articular eminence, and articular disc are directly viewed from ×1 to approximately ×30 magnification. The posterior attachment and disc-pterygoid attachment areas are, also, directly viewed. Early changes in synovium and chondromalacia are often appreciated earlier than with any other imaging technique. Additionally, arthroscopy offers therapy as well as diagnosis. Joint lavage, disc reduction, lysis of adhesions, biopsy, and other advanced arthroscopic techniques can be performed by the trained arthroscopist. Currently, arthroscopy is applied mostly to the upper joint space, lower joint space investigation and therapy being practiced by only a few investigators on a limited basis. This is because of the technical difficulties presented by lower joint space puncture owing to its small volume and anatomy. For example, it is very likely that the disc itself would have to be perforated to enter the lower joint space because of attachments to the condyle.

We recently reported a clinical study comparing MRI, arthroscopy, arthrography, and open joint surgery to assess the diagnostic accuracy of these techniques, using open joint surgery as the gold standard for accuracy (10). The study revealed that MRI is superior in assessing disc position and shape, arthrography was most useful in detecting perforations of the disc or its attachments, and arthroscopy was the most sensitive indicator of early chondromalacia or degenerative joint disease. We concluded that these tests are complementary. Depending on the specific abnormality of interest, one test can be chosen over another. In some cases, triple correlation may be needed (MRI, arthrography, arthroscopy).

Therapy

Rehabilitation of patients with TMJ disorders is multifaceted (Fig. 11.10). Specifically, treatment depends on whether the patient has MPD, internal derangement, or both. However, the goals of therapy are the same, namely, restoration of normal jaw function, elimination of pain, elimination of the need for analgesics—especially narcotics, restructuring of habits, abnormal jaw posture, or an abnormal skeletal relationship of the maxillomandibular complex that may be con-tributing factors to the TMJ disorder.

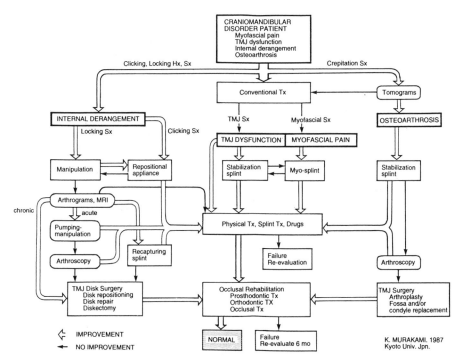

Fig. 11.10. Craniomandibular disorder patient. Reprinted with permission of K. Murakami, Kyoto University, Japan.

Management of pure MPD, once diagnosed, is non-surgical. If the clinician is reasonably certain that no structural abnormalities are present, radiographic or other diagnostic imaging need not be done. However, it is often prudent to obtain a inexpensive screening radiograph like a panoramic x-ray or TMJ spot film. The film can be used as a baseline pre-treatment or documentation radiograph so that if structural changes to the joint do eventually occur, the deviation from the starting film can be appreciated. Identification of emotional stress factors that may be contributing to parafunctional habits like clenching or bruxism is made. If necessary, referral to a behavioral specialist, psychologist, or psychiatrist can be made. Modalities like biofeedback, guided imagery, or psychotherapy may be applied. In the patient suffering acute pain, nonsteroidal anti-inflammatories (NSAIDS; e.g., ibuprofen, naproxen, aspirin) are prescribed. Usually NSAIDS are prescribed for a short duration—less than two weeks. In general, psychosedatives and/or muscle relaxants are not often prescribed. However, diazepam 2 mg or cyclobenzaprine 5 to 10 mg can be useful for the reduction of acute myospasm. Diazepam is especially useful as a nocturnal muscle relaxant, reducing the inci-

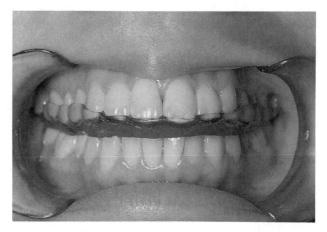

Fig. 11.11. One type of TMJ orthotic used in treating TMJ dysfunction.

dence of bruxism. These medications, like the NSAIDS, are prescribed for short-term use only, until the factors that lead to MPD can be identified and managed. Neck strain or abnormal head posture positions are identified as potential sources of referred pain and abnormal jaw posture that can contribute to MPD. If the patient cannot self-correct these problems, referral to the appropriate specialist and/or physical therapist is made. Often work habits, sleep habits and sleep posture, or previous trauma leading to cervical pathology is identified. Bite appliances can play a very important therapeutic role in pain reduction and functional rehabilitation of MPD. The appliances are described by various names, sometimes corresponding to their function. They can be referred to as splints, night guards, orthotics, mandibular repositioners, or other descriptive terms. They are made from stone or plaster molds of the dentition and are most often cast from hard acrylic (Fig. 11.11) these devices are constructed to fit much like an orthodontic retainer and are modified to accomplish specific goals in bite modification and/or to effect a relaxation pattern of the jaw musculature. Often they are prescribed for 24-hour use (except when eating or brushing). Some may be worn only at night. The general goals of a splint for MPD are to—

1. Eliminate muscle spasm cycling
2. Eliminate destructive forces on the attachment apparatus
3. Reposition the condyle into the most physiologic position
4. Allow the clinician to determine if the craniomandibular relationship can be stabilized

The MPD patient may be "cured" with one-time therapy and slowly weaned from the multifaceted treatment program. He or she may,

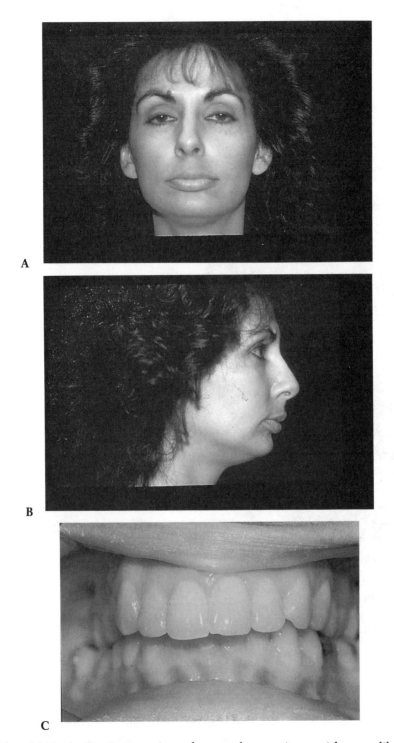

Fig. 11.12. A–C: Preoperative photos of a patient with mandibular hypoplasia over with characteristic facial and occlusal pattern. **D–F:** Postoperative photos of same patient showing improved facial and occlusal form that will help to stabilize jaw musculature and TMJ apparatus.

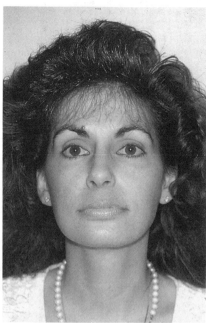

Fig. 11.12 *Continued*

D

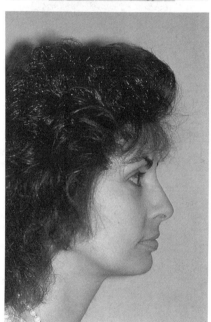

E

however, have recurrent bouts that may be self-controlled or need continued therapy or restructuring through return visits. If an underlying structural abnromality coexists, the pattern of recurrent MPD will not be eliminated until the structural abnormality is corrected.

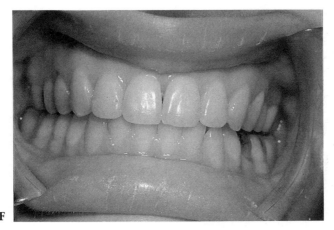

F

Fig. 11.12 *Continued*

Maxillary and/or mandibular osteotomies with repositioning of the jaws into normal structural relation is one example of a secondary correction that may be needed (Fig. 11.12).

Internal derangement, when causing functional impairment or pain, is often treated surgically. This problem can be caused by repetitive micro-or macrotrauma. Examples of repetitive microtrauma include bruxism, clenching, and unequal distribution of forces causing disproportionate joint loading as occurs in some dentoskeletal malocclusions. Congenital, developmental, post-traumatic and post-tumor resection jaw deformities (continuity defects) can also induce internal derangements. Macrotrauma causing direct or indirect (contra coup) structural joint damage is usually a one-time event as opposed to the *repetitive* microtrauma required for internal derangement to occur. Trauma from direct blows (fists, sports injuries, falls, striking the dashboard or steering wheel with the jaw) and indirect injuries, such as whiplash, have been associated with the development of internal derangement. Current surgical intervention includes open TMJ surgery (arthroplasty, arthrotomy, arthrectomy) and arthroscopy, the latter being a more recent development in the history of surgical management (11).

Temporomandibular Joint arthroplasty is performed to correct the structural pathological changes present. Disc repositioning, discectomy, repair of ligament rupture, bony recontouring in the case of advanced degenerative joint disease, gap arthroplasty in the case of ankylosis, and total joint replacement with either autogenous or prosthetic (alloplastic) reconstruction may be required (Fig. 11.13). Postoperative physical therapy is always a part of postoperative rehabilitation. Splints may also be used. A relatively new modality in TMJ rehabilitation, continuous passive motion (CPM) is currently

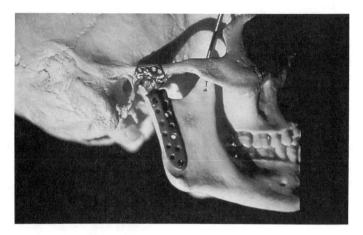

Fig. 11.13. A type of total joint replacement prosthesis used in advanced cases of TMJ pathology.

used in our institution. Our preliminary clinical trials have been very encouraging. Our protocol follows that of Salter (12,13), who performed both the original animal investigations and later clinical trials and use of the concept of continuous passive motion (CPM). He challenged the traditional concepts of placing joints at rest after surgery and proved that articular cartilage damage healed quicker and more completely when CPM was applied. He showed this to be true in observations of gross anatomical and histological sections. As a result of his 25 years of research in the orthopedic field, the CPM machine is now available for use in the knee, elbow, hip, finger, shoulder, and TMJ.

All of our patients that used the CPM device reported an increase in range of motion, no pain during use, and a reduction in muscle spasms. We find it particularly useful in hypomobile joints as may occur in fibrous or bony ankylosis. The CPM unit is applied immediately after surgical corrections and thereafter for two to four weeks. It should be noted that CPM has not proven to be useful without surgical correction of joint pathology (internal derangement). To date, it has not been shown to overcome structural articular derangements. Therefore its use is only recommended as an adjunct to surgical correction of joint pathology (Fig. 11.14).

Temporomandibular Joint diagnosis and therapy has and will continue to challenge researchers and clinicians. Continued interest, research, and clinical experience continues to improve the care of patients with TMJ disorders. Knowledge of the signs and symptoms of TMJ disorders by all clinicians will result in early detection and proper management of the underlying problem. Advanced disease can,

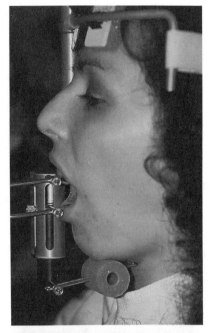

A

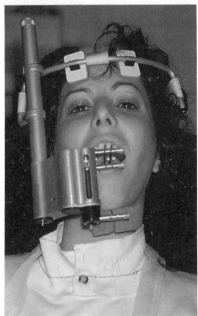

B

Fig. 11.14. Photograph of patient using continuous passive motion (CPM) device after TMJ arthroplasty surgery. Side (**A**) and front (**B**) views.

therefore, be prevented in many cases. Just as it is important for us to recognize when a TMJ disorder exists, it is equally important to recognize when it does not. Earlier in this chapter other mimickers of TMJ disorders were mentioned. Proper referral to other specialists should avoid a false diagnosis and arrive at an accurate one. Current research in TMJ disorders includes 1) investigation of a viscoelastic fluid (sodium hylaronate) for use in TMJ arthroscopy; 2) sampling of synovial fluid and quantification of pain mediators, prostaglandin, leukotrines, etc.; and 3) alloplastic, autogenous, and allogeneic disc replacements for use when discectomy is required. Most importantly, the multidisciplinary approach has resulted in better patient care in cases where adjacent or distant disorders are hindering successful TMJ rehabilitation.

References

1. DeBont LGM: Cartilage of the temporomandibular joint Ned Tijdschr Tandheelkd, 1985; 92:184–189.
2. Grant PG: Lateral pterygoid: two muscles? Am J Anat, 1973; 138:1–10.
3. Lipke DP, Gay T, Gross RD, et al.: An electromyographic study of the human lateral pterygoid muscle (Abstract 713). J Dent Res (Special Issue B), 1977; 56B:230.
4. McNamara JA Jr: The independent functions of the two heads of the lateral pterygoid muscle. Am J Anat, 1973; 138:197–206.
5. Farole A, Manalo A: Lesion of the Temporomandibular Joint-Clinicopathologic Conferences. J Oral Maxillofac Surg, 1992; 50:510–514.
6. Laskin DM: Etiology of the pain-dysfunction syndrome. JADA, 1969; 79(1):147–153.
7. Sacks H, Zelig D, Schabes G: Recurrent Temporomandibular Joint Subluxation and Facial Ecchymosis Leading to Diagnosis of Ehlers-Danlos Syndrome. J Oral Maxillofac Surg, 1990; 48:641–647.
8. Rugh JD, Solberg WK: Psychological implications in temporo-mandibular joint pain and dysfunction. Oral Sci Rev, 1976; 7:3.
9. Markoff M, Farole A: Reflex sympathetic dystrophy syndrome. Oral Surg, 1986; 61(1):23–28.
10. Rao VM, Farole A, Karasick D: Correlation of MRI, Arthrography, and Arthroscopy in Temporomandibular Joint Dysfunction. Radiology 1990; 174:663–667.
11. Buttram JR, Farole A: Arthroscopy of the temporomandibular joint. Compend Contin Educ Dent, 1989; 10(12):652–656.
12. Salter RB: Regeneration of Articular Cartilage Through Continuous Passive Motion: Past, Present, Future In Straub R, Wilson PD (eds) Clinical Trends in Orthopaedics. 1982 Ch. 12 101–107 New York.
13. Salter RB: The biological concept of continuous passive motion of synovial joints: The first 18 Years of basic research and its clinical application. Clin Orthop, 1989; 242:12–25.

— 12

Olfactory Consequences of Minor Head Trauma

Joseph R. Spiegel and Mark Frattali

Introduction

Disturbances of taste and smell frequently result as sequelae of head trauma. These deficits are commonly overlooked during the initial evaluation and may be noted by the patient months or years after the traumatic incident. This is especially so in cases of minor head trauma in which the patient may undergo little or no medical evaluation in the immediate post-traumatic period. Olfactory loss has been found in as many as 60% of patients after severe head injuries, but has also been noted in up to 8% of those with minor head trauma (1).

Loss of smell is both a physical and psychological insult. The patients must cope with the reduced sense of their world around them in general, decreased appreciation of food, an altered sense of their own physical hygiene, and increased exposure to safety hazards caused by the inability to smell smoke or natural gas. These deficits are substantial and can occur as a result of minor head trauma with few, or no, other sequelae. To appreciate the full implications of minor head trauma, it is necessary to have a complete understanding of the potential of olfactory injury.

Pathophysiology

There are three possible sites of injury that could lead to olfactory loss in head trauma: the olfactory epithelium in the nasal passages, the olfactory nerves, and the central olfactory connections.

The olfactory epithelium lies in the posterosuperior portion of the nasal vault, occupying approximately $1\,cm^2$ of mucosa on each side. Most complaints of anosmia or hyposmia after nasal trauma are a result of damage to the nasal structure that reduces nasal airflow, or are a result of secondary infection. Since minor head trauma can be associated with a facial blow, it is important to differentiate disturbances of smell that result from nasal trauma from those that are due to the more central sequelae of minor head injury. Loss of smell owing to nasal airflow obstruction can occur because of mucosal edema initially and may persist as a result of anatomical obstruction from bony or cartilaginous deformity. Sinusitis is a frequent complication of facial trauma, and both acute and chronic sinusitis can cause anosmia on a temporary or permanent basis [2]. Most patients who suffer olfactory loss as a result of nasal trauma will recover part or all of their sense of smell, or have smell disturbances on an intermittent basis. In patients who suffer total, permanent anosmia after nasal trauma, even without an additional blow to the head, the site of injury is probably at the olfactory nerves or central connections, and not in the nasal tissues. In patients who develop secondary sinusitis as a result of their traumatic nasal injury, the exact etiology of the smell disturbance may never be determined.

Probably the most common site of injury leading to post-traumatic anosmia in minor head trauma is the olfactory nerves. These tiny fibers travel from the neural epithelium in the nose through small holes in the cribiform plate to direct cortical attachments in the olfactory bulbs on the floor of the anterior cranial fossa. The olfactory bulbs are attached to the undersurface of the frontal lobes, and thus any rapid motion of the brain tissue within the cranium results in the potential for shearing forces across these fibers at the cribiform plate. Severance of these fibers leads to retrograde degeneration of the olfactory nerves. Results of this denervation have been seen in degeneration of the olfactory cilia in patients who have suffered head injuries when studied by Moran et al. [3], These shearing forces can be created by frontal, occipital, and tangential blows. Frontal trauma can lead to olfactory injury both by direct force leading to fracture of the floor of the anterior cranial fossa, and by the posterior, linear acceleration force applied to the brain tissues, leading to shearing across the nerve fibers. Occipital blows lead to contrecoup injuries in the anterior cranial fossa and can result in anosmia even when no fracture occurs. Schecter and Henkin [4] noted a preponderance of occipital injuries in patients with post-traumatic anosmia, and Sumner [5] found that occipital blows more commonly caused anosmia than frontal blows in those patients who incurred head trauma that resulted in little or no amnesia. Although there have been cases reported of late recovery of olfactory function after traumatic loss, regeneration of the olfactory nerves has never been documented. It is unclear whether these patients are demonstrating regeneration of neural tissue, repair of partial nerve damage, or healing of central contusions.

Minor head trauma can result in a generalized brain injury that is presumed to be the result of small areas of cortical hemorrhage, contusion, and edema. If these central lesions involve the olfactory brain centers (the orbitofrontal cortex, pyriform or prepyriform cortices, or the olfactory bulbs and tracts) a disturbance in smell may result. These injuries may result in parosmia or dysosmia (problems in odor recognition and odor memory) more than in loss of smell sense. Levin et al. (6) found deficits in olfactory naming and recognition in a large number of non-anosmic head-injury patients. The deficits were more common in patients with severe injuries and with frontotemporal mass lesions. These types of injuries may also have a better prognosis. However, injury to the central olfactory pathways has only been documented in patients with quite severe head trauma and in most cases is only inferred in those with less severe injuries.

Epidemiology

In 1864, Hughlinges Jackson made the first reference in the medical literature to post-traumatic anosmia (7): "In 1837 a gentleman of Sheepwash in Devon was struck from his horse. All the worst effects of concussion resulted and the sense of smell was lost forever." Ogle, in 1870, was the first to describe loss of taste in patients with smell disorders (8). He also suggested that blows to the occiput were the most likely to produce anosmia. Notta, in 1870, pointed out that anosmia could follow head injuries unaccompanied by loss of consciousness (9). He proposed that recovery from anosmia might be possible in the first eight weeks to seven months following head injury. It was not until several years later that the notion of smell recovery received much attention. Legg, in 1873, was the first to report dysosmias or distortion in the sense of smell (10). He reported a case of a 36-year-old man who, after falling off his cart and injuring his head, described everything he ate as having the flavor of "gas or paraffin." He confirmed Olga's contention that patients with dysosmias often confuse problems of smell with those of taste. He also observed that most dysosmias involve foul or unpleasant smell sensations.

Case reports continued to appear with statistical estimates of post-traumatic anosmia, but they were obviously flawed by small sample size and methodologic problems. For example, in most patients it was impractical to administer olfactory tests, and therefore assessment

Table 12.1. Incidence of anosmia in head injury patients.

Study (Ref.)	No. of patients	Patients with anosmia
Leigh (11)	1,000	72 (7.2%)
Sumner (5)	1,167	87 (7.5%)
Zusho (12)	5,000	212 (4.2%)
Rutherford (13)	145	4 (2.8%)

often relied on self-reports and medical records. Also, olfactory impairment or partial loss of olfactory function, which is probably more common than most suggest, usually went undetected by both patient and physician. According to Costanzo and Becker, when partial impairment of olfactory function is considered in an assessment, the incidence of olfactory loss following all head injuries may approach 20% to 30% (1).

It was not until 1943, when the first large-scale and relatively unselected series appeared, that Leigh found 72 patients with anosmia in 1,000 consecutive head injuries (11). Leigh did not correlate the incidence of anosmia with a severe head injury, but he suggested that post-traumatic anosmia increases with severity of injury.

Sumner reported on 1,167 cases of head injury (5). He found 7.5% (87 patients) with anosmia and that the incidence increased with the severity of head injury. He also found that the occurrence of anosmia increased to 32% in patients who suffered amnesia lasting one to seven days. Sumner's results also suggest that while frontal impact injuries may be more common, occipital impact is more likely to result in anosmia.

We now know that head trauma is one of the leading causes of olfactory disturbance. In a recently published evaluation of 750 patients through the University of Pennsylvania Smell and Taste Center, head trauma accounted for 18% of those with measurable loss of smell, ranking third behind the categories of upper respiratory infection and idiopathic cases (2). When averaged, the results of a total of 7,312 patients in four large-scale studies suggest that about 5% of patients with head injury have olfactory disorders (Table 12.1) (12,13). However, in all instances the investigators fail to report on the percentage of patients who were not tested for olfactory disorders. Untested patients would not be classified as having olfactory disorders, and thus the incidence of 5% is probably not valid.

Patient Evaluation

In cases of olfactory disturbance after minor head trauma, the patient often does not voice complaints immediately after the traumatic episode. Thus, by the time evaluation occurs, even though the patient may relate the deficit to the traumatic incident, it is critical to rule out other factors that may cause disturbance in the olfactory mechanism. All patients should have a comprehensive history taken that specifically delineates any history of nasal or paranasal sinus disease, prior facial surgery, prior head or facial trauma, or a history of chronic respiratory disease. The history must also include a nutritional evaluation and a complete list of all current and recently prescribed medications. Certain antibiotics (neomycin and streptomycin) and calcium channel blockers can lead to olfactory disturbances. Multiple medications, including aspirin, catopril, lithium, metronidazole, amphetamines, levadopa, dipyridamole, baclofen, carpamazepine, phenytoin, and doxipen can all cause disturbances in taste. Additionally, cigarette smoking has been noted to have a dose-related negative effect on olfaction (14).

The physical examination must include complete head and neck, and neurologic evaluations. Fiberoptic or rigid endoscopic examination of the nasal cavity is utilized to evaluate the patency of the nasal airways, the integrity of the olfactory slit with the olfactory epithelium bilaterally, evidence of CSF rhinorrhea, and evidence of chronic sinus disease.

Radiologic evaluation includes a non-enhanced CT scan of the paranasal sinuses and anterior skull base to look for mucosal disease in the paranasal sinuses and fractures through the cribiform plate. Levin (6) reports a 2% incidence of CSF leak in closed head injury. The incidence increases to 25% with fractures of the paranasal sinuses. He also found that 78% of post-traumatic CSF rhinorrhea had associated anosmia. An MRI scan of the brain is utilized to evaluate traumatic sequelae and to rule out central sources of olfactory disturbance, such as frontal lobe tumors, demyelinating processes, and ischemic disease.

After initial evaluation, more detailed testing, such as an EEG, auditory, or visual evoked brainstem response tests, or a psychiatric evaluation may be indicated. Blood serum is analyzed for endocrine abnormalities, liver enzyme levels, treponemal antibody titers, Lyme titers, and other viral titers as indicated.

Assessment

Despite the important functions of smell, few physiology and medical textbooks discuss procedures for evaluating this sense. Patients who have suffered head trauma should be systematically evaluated for sensory losses including olfaction.

Recently, increasing attention has been focused on evaluation and diagnostic testing of the sense of smell. In the past, most tests of olfaction were rather crude and were based on subjective reports of the patient. Simple screening tests can be included in the initial physical examination to look for olfactory abnormalities, with comprehensive tests and evaluation ordered as indicated.

Olfactory Screening Test

The most important criteria for a good clinical screening test for olfaction are that it be easy, fast, sensitive, and available enough so that it will be used. In the past, most screening tests were cumbersome and not practical in many clinical situations. Costanzo et al. at the Medical College of Virginia developed a prototype screening test referred to as the Medical College of Virginia Olfactory Screening Test (MCV-OST) (15). They looked at 51 patients with post-traumatic anosmia of two weeks' to eighteen years' duration. Test stimuli consisted of artificial fragrances of baby powder, chocolate, and coffee which were presented to each nasal cavity separately using 20-ml plastic squeeze bottles. Scoring was based on stimulus detection and identification. The left and right nasal cavity were considered separately and also together.

The results were correlated with the severity of head injury using the Glasgow Coma Scale (GCS). For mild head injury, 60% had normal olfactory function, 27% were impaired, and 13% were anosmic. However, for severe head injury, only 8% had a normal screening test, 67% were impaired, and 25% were anosmic. The MCV-OST is an easy test to administer and sensitive for post-traumatic olfactory dysfunction. The OST identifies patients with normal olfactory function, those in need of more comprehensive olfactory testing, and those who are completely anosmic.

Comprehensive Olfactory Test

Appropriate selection of standardized smell tests is vital for the clinical evaluation of olfactory function. Quantitative and qualitative olfactory function testing provide objective measurement of the extent of sensory olfactory loss. These tests can be helpful in identifying brain lesions and are useful in monitoring patient progress during recovery and rehabilitation. Two tests most commonly used are the Connecticut Chemosensory Clinical Research Center Test (CCCRC) and the University of Pennsylvania Smell Identification Test (UPSIT) (16).

The CCCRC includes both detection threshold and odor identification assessment. Threshold detection involves a two-bottle forced-choice task using a series of eight plastic squeeze bottles. Bottle 8 contains the most dilute concentration (normal detection), while bottle 1 contains the strongest concentration (4% butanol). The subjects' detection threshold is defined by the correct selection of odor bottles over the controls in four successful trials. Right and left nasal cavities are tested separately or together. Odor identification testing consists of discrimination of familiar odors contained in seven jars. Odor identification involves integration of olfactory information and is thought to involve olfactory brain centers. Threshold scores usually give an indication of olfactory function and may correlate intranasal or sensory receptor dysfunction. Identification scores may identify cortical lesions (i.e., closed head injury) or dysfunction in olfactory brain centers. Costanzo's data in 23 of 52 patients suggest that focal lesions involving the frontal and temporal lobes are more likely to result in olfactory disorders, specifically odor naming and recognition (17).

Also incorporated into the CCCRC is a screening test for psychological problems or functional smell disorders. Ammonia is often employed to test the trigeminal nerve (C V). A patient who denies sensation of this odor may be malingering or have a psychological impairment.

The development of the first standardized "scratch and sniff" olfactory test was described by Doty et al. at the University of Pennsylvania in 1983 (16). Over 1,600 subjects participated in five experiments. The technique of microencapsulation has the advantage of evaluating olfactory function without the problems of stores of chemical or cumbersome equipment. To our knowledge evaluation of olfactory dysfunction in closed head injury with UPSIT has not been reported. Unlike the CCCRC, the UPSIT quantitates bilateral olfactory function. Differential olfactory testing for each nostril may not be necessary in patients following head trauma because most cases of olfactory dysfunction involve both nostrils, and many patients do not notice subtle unilateral problems. Also change in nasal airflow from one nostril to the other makes testing of such discrimination problematic.

Finally, the physician evaluating the olfactory function should not lose sight of the overall clinical picture. Information pertaining to neuropsychologic as well as premorbid olfactory, mental, and psychological status should be assessed along with olfactory function scores.

Outcome

Most post-traumatic anosmia is irreversible. Leigh was the first to report recovery of patients who suffered total loss of smell after head trauma, but this was only in 6 of 72 patients that were evaluated (11).

Sumner reported recovery in approximately 50% of all patients who suffered anosmia after head trauma that resulted in amnesia of less than 24 hours, and much lower rates of recovery (7–14.5%) in those with more severe injuries (5). These high recovery figures may be influenced by more aggressive, early testing in head trauma patients and thus may be a truer demonstration of the head trauma population. Thirty-nine percent of these patients recovered within the first ten weeks of the injury, and the chance of recovery declined significantly after six months. Similarly, Costanzo and Becker found that the prognosis for any recovery beyond one year after the injury is very poor (18).

It is presumed that those patients who experience recovery of olfaction are demonstrating resolution of central lesions, such as cerebral hemorrhage, contusion, and edema. However, although it has not been demonstrated in humans, regeneration of nerve fibers across the cribiform plate has been demonstrated in laboratory animals (18). Sumner proposed that those patients experiencing early recovery do so on the basis of resolution of central lesions, and those that recover in the late phase do so owing to neural regeneration (5). Further laboratory and clinical research will be necessary to make this determination accurately.

Effects of Anosmia

There are four basic concerns for a patient who suffers total anosmia: safety risks, appetite, personal hygiene, and psychological disturbances. Patients' responses to anosmia are very variable, and the appropriate evaluation and treatment must vary accordingly. All patients must be counseled on specific safety risks associated with anosmia. An adequate number of well-located smoke detectors must be installed in the patient's home, and they must be kept in good working condition. Additionally, patients with gas appliances must be advised to either make sure they do not live alone or they must change to electrical devices. Other patients may have certain occupational risks or requirements relating to toxic chemical odors, fire or explosive hazards, or the need to smell certain foods (i.e., as a chef or baker) that may demand an adequate olfactory sense.

Alteration of taste related to post-traumatic anosmia is extremely variable. Taste alteration has not been discussed specifically because all patients who suffer post-traumatic taste disturbance after head trauma are found to have an olfactory deficit that is presumed to be the ultimate cause. Most anosmic patients complain that their food does not "taste the same," but some will have a surprisingly normal sense of taste. Most patients will be able to maintain an adequate level of nutrition, but they may require counseling so that they can choose foods that provide other sensory enhancement with heat, cold, or spices that will help with appetite stimulation. However, because the sense of smell is such a powerful stimulus driving hunger, it is sometimes impossible to avoid problems with loss of appetite and subsequent eating disorders.

The anosmic patient must be actively counseled about maintaining personal hygiene. Without the ability to self-monitor odor, it is important that the patient both develop standard, daily personal hygiene, and have people that he can depend on to help monitor his personal care, as well.

There is no way to quantify the loss of "quality-of-life" that results from anosmia. Olfaction is one of the most primitive, basic senses and is related to sexual drive, appetite, general mood, and the sleep cycle. The sense of smell adds to our perception of the world around us but has become almost unconscious as our surroundings have become dominated by visual and audible stimuli. Patients' responses to the deficit can range from total ignorance of the loss to severe clinical depression (19).

Summary

Olfactory disturbances are common in patients after head injuries and can affect as many as 3% to 8% of people who have suffered minor head trauma. Many of the deficits are temporary, but at least half will result in permanent anosmia. The olfactory injury can occur from any type of blow, but it appears that occipital trauma may be more important in those cases where there is no fracture. A comprehensive evaluation is necessary to delineate fully other factors that may influence olfaction, and follow-up for at least one year after the injury is required. Prognosis for recovery is poor beyond six months after the injury and remote beyond one year. Significant hyposmia and total anosmia can result in significant life-style changes for many patients and a health hazard in some. Patient education and counseling remain most important in the care of patients with post-traumatic olfactory loss.

References

1. Costanzo RM, Heywood PG, Ward JD, Young HF: Neurological applications of clinical olfactory assessment. NY Acad Sci, 1987; 510:242–244.
2. Deems DA, Doty RL, Settle RG, Moore-Gillon V, Shaman P, Mester AF, Kimmelman CP, Brightman VJ, Snow JB: Smell and taste disorders, a

study of 750 patients from the University of Pennsylvania Smell and Taste Center. Arch Laryngol, 1991; 117:519–528.

3. Moran DT, Jafek BW, Rowley JC, Eller PM: Electron microscopy of olfactory epithelia in two patients with anosmia. Arch Laryngol, 1985; 111:122–126.

4. Schecter PJ, Henkin RJ: Abnormalities of taste and smell after head trauma. J Neurol Neurosurg, Psychiatry, 1974; 37:802–810.

5. Sumner D: Post-traumatic anosmia. Brain, 1964; 87:107–120.

6. Levin HS, High WM, Eisenberg HM: Impairment of olfactory recognition after closed head injury. Brain, 1985; 108:579–591.

7. Jackson JH: Illustration of diseases of the nervous system. London Hosp Rep, 1864; 1:470–471.

8. Ogle W: Anosmia of cases illustrating the physiology and pathology of the sense of smell. Med Chir Tran, 1870; 53:263.

9. Notta A: Recherches sur La perte de 1 Oddsat. Arch Gen Med, 1870; 15:385–407.

10. Legg JW: A case of anosmia following a blow. Lancet, 1873; 2:659–660.

11. Leigh AD: Defects of smell after head injury. Lancet, 1943; 1:38–40.

12. Zusho H: Post-traumatic anosmia. Arch Otolaryngol, 1982; 108:90–92.

13. Rutherford WH, Merrett JD, McDonald JR: Sequelae of concussion caused by minor head injuries. Lancet, 1977; 1–4.

14. Frye RE, Schwartz BS, Doty RL: Dose-related effects of cigarette smoking on olfactory function. JAMA, 1990; 263(9):1233–1236.

15. Costanzo RM, Zasler ND: Head trauma. In Getchell TV, et al. (eds): Smell and Taste in Health and Diseases. New York: Raven Press, 1991; 711–730.

16. Doty RL, Shaman P, Dann M: Development of the University of Pennsylvania Smell Identification Test. *Physiology and behavior.* 1984; 32:489–502.

17. Costanzo RM, Becker DP: Smell and taste disorders in head injury and neurosurgery patients. In Meiselman Hl, Rivlin RS (eds): Clinical Measurement of Taste and Smell. New York: Macmillan, 1986; 565–578.

18. Costanzo RM: Nerval regeneration and functional reconnection following olfactory nerve transection in hamster. Brain Res, 1985; 361:258–66.

19. Levenson JL: Dysomia and dysgeusia presenting as depression. Brief Rep, Gen Hosp Psychiatry, 1985; 7:171–173.

— 13

Visual Sequelae of Closed Head Trauma

Edward W. Gerner

Introduction

With direct trauma to the orbit or globe, or penetrating injuries of the cranio-cerebral cavity, the etiology and extent of injury to the visual system is frequently obvious. With blunt trauma or minor head trauma, however, where the cranium and dura are not penetrated, the extent of the injury is frquently more difficult to ascertain, and external evidence of injury may be slight.

Head and neck injuries account for as many as 70% of all injuries sustained in automobile accidents, one of the most frequent types of accidents (1). Bicycle-related head injuries have increased as the popularity of this sport has flourished (2). In one series, falls from bicycles accounted for the majority of indirect injuries to the optic nerves (3). In addition, assaults, contact sports, and the numerous vicissitudes to which modern man is heir also subject us to potential injury. It therefore behooves the ophthalmologist to be aware of the visual sequelae of head trauma—as well as direct trauma to the globe and orbit. Not only is this important from a medical standpoint, but also from a medico-legal one.

Closed head injuries are classically described as concussion, contusion, or laceration. A concussion is defined as a loss of consciousness without focal neurologic signs or demonstrable pathology. It is due to a transient physiologic disruption, although long-term sequelae may follow. Contusion and laceration, on the other hand, are accompanied by demonstrable pathology, with the former demonstrating hemorrhages into the superficial cortex, while the latter is an actual tearing of central nervous system tissue (Table 13.1).

The changes within the eye accompanying head trauma may or may not present immediately following the injury. Once the acute phase is passed the visual sequelae may be the greatest handicap the patient faces.

Intraocular Changes

Trauma to the globe results in a myraid of changes within the eye itself, including hyphema, iris sphincter tears, detached retina, etc. (4). With closed head trauma there may be evidence within the eye of central nervous system derangement. Scattered retinal hemorrhages usually nasal to the disc have been observed, presumably from a mounting sharp rise of intracranial pressure at the time of impact (5). In addition, there may be "low-grade" edema of the optic disc and surrounding retina, not necessarily associated with increased intracranial pressure (6). This usually subsides without visual impairment or optic atrophy. However, papilledema may also signify an expanding intracranial process and is an important sign in all patients with head trauma. The sequelae of papilledema may ultimately prove to be most injurious to the patient. Patients with papilledema may complain of transient obscurations of vision. Long-standing high-grade papilledema may lead to pallor with atrophy and deterioration of vision (7). Closed head trauma may also lead to a partial cross-tearing of the optic nerve at the junction of the globe and nerve. This results in hemorrhage at the site where Bruch's membrane terminates and leads to a characteristic hemorrhage at the disc which Loewenstein has termed an arcuate hemorrhage (8). Complete avulsion of the nerve is, of course, catastrophic to vision.

Optic Nerve

The optic nerve is approximately 50 mm in length. Of this, the intraocular segment is only about 0.7 mm and is not frequently involved with closed head trauma. The remainder of the nerve is divided into an intra-orbital part (33 mm), intracanalicular or intraosseous part (6 mm), and intracranial portion (10 mm); and it ends when the two nerves join together to form the optic chiasm. The optic nerve within the orbit is mobile, cushioned by fat, and is thereby usually spared all but direct trauma. The intracanalicular portion, on the other hand, is immobile and constrained within a bony canal. It is this portion of the nerve which is most susceptible to injury.

Table 13.1. Closed head injuries.

Concussion	Brief loss of consciousness
	No focal signs
Contusion	Loss of consciousness
	Hemorrhage in cortex
Laceration	Rupture of CNS tissue
	Focal neurologic signs

Blows to the forehead, frontal convexity, and anterior temporal region are the most common sites of head injury producing loss of vision. However, injury to any area of the head may result in visual loss (9). The most common causes of injury to the frontal area of the head are automobile accidents, with forehead trauma against the windshield (1). Falls from bicycles are also a common source of injury resulting in traumatic optic neuropathy (3).

While the blow necessary to cause loss of vision is usually severe (with loss of consciousness) this is not always the case. Duke-Elder cites a report of optic atrophy following a blow on the eyebrow by a potato (7)! In general, however, the clinical picture varies with the severity of the trauma.

With very mild injuries, the visual impairment may be transitory immediately following the trauma and last several seconds to minutes. The patient may only complain of "seeing stars." The loss of vision, particularly in children, may last as long as 12 hours with full recovery of vision taking as long as four weeks (10). Furthermore, during the recovery phase there may be attacks of transient (one to ten minutes) blindness without headache. Presumably this phenomenon is on a vascular (spasm) basis (10). However, in this syndrome of transient visual loss with complete return of function, the retina is normal in all cases. With mild trauma there may also be delayed onset of visual impairment. In these instances callus formation of bone impinging on the optic nerve, and arachnoiditis, have been proposed causes (7). There have been reports of cases where vision has improved markedly with the freeing of adhesive arachnoiditis (11). In those cases in which vision is only transiently impaired, concussion of the optic nerve appears to be the most likely explanation (12).

With more severe head trauma, a more discrete clinical entity (indirect optic atrophy or traumatic optic neuropathy) has been described. Duke-Elder states that 1.7% of all head injuries suffer this complication (7). The blow to the head is usually, but not necessarily supraorbital, and vision may be impaired immediately (13). Rarely is this bilateral (10). Recovery of vision, if it should occur, begins three to four days after the injury and progresses until three to four weeks later, after which time further improvement usually does not occur.

Depending on the site of the lesion along the optic nerve atrophy may be observed as early as three to six days following the injury, but it is seen more usually at around the end of the third week (7). Loss of consciousness, again, is not a constant finding.

Closed head injuries may result in transection of the optic nerve. If the injury results in partial interruption, the pupillary response may be normal (14); if complete interruption occurs, the pupillary light reflex is lost.

The field defect most commonly observed with indirect traumatic optic atrophy is an inferior altitudinal defect without macular sparing. According to Harrington this occurs as a result of a shearing force in the optic canal which separates the vessels supplying the upper half of the nerve. He states that these vessels are shorter than those supplying the lower half and are therefore more vulnerable to shearing action (15). However, the blood supply to the intracanalicular portion of the optic nerve (the site where injury to the nerve is most common) is in dispute, and the exact reason for this type of field cut with both trauma and ischemia is not completely understood (16). Other types of defects not infrequently seen with trauma are scotomata which are small and peri- and paracentral in location (14). Superior altitudinal hemianopsias, sector defects, and lower hemianopsias with upper temporal field loss in the contralateral eye have also been described. Therefore, it is important to check the visual fields carefully in all patients with head trauma—particularly those who complain of alterations of vision.

Radiologic evidence of fracture is lacking in most cases of indirect traumatic optic atrophy (14). A combination of plain x-rays and CT scanning has been more successful at identifying skull fractures than either technique alone (17). Even when both techniques were employed it was rare that a fracture of the optic canal, a bony spicule pressing on the optic nerve, or fracture of the anterior clinoid could be demonstrated (17).

There is much controversy as to the exact mechanism of injury in indirect traumatic optic atrophy. Prior to the discovery of the ophthalmoscope in 1848 by Babbage and its rediscovery in 1851 by Helmholtz, it was generally believed that the traumatic event led to reflex ischemia of the retina and this caused the visual loss. When the ischemia was not confirmed ophthalmoscopically many theories were proposed as to the pathophysiology of the visual loss. Since few of these injuries resulted in death, the number of pathologic studies have been few; and most publications consisted of a single case report. Walsh summarized the literature on the subject and classified lesions of the optic nerves and chiasm due to indirect trauma (12). This classification is summarized in Table 13.2. Attempting to determine the pathophysiologic process involved in an individual case

Table 13.2. Classification of lesions of the optic nerves and chiasma.

Primary lesions
    Hemorrhages in nerve, dura and sheath spaces
    Tears in the nerve or chiasm
    Contusion necrosis of nerve or chiasm
Secondary lesions
    Edema
    Necrosis from cirulatory failure
    Infarction from vascular obstruction

can be important from a therapeutic standpoint. The history is particularly valuable when attempting to determine the sort of lesion involved. Distinguishing whether the visual loss occurred *immediately* after the accident or had a *delayed onset* is the most important factor. With immediate loss, the etiology is either 1) concussion of nerve, 2) contusion, or 3) a tear of the nerve. In any event, no therapeutic possibilities exist for any of these. However, when there has been a delay in the onset of visual loss, or when some vision is retained after the trauma but is deteriorating, the possibility of medical and/or surgical therapy is raised. Edema and swelling of the optic nerve within the optic canal may lead to ischemia of the nerve. In this instance, the use of osmotic agents and megadose steroids to reduce the swelling may preserve the patient's vision (18) but is controversial (19). Surgical decompression of the optic nerve has also been proposed, but the value of this is in dispute. The studies by Fukado (20) and Fujitani (21) support a surgically aggressive approach, while Anderson (18) suggests an "individualized" approach to this therapeutic modality. Walsh suggests waiting four to six days before surgical intervention since spontaneous improvement does occur (12). While, statistically speaking, conservative management is probably the indicated course, every study on the subject invariably reports cases in which decompression of the optic nerve has restored vision (22) even when visual loss was immediate (23). An extracranial approach for surgical decompression (transantral-ethmoidal) would seem to be safest in a patient with head injury (22). The third therapeutic modality that should be considered is used anticoagulants and antispasmodic agents if it appears that vascular obstruction and thrombosis are the primary factors. There have been several reports of central retinal artery occlusion following closed head trauma; and since this diagnosis can be made from fundoscopic assessment and treated, it is especially important to keep it in mind early in the evaluation process.

It has been suggested from physiologic studies that, in cases in which loss of vision has been transient and the patient later shows

Table 13.3. Distribution of lesions.

Location of lesion	Percentage of cases
Anterior marginal	13
Anterior optic nerve	12
Canalicular	63
Opto-chiasmal	8
Chiasmal	4

optic atrophy, the defect is due to a focus of necrosis or demyelination surrounded by edema. Therefore, steroids appear to be indicated early in traumatic loss of vision to help relieve the area of localized swelling and prevent permanent damage to the optic nerve (25).

With regard to prognosis of indirect traumatic optic atrophy, two factors seem to be crucial: 1) the type of lesion (as noted above) and 2) the site of the lesion. Hughes (11) reviewed 90 cases of optic nerve and chiasmal injury and found the distribution of lesions to be as noted on Table 13.3. The vast majority of optic nerve injuries occurred in the intracanalicular portion, in spite of the fact that this constitutes a relatively short portion of the nerve. This is due to the confined space in which the nerve is contained in that segment, as noted previously. With anterior marginal tears, the fundus usually, but not always, showed a marginal hemorrhage following the contour of the disc with a sector or nerve fiber bundle defect (8). This group had a poor prognosis. Similarly, when the lesion was anterior to the entrance of the central retinal artery and there was funduscopic evidence of occlusion of that artery, the prognosis was poor. In this latter group the average time for pallor of the optic disc to appear was only 2.7 days (11).

If the injury is intracanalicular, the prognosis for return of vision appears to be better than with any other lesion along the course of the optic nerve. Fifty-six percent of patients had some return of vision when the lesion was intracanalicular, with the prognosis being better in those that did not lose all vision immediately following the accident (11). Pallor of the disc appeared in 12 to 32 days following intracanalicular injuries.

The prognosis for final visual acuity in optic nerve injuries varies (14). In 46 cases studied, Turner found 28% remained with no light perception but 26% had acuities in the 6/12 to 6/9 range (Table 13.4).

Chiasm

Lesions at the opto-chiasmal junction and chiasm (as determined by field defects) have a poor prognosis for return of vision; but, fortunately, these injuries are rare. Most commonly the site of injury

Table 13.4. Final visual acuity in optic nerve injuries.

Final acuity	No. of cases
No light perception	13
Less than 6/60	10
6/60–6/36	3
6/24–6/18	6
6/12–6/9	12
6/6	2

with chiasmal lesions is forehead or convexity. Chiasmal injury may be due to stretching and/or tearing of the chiasmal fibers themselves or ischemia of the chiasm (13,26). Disruption of the central chiasmal artery of Francois appeared to be responsible in several cases (27). Occlusion of this vessel leads to a superior bitemporal field defect (11). A junctional-type scotoma has also been reported secondary to trauma (28).

Optic Tract

Optic tract lesions secondary to closed head trauma are rare (11). Walsh and Hoyt state that they have never clinically recognized an isolated lesion of the optic tract owing to trauma (6). Hughes concurs in this and believes that this is due to the fact that since the lateral geniculate bodies and optic tracts are relatively deep within the brain, any traumatic destruction in this area would be fatal (16).

Optic Radiations and Visual Cortex

Injury to the geniculo-calcarine portion of the visual system is not uncommon, particularly after large contusion injuries of the cerebral hemispheres (13). If the patient suffers increased intracranial pressure (e.g., owing to edema or subdural hematoma) the posterior cerebral artery may be compressed along the edge of the tentorium causing cerebral infarction (29,30). Initially, it was thought that the lesion produced was due to venous stasis, but Lindenberg showed in a classic neuropathologic study that the lesion was, in fact, due to compression of the posterior cerebral arteries (31). This results in an homonymous hemianopsia or, if bilateral, cortical blindness (Anton's syndrome). The remainder of the neurologic examination in such cases may be normal; and the patient, because of macular sparing, retains good visual acuity (29). Homonymous hemianopsia with macular sparing helps make the diagnosis of an occipital lobe lesion.

In addition, the Riddoch phenomenon may be elicited (32). In this phenomenon the patient can detect moving objects but not stationery objects in the involved field.

Transient blindness from a blow on the head without loss of consciousness or other neurologic signs has been described (9,33). In these instances most of the reported cases were children, and the blindness lasted only a matter of hours (1–3 hours). In most cases no pupillary or extraocular muscle abnormalities were noted. No cases of permanent blindness were reported. This type of lesion is probably caused by concussion. Bodian believed that the blindness was due to vasospasm of the vessels supplying the optic nerve, chiasm or tract (9). Griffith and Dodge in a more comprehensive study involving cerebrospinal fluid and electroencephalographic (EEG) results felt that the blindness was due to a localized concussion of the visual cortex. Posterior slowing observed on the EEG, they felt, supported this idea (33).

Differential Diagnosis

The ophthalmologist confronted with a patient complaining of impaired vision following head trauma should be aware of the many possibilities to account for this. Small scotomata and other field changes, as emphasized previously, should be looked for in all patients. Visible lesions, such as macular hemorrhage, avulsion of the optic nerve, and choroidal tears will be obvious on careful examination. It is also possible that the patient, prior to the trauma, had a refractive error which became "unmasked" followed the injury (14).

In addition to the entities and lesions described above, the question of hysterical amblyopia and/or malingering is often raised. It should be noted that the presence of a normal pupil does not rule out a partial injury to the optic nerve (14). Physiologic testing such as visual evoked response may help to determine the facts, but more often than not careful clinical evaluation with a thorough knowledge of the ophthalmic and neurologic factors involved will suffice.

Summary

Closed head trauma may affect any part of the visual system with or without accompanying neurologic signs. It is incumbent on the ophthalmologist to determine the site and type of lesion which has led to the loss of vision, as in some instances medical and/or surgical intervention may be indicated to preserve vision.

References

1. Nauhm AM: Facial trauma in automobile collisions. Trans Am Acad Ophthalmol Otolaryngol, 1965; 69:396–404.
2. Thompson RS, Rivara FP, Thompson DC: A case-control study of the effectiveness of bicycle safety helmets. N Engl J Med, 1989; 320:1361–1367.
3. Lessell S: Indirect optic nerve trauma. Arch Ophthalmol, 1989; 107: 382–386.
4. Scheie HG, Albert D: Adler's Textbook of Ophthalmology. 9th ed. Phila: Saunders Co., 1977; pp 554–576.
5. Kearney JA: The value of eye observations in fractures of the skull and severe head injuries. NYJ Med, 1922; 22:341–344.
6. Walsh FB, Hoyt WF: Clinical Neuro-Ophthalmology. 3rd ed. Balto: Williams & Wilkins, 1969; pp 2331–2518.
7. Duke-Elder S: System of Ophthalmology. Vol. XII. St. Louis: Mosby Co., 1972; pp 273–280.
8. Loewenstein S: Marginal hemorrhage on the disc. Partial tearing of the optic Nerve. Clinical and histological Findings. Br J Ophthalmol, 1943; 27:208–215.
9. Bodian M: Transient loss of vision following head trauma. NYJ Med, 1964; 64:916–920.
10. Russell WR: Injuries to cranial nerves and optic chiasm. In Brock S (ed): Injuries of Brain and Spinal Cord and Their Coverings. 3rd ed. Balto: Williams & Wilkins, 1949; p 62.
11. Hughes EBC: Injury to the optic-chiasmal junction. Brit J Ophthalmol, 1943; 27:367–371.
12. Walsh FB: Indirect trauma to the optic nerves and chiasm. Invest Ophthalmol 1966; V:433–449.
13. Symonds CP: Discussion of the ocular sequelae of head injuries. Trans Ophthalmol Soc UK, 1945; 65:3–19.
14. Turner JWA: Indirect injuries of the optic nerve. Brain, 1943; 66: 140–151.
15. Harrington DO, Drake MV: The Visual Fields. 6th ed. St. Louis: Mosby, 1990; pp 85–93.
16. Hughes B: The Visual Fields. 1st ed. Springfield, IL: Charles C. Thomas, 1954; pp 76–79.
17. Noble MJ, McFadzean R: Indirect injury to the optic nerves and optic chiasm. Neuro-Ophthalmology, 1987; 7:341–348.
18. Anderson RL, Panje WR, Gross CE: Optic nerve blindness following blunt forehead trauma Ophthalmology, 1982; 89:445–455.
19. Wolin MS, Lavin PJM: Spontaneous visual recovery from traumatic optic neuropathy after blunt head injury. Am J Ophthalmol, 1990; 109:430–435.
20. Fukado Y: Results in 400 cases of surgical decompression of the optic nerve. Mod Probl Ophthalmol, 1975; 14:474–481.
21. Fujitani T, Inoue K, Takahashi T, Ikushima K, Asai T: Indirect Traumatic optic neuropathy—Visual outcome of operative and nonoperative cases. Jpn J Ophthalmol, 1986; 30:125–134.

22. Kennerdell JS, Amsbaugh GA, Myers EN: Transantral-ethmoidal decompression of optic canal fracture. Arch Ophthalmol, 1976; 94:1040–1043.
23. Spoor TC, Muthog RH: Restoration of vision after optic canal decompression. Arch Ophthalmol, 1986; 104:804–806.
24. Cullen JF: Occlusion of the central retinal artery following a closed head injury. Am J Ophthalmol, 1964; 57:670–672.
25. Ticho U, Feinsod M: Traumatic Optic Neuritis. Ann Ophthalmol, 1973; V:430–432.
26. Logan WC, Gordon DD: Traumatic lesions of the optic chiasm. Br J Ophthalmol, 1967; 51:258–260.
27. Francois J, Neetens A, Colette JM: Vascularization of the optic pathway. No. V. Chiasma Br J Ophthalmol, 1956; 40:730–741.
28. Hughes B: Injury to the optico-chiasmal junction. Br J Ophthalmol, 1943; 27:367–371.
29. Hoyt WF: Vascular lesions of the visual cortex with brain herniation through the tentorial incisura. Arch Ophthalmol, 1960; 64:78–87.
30. Meyer A: Herniation of the brain. Arch Neurol Psychiatry; 1920; 4:387–400.
31. Lindenberg R: Compression of the brain arteries as pathogenetic factor for tissue necroses and their areas of predilection. J Neuropathol Exp Neurol, 1955; 14:223–243.
32. Haymaker W: Bing's Local Diagnosis in Neurological Diseases. 15th ed. St. Louis: Mosby, 1969; pp 349–378.
33. Griffith JF, Dodge PR: Transient blindness following head injury in children. N Engl J Med, 1968; 278:648–651.

— 14

Cervical Spine Injury Associated with Minor Head Trauma

Donald L. Myers, Francisco Batlle, Sanford Davne, and Steven Mandel

The patient who has sustained minor head trauma has almost certainly also experienced unusual force delivered to the cervical spine. With the possible exception of direct crushing trauma, head injury is associated with rotation, flexion, extension, compression, or other force vectors applied to the neck. While the most extreme failures of the cervical spine may manifest as fractures, dislocations, and acutely ruptured discs, other injuries can be more subtle, resulting in "chronic" conditions, such as neckache, headache, musculoligamentous sprain, cervical radiculopathy, thoracic outlet syndrome, and other problems. A brief review of some of these problems highlights the importance of their consideration in the evaluation and management of patients with head trauma.

The head and cervical spine should be considered as a functional unit and should be evaluated concomitantly. In general, the degree of head injury parallels more-or-less the severity of cervical spinal injury [1]. However, in any specific case, head or brain trauma varies widely in severity, as does cervical spinal trauma, and no assumptions can be made about the correlations between them. Minor head trauma does not indicate that the spinal trauma must also be minor. Any patient who has sustained head or brain injury must be thoroughly evaluated for cervical spinal injury and other spinal injuries as well. The patient with obvious cervical fracture(s) as evidence of spinal cord injury represents a complex, emergent clinical picture. Diagnosis and treatment of these conditions is beyond the scope of this discussion. If these problems are suspected, immediate evaluation by a spinal specialist is mandatory.

Presentation

The patient presentation and history encompass a wide range of possible variables and perspectives. The views from the emergency room physician, family doctor several days post-injury, or the spinal specialist several months later are all considerably different. Some of the salient details of each viewpoint are contained in this discussion. The presentation, history, and examination allow one to form initial impressions as to the nature of the problem. The decision whether to obtain roentgenograms has given rise to extensive controversy. Treatment options vary depending on the severity of the problem and the duration of symptoms.

Most patients will present to an emergency room soon after trauma. They may be brought in by the rescue squad, relatives, a friend, or even their lawyer. Some authors (2,3) have observed that up to 3% of the spinal cord injuries may occur after the patient has come under medical care. Upon initial contact with the patient in the emergency room, if any history of cervical pain or trauma is given, the neck should be immobilized until evaluation can be completed. The basics of good trauma management are essential, and the patient must have an airway and appropriate resuscitative measures to achieve medical stability. The seriously injured or comatose patient should receive the benefits of full spinal precautions and immobilization until the questions of spinal injury and stability can be satisfactorily resolved. Decisions then need to be made about the timing and nature of further evaluation efforts and studies. Early, rapid, limited examination must be closely followed by thorough and complete examination when the patient is sufficiently stable. The patient with an altered sensorium or with a concomitant serious and/or painful distracting injury presents a special set of clinical problems and, with respect to the cervical spine, should be treated as a comatose patient.

The patient may present several days, weeks, or even months after the traumatic episode. Delay in presentation should in no way reassure the examiner as to the relative safety or stability of the spine (4–6) and all patients must be carefully and completely evaluated. The examiner must also be particularly cautious when he first evaluates a patient, even days or weeks after the trauma. One cannot make the assumption that proper and complete medical evaluation has ever been accomplished. Review of all films, documents, history, and examination are essential for thorough initial evaluation of a patient at any time. If the roentgenograms are substandard, lost, or not available, they must be repeated.

Of great concern is the missed, or unrecognized, or "occult" cervical spine fracture, which could result in neurologic catastrophe if not recognized. Careful review by several authors (4–10) indicates that in virtually all of these cases, the patient did have either associated neck pain, tenderness to palpation, stiffness, distracting injury, or had an altered sensorium from alcohol, drugs, or head trauma. One should keep in mind the fact that the majority of "occult" cervical spinal injuries occur in patients with altered mental status or with severe masking injuries. Awareness of cervical pain or symptoms can be altered in patients who do not have completely clear mental status because of head trauma, or with altered sensorium because of intoxication with alcohol or illicit or prescription drugs. Patients with severe injuries such as hip, pelvic, multiple rib fractures, long bone fractures, or with major abdominal injuries may be in so much pain that they may not even perceive cervical discomfort. The patient may be the focus of a major resuscitative effort and may not be able to recognize or verbalize his discomfort. Patients in these categories must be treated with extreme caution and thoroughness, as an unconscious patient would be. Cervical spinal roentgenography should be strongly considered if there are any symptoms or pain associated with the cervical area, if there is any alteration of sensorium, or if there are other serious injuries which might mask the symptom of neck pain (7,9–12).

Patient History

Aside from discussing the mechanism of injury, history-taking immediately after an injury is often not particularly helpful, although an effort should be made to determine whether the patient has had previous head or neck trauma, disease, or surgery. Sometimes the patient is unable to remember the incident or exact mechanisms of the injury. The patient should be asked about his perception of the incident, pain in and about the neck, numbness, tingling, electric-shock-like sensations, and function of the extremities. Pain with movement and the less tolerated positions should be noted. The patient who presents acutely may be aware of stiffness, immobility, and discomfort in his neck immediately. Sometimes patients may be locked so stiffly in spasm that they appear to have torticollis or may suffer very severe and intractable pain in the neck. The examiner should question the patient about the position(s) which initiate or aggravate the symptoms. Different motions and the limitations thereof, such as rotation, tilting, or flexion, may give clues to the origin of the problem. Pain radiating up the back of the neck may be related to spasm, craniovertebral fracture or instability, spinal stenosis, C2 or C3 root injury, or compression. Pain radiating up the side of the neck made worse when tilting to the affected side may be indicative of a facet joint or lateral mass injury. Pain on flexion may indicate a disc or vertebral body injury. Pain radiating to the jaw may indicate craniovertebral fracture.

Historical information generally becomes more available later on, and the patient who presents to the physician's office days, weeks, or months after an injury can hopefully give a substantial amount of information which may help lead to the diagnosis. Some patients will feel worse several days following the injury. The confusion surrounding the episode will begin to clear, and the reality of their pain syndrome will become apparent as they try to resume normal activity or work. Over several weeks, they may begin to see the patterns and rhythm of their pain. Hopefully, the condition will begin to resolve over this time; however, it may not. If they have a persistent problem, reevaluation and further study are appropriate.

Headache and neckache are two of the most common symptoms which may arise from a cervical spine injury. Some of the general questions to ask about onset and the daily course of symptoms include whether it is sudden, explosive, related to certain types of activity, related to time of day, or related to sleep. Ask if the patient wakes up with the problem, and whether it gets a little better during the day as they become active. The pain may get worse in the afternoon after the patient has been concentrating or leaning forward through the day, or in the evening after a day of stress. In some patients, the headache may be fairly constant throughout the day. If the headaches and/or neckaches are cyclic, the manner and mode of onset can give clues to the underlying mechanism. Patients whose problems are more activity related could be said to be mechanical in nature, and thus may be indicative of an underlying structural problem. The description of the pain can be important with reference to whether the pain is coming up the back of the head; up the side of the head; beneath the ear; or whether it is a dull ache, a sharp ache, or a cramping sensation. All of these details should be recorded, including the specific areas that are affected. The discomfort is generally distributed throughout the neck; however, discomfort in the specific area of the rhomboids or trapezius, or radiating down the arm, may be indicative of an underlying cervical radiculopathy.

Weeks or months after the onset, it is important to decide whether the symptoms are progressing, stabilizing, plateaued, or improving. In the majority of patients, these problems will improve spontaneously over time. However, a patient who continues to deteriorate months after the injury is in need of specific attention. At this point, the patient should then be evaluated by an experienced spinal specialist.

Examination

Careful examination of the cervical spine is fairly simple and essential in evaluation of minor head trauma. One should exercise great care in a patient with obvious neurological deficits or severe pain. These patients should have a limited examination and immediate roentgenograms. For the complete examination, observe the general position and carriage of the spine and watch the patient's head as you or the patient moves around. Check for tilting, reduced motion, voluntary guarding, or torticollis. In performing the examination, ask the patient to move voluntarily and do not apply any force to the spine. Have the patient go through rotation, tilting, and flexion and extension of the spine, moving as far as is comfortable. Gently palpate the major paraspinal muscle groups for muscle tone and spasm. Specific patterns of spasm may be an indication of radiculopathy, such as in the rhomboids, where the upper section is innervated by C5, the middle by C6, and the lower by C7. The other major muscle groups include trapezius and sternocleidomastoid muscles for shoulder shrug and head turning innervated by the spinal accessory nerve and C2–3; deltoid for shoulder abduction and biceps for forearm flexion (C5–C6); triceps for forearm extension (C7); and hand intrinsic muscle function (C8–T1). Sensory evaluation to pin prick is generally considered subjective and unreliable. However, in clinical practice, this is probably the single most revealing exam when performed and interpreted properly. Ask if there is a difference in the sharpness of the pin-prick sensation, not just whether it can be felt. Move from one dermatome to another, right to left, back and forth. Test the face during this procedure to establish what is "normal." The back of the head and sides of the neck should also be included in the evaluation, as well as the upper extremity sensory areas. Craniovertebral and upper cervical injuries may show only subtle sensory radicular abnormalities along the side of the neck. Check the biceps, triceps, and brachioradialis reflexes for activity and symmetry. Evaluate for Hoffman's sign by flicking the fingertip and looking for the thumb and fingers twitching into a slight grasp. This may be an indication of myelopathy, especially if the response is unilateral. Check the lower extremities for gross motor strength, gait, reflexes, and for Babinski's sign, which may indicate spinal cord dysfunction or myelopathy.

The acutely injured patient may be anywhere in the spectrum of consciousness when first examined and should probably be examined initially and then again briefly at least once within the first few hours. If it is decided that the patient can be discharged, the patient should be properly advised and cautioned about possible sequelae of trauma, including both head and neck symptoms. Injury to a disc might be fairly obvious, with severe pain, cervical radiculopathy, and perhaps even focal changes or interspace collapse seen on x-rays. Pain is seen much more commonly, with the other symptoms becoming apparent later on. Sometimes even the cervical pain is not really prominent until days or weeks later. For these and other reasons, follow-up is very important. Written instruction should be given to the patient or a family member or friend because the patient's concentration, judgment, and memory may be impaired. Appropriate instructions include severe limitation of activity, no driving, intermittent use of a collar, rest, symptomatic treatment for spasm, and medication for pain and/or spasm. The patient should be specifically advised to return for reevaluation if numbness or weakness develops, if the pain continues or worsens, if the pain begins to radiate with movement of the neck, if swelling develops, or if the patient experiences difficulty breathing or swallowing.

Cervical Spine Radiological Evaluation

The role of cervical spine roentgenography (CSR) has remained controversial and is always a primary consideration with trauma in general. The primary purpose of CSR is to exclude the presence of fractures, dislocations, or other structural problems. There are several levels of considerations, including the rationale of when to obtain films, the logistical problem of the number of patients to evaluate, the sometimes suboptimal views obtained in emergency settings, and the availability of properly trained staff to interpret (and take responsibility for) the films. This is of course to be weighed against the risk that even one unrecognized fracture might slip by and allow a neurological disaster to occur.

A patient with any symptoms referable to the neck, with any conceivably cervically related abnormalities, with prolonged loss of consciousness, with an altered sensorium, or with any other serious "masking" injury should have a set of cervical spine x-rays as part of the early evaluation. Multiple reports (7–10,12,13) exist regarding minimal cervical symptoms, intoxication, altered sensorium, hip fractures, flail chest, and other injuries associated with "occult" fractures missed initially because the patient could not perceive the cardinal symptom of cervical pain. Patients who complain of any cervical symptoms, even moderate or minor spasm or stiffness in the neck, should be strongly considered for evaluation by CSR. The comatose patient fared better in one series (1) because the full evaluation and precautions became mandatory. The presence of a cervical spine fracture in an alert asymptomatic patient without at least one of these findings, or other major injuries, would be very rare.

One author (10) observed a less than 1% chance of a cervical spine fracture in this group of patients, with a 90% confidence level. It is generally accepted (7,9,14,15) that CSR can be deferred in these patients.

Some authors have seen a correlation of facial fractures with cervical spine fractures. Mandibular fracture has been associated with upper cervical spine fractures by several observers (16–19). Zygomatic fractures can have an association (20) with hangman's fractures. Some authors (20) feel there are general, but not specific, correlations between cervical and facial fractures. Patients who have been in motor vehicle accidents (MVA) and have facial fracture(s) quadruple their incidence of cervical spine fractures (20,21) from 1.3% to 4%–5.6% when compared to the general group of facial fractures. If facial fractures become evident in the course of evaluation, particularly after MVA, CSR is probably advisable even in the absence of neck complaints.

When interpreting plain films of the cervical spine, at least the following thoughts should be addressed. Check the lateral view for general alignment, subluxation, lineup of the facets, the base of the odontoid, the arch of C1, basilar invagination, and the pretracheal air shadow. The oblique views show the foramen, pedicles, and facets. The anteroposterior (A-P) view shows the vertebral bodies. The open-mouth A-P view shows the lateral masses of C1 and the base of the odontoid process. We frequently see straightening of the spine or loss of the normal lordotic curve on lateral cervical spine x-rays. This is generally associated with muscle spasm and must be considered but is probably of no specific consequence (22).

Odontoid fractures may be minimally symptomatic, and open-mouth odontoid views may be advisable if misalignment, increased prevertebral soft tissue, or symptoms suggest upper cervical fracture. The lower cervical spine (C6–C7 level) is a common site for fractures or dislocations, and a lateral cervical spine roentgenogram cannot be considered acceptable for evaluation without good visualization of C7–T1 junction. A swimmer's view may be of value in visualizing the lower cervical spine. If satisfactory films cannot be obtained, CT scanning should be used to resolve the issue. Cervical flexion-extension x-rays can be of value if subluxation is seen on screening films, if soft tissue swelling is seen on films, or if severe persistent neck pain is present (11). These views are particularly helpful in evaluating the craniovertebral junction and the odontoid. To be performed safely, these films must be taken in a carefully controlled setting by experienced technicians.

The diagnostic accuracy of CSR is a matter of some concern. A lateral view alone can miss critical pathology 15% of the time (6,14,23,24). A five-view study can reduce this rate to 8% (25). Some authors feel that by increasing general awareness of some of the more subtle signs of cervical fracture or dislocation on CSR, and by following through on these patients with CT scanning, the rate of missed lesions can be reduced to less than 1% (6). Although a posterior disruption such as a facet bony or ligamentous injury may be relatively stable initially, it may later lead to angulation deformity and canal compromise. A missed anterior vertebral body fracture may lead to an analogous picture. An excellent discussion of the subtle signs of fracture, disruptions, and the ramifications thereof is given by Harris and Yeakley (26) and includes essential information for physicians called upon to evaluate CSR on an emergent basis.

Unfortunately, many "soft tissue," musculoligamentous, discal, and other injuries to the spine are just not apparent on plain film evaluations of the cervical spine. Computed tomography scanning is the next line of resolution in defining bony spinal injury (6). If laminar, facet, or vertebral fractures are suspected, or if the spine cannot be visualized readily on plain roentgenograms, CAT scanning has a high probability of resolving the diagnostic problems (6,27) and should be used liberally. Preexistent cervical spondylolysis is commonly seen, and in general is not felt to be a factor in the outcome of these patients (22). However, if significant spondylolysis is apparent, CT scanning is advisable for the best possible evaluation (6).

Hypocycloidal polytomography was the most definitive study available for clinical use for a long time but has now been largely supplanted by the CT scan for visualization of bony elements. Polytomes are still particularly useful in defining the base of the odontoid, if facet fractures are suspected, with very heavy patients, or if metallic artifacts are present (11). Polytomes can also be taken in certain planes and orientations (coronal and sagittal), which can only be approximated by reconstructed CT scanning. When performing the CT scan, the neck should be maintained in a neutral position because one must presume the presence of spinal fractures. Direct CT scanning of the neck in unusual planes is therefore not generally advisable if any possibility of instability exists. Magnetic resonance imaging scanning has proven to be a powerful tool (28) and can be helpful in evaluating cervical discs, the relative degree of spinal stenosis, the spinal cord, the brachial plexus, and other soft tissue structures. However, MRI cannot be considered as a screening tool in the emergency room and is not generally available in the middle of the night.

If you are evaluating a patient in severe cervical pain, caution and careful consideration are essential, particularly if the best possible roentgenographic facilities, including CT, MRI, and polytomes, are not immediately available. As an example, I evaluated a patient with minor head trauma and fairly severe cervical pain in the emergency room who had "normal" x-rays and a normal neurological exam. The radiologists later agreed that the plain films appeared "normal." Fortunately, the patient was admitted for observation because of his severe cervical pain. Hypocycloidal polytomes (before CT scans were readily available) the next day revealed eight individual fractures throughout the cervical spine. Other similar reports have appeared in the literature. If sufficient concern exists, admit and immobilize the patient until more definitive studies can be obtained.

Headache Related to Cervical Injury

Minor head trauma may cause headache for many reasons; one of the more common etiologies is cervical spinal problems. Frykholm (29) states that cervical headache is "the type of headache most frequently seen in general practise and also the most frequently misinterpreted." There are numerous pain-generating structures in the spine, including ligaments, muscles, discs, and nerves. However, one of the more common pain syndrome mechanisms involves the indirect or secondary physiologic response of muscle spasm, which is a common response to an underlying spinal problem. In the cervical spine, this in effect produces an internal splint or collar and can be quite uncomfortable, both initially and over time. Spasm in the upper cervical musculature can compress the greater occipital nerves (which provide sensory innervation to the back of and top of the head), producing headache and/or hypoesthesia radiating generally up the back of the head toward the vertex. The muscles in spasm may develop lactic acid buildup secondary to relative ischemia, leading to severe pain or cramping, as well. The patient may not even be aware of the degree of cervical spasm underlying the problem. Almost any of the structures in the cervical spine can serve to trigger spasm. Musculoligamentous strain, ligaments, facet injury, and disc injuries can all cause muscle spasm. In clinical evaluation, this symptom complex or parts of it underlie almost every cervical pain syndrome. There are multiple possible radiations of cervical pain leading to or perceived as headache. Pain may radiate up the posterior aspect of the neck to the base of the skull and vertex, up the side of the neck to the skull base, up the shoulder to the neck and to the ear, up the anterolateral aspect of the neck along the facets, or anteriorly to the skull base and jaw.

Edmeads (30) divided the causes of cervical headache into two groups. In the first group, the lesion is demonstrable and the headache is helped by treating the underlying condition; in the second group, the lesion is not apparent. Examples of the first group include congenital and acquired craniovertebral junction disorders, rheumatoid arthritis and ankylosing spondylitis of the upper cervical spine, and carotid or vertebral arterial injury. Examples of the second group are whiplash syndrome, segmental hypomobility-hypermobility syndrome, the posterior cervical sympathetic syndrome, cervical migraine, third occipital nerve headache, and cervicogenic headache. Symptoms suggestive of cervical origin of headache include abrupt onset following sudden excessive movement of the head, persistent unilateral suboccipital or occipital pain, consistent reproduction by neck movements only, abnormal postures of the head or neck, significant painful limitation of movement of the cervical spine, abnormal mobility at the craniovertebral junction, C2 sensory abnormalities, and lower medulla or upper cervical cord symptoms.

Cervical spinal fracture or ligamentous injury can be headache generators, particularly at the craniovertebral junction, where the pain may radiate down along the jaw and up toward the temple and/or locally. Cervical disc injuries may cause headache through the previously mentioned mechanism of muscle spasm, or by direct irritation of the posterior longitudinal ligament (30,31). Cervical spinal stenosis can give rise to profound headache syndromes, generally radiating up the back of the neck to the vertex. There may be very little evidence of radiculopathy and perhaps no evidence of myelopathy on exam in some cases. An electric-shock-like sensation with flexion of the neck which radiates through the body and into the legs may be present by history or on exam. This is Lhermitte's sign and can be caused by cervical spinal stenosis or spinal cord impingement. Headache can be the presenting symptom of thoracic outlet (TOS) syndrome. This headache tends to be worse in the morning as the patient arises. The headache can also be sympathetically mediated. The descending trigeminal tract can be injured in the cervical spinal cord or can be sympathetically overstimulated (32,33), leading to hypoesthesia, abnormal sensations, or pain in and about the head or face.

Whiplash

One of the more common cervical syndromes was first described by Crowe (34) in 1928 as whiplash. This is thought to be the result of violent or sudden extreme motion of the neck as might result from a motor vehicle accident, fall, or other accident. The motion may be flexion-extension, rotational, or acceleration-deceleration with or without clinically apparent head or brain injury. The exact anatomic nature of the injury remains obscure, although it is thought to involve musculoligamentous sprain or injury (35). Controversy exists even as to the existence of the syndrome, and financial considerations have been postulated as a possible contributory element. Clinically, the patient complains of primarily of headache, neckache, and stiffness, as well as a variety of symptoms including dizziness, temporomandibular joint (TMJ) problems, TOS problems, radicular symptoms, and other discomforts. The male:female ratio ranges from 35:65 to 29:71 across some of the different series (35,36). Of patients with whiplash, 6% can have accompanying head injury (1,37). A patient who has sustained a whiplash injury can complain of (or experience) some or even all of the symptoms exhibited by a patient who has sustained head trauma. There are no specific diagnostic tests which can confirm the diagnosis. About three-quarters of patients return to work within the first month; two-thirds are near normal at three months. About one in ten continues to suffer significantly more than a year after injury. There are numerous series and they vary widely in results and conclusions (35,36,38–42).

Thoracic Outlet Syndrome

Thoracic outlet syndrome is an irritation of the trunks of the brachial plexus, either by direct injury or stretching, or as a secondary result of cervical muscle spasm. Symptoms from the lower trunk are far more common. Numbness in the ulnar aspect of the hands, stiffness of the neck, difficulty elevating the upper arm for any length of time, sympathetic alteration or dysfunction in the arm and hand are all symptoms suggestive of thoracic outlet syndrome. The syndrome can even present primarily as headache or "migraine." Electrical studies such as EMG testing or evoked potentials can show conduction slowing through the brachial plexus if done properly and interpreted accurately. These studies must be carefully correlated with the clinical symptom complex, as both false-negative and false-positive studies occur. Possible causes of TOS include spasm through the scalenes entrapping the brachial plexus, abnormal bands or ligaments in the same area, cervical rib; abnormal or tight configuration of the thoracic outlet; or injury to or stretching of the brachial plexus. Headache is commonly seen in association with this syndrome, possibly as an indirect result of muscle spasm. Treatment may include physical therapy, exercise, medication, blocks, manipulation, or acupuncture. The more severe and refractory cases may require surgical procedures such as brachial plexus exploration, first rib resection, scalenotomy, and others. However, the timing of surgery and the selection of a specific surgical procedure remain controversial.

Other Problems

Cervical vertigo, dizziness, or hearing disturbances can be caused by cervical injuries. Several mechanisms are postulated, including muscle spasm intermittently interfering with motion of the neck, spasm interfering with the perceived orientation of the neck, compression of the vertebral artery by osteophyte, or direct compression of the spinal cord by osteophytes. Half of the proprioceptive receptors of the vestibulospinal tracts are located in the joint capsules of the C1–C3 vertebrae, and the remaining half are located in the deep cervical musculature (43). Animals demonstrated disequilibrium and nystagmus when these cervical receptors were anesthetized with procaine (43,44). These studies support the hypothesis that the majority of proprioceptive information for maintainence of equilibrium comes from the cervical joint capsule and muscle receptors (45). With whiplash-type injuries, Toglia and Rosenberg (46) and Rubin (47) demonstrated abnormalities on electronystagmography. Toglia (48) observed tinnitus and hearing loss, even with normal neurologic examinations. The significance of these observations and the frequency of occurrence of these complaints warrants their careful consideration.

Temporomandibular joint dysfunction syndromes can give rise to a variety of symptoms, some of which can be quite difficult to associate. Any condition which irritates, compresses, misaligns, or alters the TMJ relationship can serve as a triggering mechanism for the TMJ syndrome. A jaw click alone does not imply TMJ syndrome, as the syndrome represents a variety of painful complaints. Pain beneath the ear, pain on chewing, difficulty opening the jaw, and neckache and headache problems may all be part of the symptom complex. Headache may be one of the prominent initial symptoms of this disorder. The pain may even be so severe as to mimic the syndrome of tic douloureux. Trauma is the leading cause of subarachnoid hemorrhage, and symptoms may become apparent days or weeks later as neckache or headache. Consequently, the physician must remember that not all post-injury neck pain is due to simple muscle spasm, or potentially fatal conditions will sometimes be missed.

Carotid artery injury or dissection can be caused by minor trauma or even a strenuous movement. Pain radiating up the neck into the skull base and face and/or ischemic or embolic symptoms in the ipsilateral cerebral hemisphere are typical. This injury is uncommon but life-threatening. Vertebral artery injury may result from hyperextension or flexion-extension injuries to the spine. With either of these vascular syndromes, the presentation may be both sudden and disastrous. If a patient has sustained a cervical injury and there are signs of transient brain ischemia, immediate pancerebral angiography must be strongly considered.

Post-traumatic cervical autonomic dysfunction, or Barre-Lieou syndrome (49,50), can include vertigo, nausea, vomiting, gastric distress, constipation/diarrhea, hyper/hypoglycemia, anxiety attacks, visual blurring, and other problems. The origin of this complex has been discussed, and remains somewhat obscure (51–53), although it probably involves intrinsic brainstem damage or dysfunction.

Cervical spine injury of a more severe nature even in the absence of direct head trauma can be associated with lesions which may present with primarily intracranial problems. Examples of this include a diencephalic syndrome (54), which includes diabetes insipidus and hyperthermia, or even intracerebral hemorrhage. This highlights the importance of meticulous, combined evaluation of the head and neck following any episode of trauma.

Treatment

Treatment depends to a large extent on when the patient is being evaluated and the severity and nature of the complaints. Muscle relaxants and analgesics may be in order, along with intermittent local immobilization of the spine with either a soft or semi-rigid collar. In an intermediate phase, several days to several weeks following injury, if the patient continues to have symptoms, and particularly if the difficulties are worsening, x-rays should certainly be reviewed and possibly repeated. Again, medications and a collar may be helpful. Passive therapy may provide some symptomatic benefit at this point, and ultrasound, hot packs, gentle massage, and expert manipulation in selected cases may afford transient relief. There are several distinct advantages to such treatment. The patient is seeing a health care professional and is being observed and evaluated on a regular basis. The "cycle of pain" is being broken intermittently to allow the symptoms to subside. The patient is able to discuss the symptoms with a health care professional who will listen and try to help, and the patient feels as though something is being accomplished through all this. If the problem persists over time, consultation with a spinal specialist such as a neurosurgeon or orthopedic surgeon should be sought and a careful neurological examination should be obtained along with repeat x-rays and MRI scanning. Magnetic resonance imaging is probably the most helpful tool in evaluating patients with significant problems of more than a month or so in duration. It can be quite embarrassing at best to try to explain the rationale for a year of conservative management when the MRI finally obtained at the insistence of the patient reveals the presence of a massively ruptured cervical disc with spinal cord compression. I have seen this in clinical practice. If a patient is having substantial difficulties for more than six weeks after trauma, more extensive evaluation is most certainly warranted.

References

1. Steudel WI, Rosenthal D, Lorenz R, Merdes W: Prognosis and treatment of cervical spine injuries with associated head trauma. Acta Neurochir, 1988; 43:85–90.
2. O'Malley KF, Ross SE: The incidence of injury to the cervical spine in patients with craniocerebral injury. J Trauma, 1988; 28(10):1476–1478.
3. Geisler WC, Wynne-Jones M, Jousse AT: Early management of the patient with trauma to the spinal cord. Med Serv J Can, 1966; 23:512–522.
4. Cox GR, Barish RA: Delayed presentation of unstable cervical spine injury with minimal symptoms. J Emerg Med, 1991; 9:123–127.
5. Rosa L: Missed fractures of the cervical spine. Milit Med, 1989; 154(1):39–41.
6. Gerrelts BD, Petersen EU, Mabry J, Petersen SR: Delayed diagnosis of cervical spine injuries. J Trauma, 1991; 31(12):1622–1626.
7. Kreipke DL, Gillespie KR, McCarthy MC, Mail JT, et al.: Reliability of indications for cervical spine films in trauma patients. J Trauma, 1989; 29(10):1438–1439.
8. Roberge RJ, Wears RC, Kelly M, et al.: Selective application of cervical spine radiography in alert victims of blunt trauma: A prospective study. J Trauma, 1988; 28:748–788.
9. Saddison D, Vanek VW, Racanelli JL: Clinical indications for cervical spine radiographs in alert trauma patients. Am Surgeon, 1991; 57(6):366–369.
10. Neifeld GL, Keene JG, Hevesy G, Leikein J, et al.: Cervical injury in head trauma. J Emerg Med, 1988; 6:203–207.
11. Holliman CJ, Mayer JS, Cook RT, Smith JS: Is the anteroposterior cervical spine radiograph necessary in initial trauma screening? Am J Emerg Med, 1991; 9(5):421–425.
12. Ducker TG: Head trauma and cervical spine injuries. Am J Emerg Med, March, 1989; 7(2):248.
13. Soicher E, Demetriades D: Cervical spine injuries in patients with head injuries. Br J Surg 1991; 78(8):1013–1014.
14. Shaffer MA, Doris PE: Limitation of the cross table lateral view in detecting cervical spinal injuries: A retrospective analysis. Ann Emerg Med, 1981; 10:508.
15. Bayless P, Ray VG: Incidence of cervical spine injuries in association with blunt head trauma. Am J Emerg Med, 1989; 7(2):139–142.
16. Sinclair D, Schwartz M, Gruss J, McLellan B: A retrospective review of the relationship between facial fractures, head injuries, and cervical spine injuries. J Emerg Med, 1988; 6:109–112.

17. Lewis VL, Manson PN, Morgan RF, et al.: Recognition, patterns and management. J Trauma, 1985; 25:90–93.
18. Donoff RB, Roser SM: Management of condylar fractures in patients with cervical spine: Report of cases. J Oral Surg, 1973; 31:130–135.
19. Haisova L, Kramova I: Facial bone fractures associated with cervical spine injuries. Oral Surg, 1970; 30:742–748.
20. Davidson JS, Birdsell DC: Cervical spine injury in patients with facial skeletal trauma. J Trauma, 1989; 29(9):1276–1278.
21. Schultz RC: Facial injuries from automobile accident: A study of 400 consecutive cases. Plast Reconstr Surg, 1967; 40:415–419.
22. Hildingsson C, Toolanen G: Outcome after soft-tissue injury of the cervical spine: A prospective study of 93 car-accident victims. Acta Orthop Scand, 1990; 61(4):357–359.
23. Ross SE, Schwab CW, David ET, et al.: Clearing the cervical spine: Initial radiologic evaluation. J Trauma, 1987; 27:1055.
24. Williams CF, Bernstein TW, Jelenko C: Essentiality of the lateral cervical spine radiograph. Ann Emerg Med, 1987; 16:738.
25. Doris PE, Wilson RA: The next logical step in the emergency radiographic evaluation of cervical spine trauma: The five view trauma series. J Emerg Med, 1985; 3:371.
26. Harris JH, Yeakley JS: Radiographically subtle soft tissue injuries of the cervical spine. Curr Probl Diagn Radiol, 1989; 18(4):161–192.
27. Acheson MD, Livingston RR, Richardson ML, et al.: High resolution CT scanning in the evaluation of cervical spine fractures: Comparison with plain film examinations. AJR, 1987; 148:1179.
28. Flanders AE, Schaefer DM, Doan HT, Mishkin MM, et al.: Acute cervical spine trauma: correlation of MR immaging findings with degree of neurologic deficit. Radiology, 1990; 177:25–33.
29. Frykholm R: The clinical picture. In Hirsch C, Zotterman Y, (eds): Cervical Pain. Elmsford, NY: Pergamon Press, 1972.
30. Edmeads J: Headache of cervical origin. Revue Du Praticien, Feb 11, 1990; 40(5):399–402.
31. Henderson DJ, Dorman TM: Functional roentgenometric evaluation of the cervical spine in the sagittal plane. J Manipulative Physiol Ther, 1981; 4:65–68.
32. Anthony M: Migraine and its management. Aust Fam Physician, 1986; 15:643–49.
33. Siwe SA: The cervical part of the ganglionated cord with special reference to its connections with the spinal nerves and certain cerebral nerves. Am J Anat, 1931; 48:479–97.
34. Crowe H: Injuries to the cervical spine. Presentation to the Annual Meeting of Western Orthopaedic Association, San Francisco, 1928.
35. Pearce JMS: Whiplash injury: fact or faction? Headache Quarterly, 1992; 3(1):45–49.
36. Balla JI: Report to the Motor Accidents Board of Victoria on whiplash injuries, 1984, Headache and cervical disorders. In Hopkin A (ed): Headache, Problems in Diagnosis and Management. London: Saunders, 1988; pp 256–289.

37. Soderstrom LA, Brumback RJ: Early care of the patient with cervical spine injury. Orthop Clin North Am, 1986; 17:3–13.
38. States JD, Balcerak JC, Williams JS, et al.: Injury frequency and head restraint effectiveness in rear-end impact accidents. Proc 16th STAPP Car Crash Conference, Detroit, 1972.
39. Deans GT, Magalliard JN, Kerr M, Rutherford WH: Neck sprain—A major cause of disability following car accidents. Injury, 1987; 18:10–12.
40. Hohl M: Soft tissue injuries of the neck in automobile accidents; factors influencing prognosis. J Bone Joint Surg, 1974; 56A:1675–1682.
41. Norris SH, Watt I: The prognosis of neck injuries resulting from rear-end vehicle collisions. J Bone Joint Surg, 1983; 65B:608–611.
42. Gargan MF, Bannister GC: Long-term prognosis of soft-tissue injuries of the neck. J Bone Joint Surg, 1990; 72-B:901–903.
43. Hulse M: Disequilibrium caused by a functional disturbance of the upper cervical spine: clinmical aspects and differential diagnosis. Manuelle Medizin, 1983; 1:18–23.
44. Biemond A, Dejong JMBV: On cervical nystagmus and related disorders. Brain, 1969; 42:437–58.
45. Guyton AC: Textbook of Medical Physiology. 6th ed. Philadelphia: W.B. Saunders, 1981.
46. Toglia J, Rosenberg R: Post traumatic dizziness. Arch Otolaryngol, 1970; 22:485–91.
47. Rubin W: Whiplash with vestibular involvement. Arch Otolaryngol, 1973; 97:85–87.
48. Toglia JV: Acute flexion/extension injury of the neck. Neurology, 1976; 26:808–14.
49. Barre JA, Lieou CR: XXXme Congres des Medicins alienistes et neurologistes de france et des pays de lanque fraise. Paris: Masson (English translation), 1926.
50. Lenhart LJ: Post-traumatic cervical syndrome. J Manipulative Physiol Ther, 1988; 11(5):409–415.
51. Hinoki M, Niki H: Neurological studies on the role of the sympathetic nervous system in the formation of traumatic vertigo of cervical origin. Acta Otolaryngol (Stockh), 1975; 330:185–196.
52. Khurana RK, Nirankari VS: Bilateral sympathetic dysfunction in post-traumatic headaches. Headache, 1986; 26:183–188.
53. Brieg A: Biomechanics of the Central Nervous System. Chicago: Year Book Publishers, 1960.
54. Iob I, Salar G, Mattisi G, Ori C, Rampazzo A: Diencephalic syndrome following spinal cord trauma. Acta Neurochir, 1989; 97(3–4):123–7.

— 15

The Role of the Speech-Language Pathologist in the Treatment of Mild Brain Injury: A Community-Based Approach

Rhona Paul-Cohen

In 1986, the American Speech-Language Hearing Association (ASHA) formed a subcommittee to describe the role of the speech-language pathologist in the rehabilitation of the individual with cognitive impairments. The results of their efforts were published in the ASHA journal in 1987 (1). The report describes the relationship between cognition and language which provides the basis for a clinical focus on cognitive-communication deficits. The role of the speech-language pathologist in the evaluation and treatment of this population and the professional's role within the interdisciplinary treatment team is described within this report. These authors state that "the speech-language pathologist concerned with the management of cognitive-communication disorders assumes responsibility for thorough and flexible exploration of relations between cognitive deficits and their possible communicative consequences...." The phrase "thorough and flexible" cannot be underscored enough when treating a subgroup of this population: the mildly brain injured.

According to Mandel (2), "Minor head injury is a major health problem, one that is often not recognized or accepted by the patient's family and employer." The incidence of mild traumatic brain injury is staggering. Of the more than 400,000 persons each year that seek medical attention for brain trauma, 80% have mild injuries (3). Kay points out that individuals with mild traumatic brain injuries often spend a brief time, if any, in the hospital (4). These patients often make quick medical recoveries and are frequently sent home without any perceived need for formal rehabilitation. Such individuals frequently appear normal until they attempt to resume their pre-injury responsibilities at home, work, and/or school. Reports by O'Hara (5) and Conboy et al. (6) both note that the majority of mild traumatic brain injury patients are often told when they leave the hospital that everything will be fine and that all of their symptoms will clear. Unfortunately, this is not always the case. As a result of inadequate knowledge about their injury, these patients often feel confused and distressed over their "new" behaviors. In addition, they frequently possess unrealistic expectations about their abilities.

Gronwall (7) suggests that although all mild head injury patients should be screened and followed until they return to work, such a screening program would be expensive and impractical. She therefore proposes that services be provided to those patients "... at risk for longer than normal periods of incapacity." This population includes the following individuals: 1) the older patient, 2) the patient with a previous history of traumatic brain injury, 3) the patient who is a high achiever or is in a demanding occupation, and 4) the patient who has family or social stressors.

Kay states that deficits resulting from mild diffuse brain injury are not specific to particular areas of cognition (4). Rather, there is a general disruption in speed, efficiency, execution, and integration of mental processes. According to Mateer (8), the most frequent cognitive complaints following mild traumatic brain injury include problems with memory, new learning, and concentration. Patients often describe that they cannot do more than one thing at a time and that they frequently experience "information overload." Many will report being sensitive to noise or to hectic environments. They often state that common tasks take longer and require more effort. Hagen notes that subtle communication problems after traumatic brain injury are "heavily influenced and in some instances created" by underlying cognitive deficits which include attention, inhibition, memory, integration/organization of information, and speed of information processing (9).

Although several researchers report that recovery from mild traumatic brain injury typically occurs within three months (10–12), Leininger and Kreutzer point out that these studies contain problems in their methodology that "... systematically reduced the likelihood of detecting impaired functioning among their mild traumatic brain injury samples" (13). Neuropsychological deficits may be detected beyond one year following injury (14). Longer recovery periods are associated with persons who are 40 and above at the time of injury, those injured in a motor vehicle accident, and those with a previous brain injury. In trying to answer the question of why some patients "recover" and others who experience similar degrees of injury have long-term problems, Kay concludes that it is a case of "individual vulnerability" (15). He adds that functional outcome is determined by a combination of underlying neurologic and overlying personality, environmental, and psychological factors.

Assessment Techniques

Because impairments in cognitive-communicative functioning are often subtle, neuropsychological assessment coupled with behavioral observations of the individual in his/her own environment(s) are recommended in order to identify the nature and extent of problems that affect daily functioning. Kay warns, however, that traditional neuropsychological assessment and interpretation, especially if one uses a "fixed-battery approach," will not necessarily be sensitive to cognitive impairments after mild traumatic brain injury (15). He suggests that neuropsychologists use a specialized battery of tests that focus on the constellation of deficits that are commonly seen in this population as discussed elsewhere in this book.

Milton (16) and Mayer et al. (17) advocate the use of behavioral observations of the individual in his/her own natural settings coupled with questionnaires and interviews of the client and family/significant other. Mayer et al. developed a tool which they call the Activity Pattern Indicator (API). The API consists of 148 questions, divided into nine categories. Information gathered through the API provides data regarding both premorbid and current activity patterns. Milton calls on speech-language pathologists to shift their focus from an isolated stimulus-response framework to a more functional perspective. She points out that the environment in which the assessment takes place will influence the results. She advocates evaluation in real-life communication situations in order to challenge attention, integration of functional skills, and frustration control. Milton stresses a "program without walls" approach to service delivery. In this model of treatment, therapy takes place in the client's own home and community. The clinician works one-to-one with the client in these real-life settings. This approach promotes generalization and provides actual situations that require skill integration. In addition, observations made in these settings provide a better understanding of the interactions between family members/significant others and the client. The program typically extends to include family, friends, community members, etc.

Miller et al. also recommend using informal observations in assessing cognitive-communication impairments secondary to brain injury (18). Clinicians are able to evaluate the client's skills in more functional, natural settings. Informal assessment can be tailored to each client's unique set of needs and interests. It allows the clinician the ability to manipulate cues and to determine which ones maximize performance. The authors caution that responses should be measured and documented in a consistent manner over time so as to measure progress accurately. The Good Samaritan Hospital's Cognitive Behavioral Rating Scale, developed by Sohlberg and Mater (19), is a tool used to document observations of clients' functional performance. The scale divides performance into four levels. Areas addressed include attention/concentration, memory, visual processing, reasoning/problem-solving, executive functions, and language.

This author recommends assessing the client's cognitive-communication status in his/her natural environments (home, community, work, school). In addition to a behavioral assessment, questionnaires, checklists, and rating scales that focus on day-to-day issues are useful diagnostic tools. Using the same tool with both client and family member/significant other can provide an important comparison regarding such areas as insight, understanding, and expectations. It is also necessary to determine the level of support that family members/significant others provide to the individual with the brain injury. When both parties describe, in detail, a typical day both pre- and post-injury, changes in activity patterns, efficiency, energy level, etc., will become more apparent.

The speech-language pathologist should observe the client in multiple situations and various activities, and should try to spend several hours, at varying times in the day, in order to gain a realistic assessment of functioning. If the client has returned to work, the therapist should try to arrange a time to observe him/her in that setting. This may not be possible or advisable if there are security, safety, or other extenuating circumstances in the workplace.

In addition, the therapist should provide ongoing feedback and suggestions for compensatory strategies and note how the client receives constructive comments, as well as how well he/she is able to integrate therapeutic suggestions. These data are helpful in predicting the future effectiveness of treatment.

Another factor that will correlate with treatment effectiveness is the ability to develop a professional rapport between client and clinician. This author advocates informing the client from the outset that they are beginning a "professional partnership." The clinician brings his/her expertise about cognitive-communication deficits secondary to mild traumatic brain injury and the client shares his/her knowledge about his/her skills, strengths/weaknesses, interests, etc. The two dovetail and help to create a sound, trusting working relationship. This approach has been successful with a significant number of clients and has been especially advantageous when working with professionals who have sustained mild brain injuries. These individuals often enter treatment leery of what the clinician has to offer. They are often struggling to regain control over their lives and feel threatened by clinicians who "tell them what to do and when to do it." Clients should be reassured, not only in words but in actions, that they are indeed regaining control in their rehabilitation efforts.

Once the clinician has completed his/her assessment, a prioritized list of goals should be generated. The client and clinician need to work together to arrive at this list. Criteria to consider when prioritizing the objectives should include—

1. The degree to which behavior influences daily functioning
2. The ease with which behavior may be modified/improved using various therapeutic strategies/techniques
3. The client's overall awareness and insight regarding the occurrence of the targeted behavior
4. The client's motivation to improve targeted behavior

With the client's permission, goals of treatment should be shared with family members/significant others so that objectives of therapy may be reinforced and carried over, and so that feedback may be provided regarding the effectiveness of various treatment strategies. If possible, the client should identify an individual at the workplace who can be apprised of the treatment issues. The choice of whether this individual is a supervisor, employer, or co-worker will depend on the client's individual circumstances, as well as such factors as rapport, trust, personality, etc. Involving an individual at the work-place often enhances support and understanding as the client attempts to re-enter a work situation.

The clinician may also assist the client in determining how and what to say about his/her cognitive-communication impairments. Some clients have a tendency to be highly focused on their problems, no matter how subtle those problems may be. It is therefore important to discuss common scenarios and what, if any, information about their deficits should be given.

Approaches to Intervention

Kay outlines intervention for clients with mild traumatic brain injury to include the following: education and information, identification of problems, support, neuropsychological rehabilitation, and accommodation ("the process of recognition, acceptance and adjustment to a new set of limitations.") [4]. Conboy et al. emphasize the importance of reducing stress and demands in the environment, as well as structuring daily activities so that there are set routines [6]. They also point out that each case is unique, and therefore the clinician must take into account the client's premorbid personality and intellectual resources, present needs, motivation, etc. The authors add that "... the most effective and necessary interventions are the recognition and 'legitimization' of the true sequelae..." of the brain injury. They emphasize that failure to understand or recognize mild deficits may give rise to feelings of frustration, self-doubt, anxiety, and depression.

The use of a "fatigue-control approach" is advocated by Gronwall (20). She points to evidence in the literature that even after mild brain injury there are changes in EEG recordings. These changes may be related to disturbed sleep cycles that are often common in these cases (21). Gronwall further suggests that patients should be encouraged to take naps.

Mateer focuses treatment on attentional deficits (8). Mateer and her colleague, M. Sohlberg, developed a "process-specific" tool to train attentional capacity and control in four areas: sustained, selective, alternating, and divided attention (22). This tool, Attention Process Training (APT), has been shown to be effective in both improving attention and memory capacities (23,24). These investigators also suggest that rehabilitation efforts involve implementing compensatory strategies, as well as attention training. They emphasize the use of organizational and time management strategies, in addition to effective systems for supplementing memory.

Cicerone points out that patients with mild traumatic brain injuries are often able to self-monitor (25). This skill contributes to the increased likelihood that they will benefit from a variety of cognitive treatment techniques. It follows then that Cicerone suggests implementing a self-monitoring procedure in the context of the individual's daily routine. This involves having the client develop a routine and monitor its execution, especially instances when he/she deviates from scheduled activities. Particular attention is paid to time management, organization of tasks, and the management of multiple task demands.

Case Illustration

This case of a client with a mild brain injury will illustrate the application of the various assessment and treatment principles mentioned above.

Background Data

M.T., a 48-year-old famale, was involved in a motor vehicle accident and sustained a mild brain injury. She reportedly has no recollection of the accident and only remembers waking up in the hospital three to five hours later.

M.T. earned a two-year degree from college and was on the honor roll. She has been employed for the past ten years as a real estate agent. This client has been separated from her husband for three years. Two of her four children live with her. M.T. smokes over one pack of cigarettes a day and her caffeine intake is judged to be moderate to heavy. She denies any alcohol or drug abuse. Her past medical history is negative.

M.T. has been seeing a psychologist for one year to address stress and anxiety issues that resulted after her injury.

Neuropsychological Findings

A neuropsychological evaluation was performed approximately one-and-a-half years post-injury. Mild difficulties were noted in the areas of visual memory, attention, speed of information processing, and complex problem-solving. Intellectual abilities were found to be in the average range.

As a result of these findings, it was recommended that M.T. be enrolled in treatment for her cognitively based problems.

Treatment Approach

A "program without walls" approach was instituted. The speech-language pathologist went to M.T.'s home and worked one-on-one with her for $1\frac{1}{2}$ hours per week.

Using self-report, behavioral observations, and a functional rating scale (Table 15.1), the clinician was able to identify several problem areas. M.T. reported experiencing difficulties with word finding and short-term memory. She noted that when these deficits occurred, she would become frustrated and anxious. This, in turn, negatively affected her performance. She also reported feeling "scattered" and "out of control," which also brought on a similar emotional response.

Behavioral observations revealed that M.T. often digressed from the topic of conversation without awareness. She also appeared to have difficulty organizing her day and had seemingly large portions of unstructured time in each day.

The functional rating scale was devised specifically to target potential areas of difficulty given M.T.'s profession and the already identified impairments (Table 15.1). Keeping appointments; recalling the contents of a meeting/phone call; communicating messages in a succinct manner; meeting dealines; making smooth transitions from

Table 15.1. Functional rating scale.

Client's initials:
Date:
Directions: Read each item and circle the appropriate number (1 = no problems;
2 = mild difficulties; 3 = moderate difficulties; 4 = severe difficulties;
5 = unable to do)

1. Able to keep appointments	1	2	3	4	5
2. Able to return phone call in a timely fashion	1	2	3	4	5
3. Able to utilize free time effectively	1	2	3	4	5
4. Able to recall the contents of a meeting accurately	1	2	3	4	5
5. Able to recall the contents of a phone call accurately	1	2	3	4	5
6. Able to take constructive feedback	1	2	3	4	5
7. Able to relate to peers and co-workers	1	2	3	4	5
8. Able to communicate messages in a succinct manner	1	2	3	4	5
9. Able to meet deadlines	1	2	3	4	5
10. Able to relate to supervisors and employers	1	2	3	4	5
11. Able to transition smoothly from task to task	1	2	3	4	5
12. Able to remain even-tempered	1	2	3	4	5
13. Able to interact in a group setting	1	2	3	4	5
14. Able to succeed	1	2	3	4	5
15. Aware of own errors	1	2	3	4	5

one task to another; interacting in a group setting; taking constructive feedback; relating with peers, co-workers, and supervisors; remaining even-tempered; and feeling "successful" were all rated as mildly moderately impaired. Effective utilization of free time was judged to be severely impaired.

It should be noted that M.T. had a great deal of difficulty developing a professional working relationship. She openly admitted that having to work directly on deficit areas was very difficult for her. She also stated that she had always needed to be in control and that *any* therapy made her feel less so. However, she wanted to participate in treatment so that she would be able to function more efficiently and effectively.

With M.T.'s permission, the clinician contacted her treating psychologist. It became clear that M.T.'s premorbid personality coupled with her current stress and anxiety issues would most likely limit the gains that she could make in treatment. It was therefore decided that treatment should focus on teaching M.T. several strategies that would have the most positive impact on improving functioning. M.T.'s psychologist was going to reinforce the use of these cognitive-communication strategies in her sessions, and the speech-language pathologist would utilize relaxation techniques used in the counseling.

Given this individual's personality and emotional issues, it was determined that treatment should be conducted in an informal, nonthreatening setting (i.e., in M.T.'s living room, sitting and drinking a cup of coffee). At times M.T. would feel the need to answer the phone during a session rather than letting her answering machine get the call. This was viewed as M.T. taking control and/or needing a break. Therefore, the clinician did not try to stop this activity from occurring.

Results from the informal assessment were discussed with M.T. The clinician spoke wth M.T. about presenting her with several strategies that would most likely make a significant difference in functioning. She was in agreement with this plan. Strategies for improving memory, organization, and time management were the focus of treatment. M.T. often shared instances in which problems in these areas had affected actual functioning. Techniques were developed to help circumvent similar problems in the future. Some of the suggested strategies included—

1. Organizing each day by writing down activities on a specified sheet of paper that is kept in a central location
2. Using a checklist so as not to forget important items when leaving home or office
3. Writing a new name or phone number on the top of the weekly schedule and reviewing it several times a day to facilitate learning it
4. Identifying one hour per day that is "free" and structuring it by writing down specific activities to be done
5. Checking off activities that have been completed and at the end of the day, transferring incomplete tasks to the next day
6. Trying to stop and regroup, when feeling rushed and overwhelmed, taking time to organize thoughts before jumping in
7. Developing face sheets and other forms/checklists to organize information in real estate files

After three months of treatment, M.T. reported that she was able to utilize the strategies presented successfully. She felt as if she had learned what she needed to in order to maximize her functioning and felt that she would be able to generalize the techniques to other situations. Phone contact was maintained over the next several months, with M.T. reporting continued success in implementing the strategies. This treatment resulted in M.T.'s feeling that she had experienced an overall improvement in functioning.

Summary

The assessment and management of cognitive-communication impairments secondary to mild traumatic brain injury compels the speech-language pathologist to break away from traditional approaches and adopt a functional, community-based approach. The effects of mild and, often, subtle problems in such areas as memory, attention, information processing, and organization can have a significant impact on the individual's communication skills and on his/ her overall ability to function. Speech-language pathologists possess abilities and techniques that can help clients in this population.

References

1. American Speech-Language-Hearing Association, Sub-Committee on Language and Cognition: The role of speech-language pathologists in the habilitation and rehabilitation of cognitively impaired individuals: A report of the sub-committee on language and cognition. ASHA, 1987; 29:53–55.
2. Mandel S: Minor head injury may not be "minor." Postgrad Med, 1989; 85(6):213–225.
3. Dikmen S, McLean A, Temkin N: Neuropsychological and psychosocial consequences of minor head injury. J Neurol Neurosurg Psychiatry, 1986; 49(11):1227–32.
4. Kay T: Minor head injury: An introduction for professionals. National Head Injury Publication, 1986; 1–12.
5. O'Hara C: Emotional adjustment following minor head injury. Cogn Rehabil, 1988; 6:26–33.
6. Conboy TB, Barth J, Boll T: Treatment and rehabilitation of mild and moderate head trauma. Rehabil Psychol, 1986; 31:203–215.
7. Gronwall D: Cumulative and persisting effects of concussion on attention and cognition. In Levin HS, Eisenberg HM, Benton AL (eds): Mild Head Injury. New York: Oxford University Press, 1989; pp 153–162.
8. Mateer CA: Systems of care for post-concussive syndrome. In Horn LJ, Zasler ND (eds): Rehabilitation of post-concussive disorders. Philadelphia: Hanley and Belfus, 1992; pp 143–160.
9. Hagen C: Language disorders in head trauma. In Holland A (ed): Language Disorders in Adults. San Diego: College-Hill Press, 1984; pp 247–281.
10. Gronwall D, Wrightson P: Delayed recovery of intellectual function after minor head injury. Lancet, 1974; 2:605–609.
11. Gronwall D, Wrightson P: Cumulative effects of concussion. Lancet, 1975; 2:995–997.
12. Levin HS, Mattis S, Ruff RM, et al.: Neurobehavioral outcome following minor head injury: A three center study. J Neurosurg, 1987; 66:234–243.
13. Leininger BE, Kreutzer JS: Neuropsychological outcome of adults with mild traumatic brain injury: implications for clinical practice and research. In Horn LJ, Zasler ND (eds): Rehabilitation of post-concussive disorders. Philadelphia: Hanley and Belfus, 1992; pp 169–182.
14. Leininger BE, Gramling SE, Farrel AD, et al.: Neuropsychological deficits in symptomatic minor head injury patients after concussion and mild concussion. J Neurol Neurosurg Psychiatry, 1990; 53:293–296.
15. Kay T: Neuropsychological diagnosis: Disentangling from multiple determinants of functional disability after mild traumatic brain injury.

In Horn LJ, Zasler ND (ed): Rehabilitation of Post-Concussive Disorders. Philadelphia: Hanley and Belfus, 1992; pp 109–127.

16. Milton SB: Management of subtle cognitive communication deficits. J Head Trauma Rehabil, 1988; 3(2):1–11.

17. Mayer N, Keating D, Rapp D: Skills, routines, and activity patterns of daily living. In Uzzell B, Gross Y (eds): Clinical Neuropsychology of Intervention. Boston: Martinus Nijhoff, 1986; pp 205–222.

18. Miller TK, Halper AS, Cherney LR: Evaluation of communication problems in the traumatic brain injured adult. In Halper AS, Cherney LR, Miller TK (eds): Clinical Management of Communication Problems in Adults with Traumatic Brain Injury. Gaithersburg, MD: Aspen Publishers, Inc., 1991; pp 27–56.

19. Sohlberg MM, Mateer CA: The assessment of cognitive-communicative functions in head injury. Topics Lang Dis, 1989; 9:15–33.

20. Gronwall D: Rehabilitation programs for patients with mild head injury: Components, problems, and evaluation. J Head Trauma Rehabil, 1986; 1:53–62.

21. Gronwall D, Wrightson P: Memory and information processing capacity after closed head injury. J Neurol Neurosurg Psychiatry, 1981; 44:889–895.

22. Sohlberg MM, Mateer CA: Attention Process Training. Puyallup, WA: Association for Neurological Research and Development, 1986.

23. Mateer CA, Sohlberg MM: A paradigm shift in memory rehabilitation. In Whitaker H (ed): Neuropsychological Studies of Nonfocal Brain Damage: Dementia and Trauma. New York: Springer-Verlag, 1988; pp 204–219.

24. Sohlberg MM, Mateer CA: Introduction to Cognitive Rehabilitation: Theory and Practice. New York: Guilford Press, 1989.

25. Cicerone KD: Psychological management of post-concussive disorders. In Horn LJ, Zasler ND (eds): Rehabilitation of Post-Concussive Disorders. Philadelphia: Hanley and Belfus, 1992; 129–141.

— 16

Identification and Remediation of Cognitive-Communication Impairments Following Mild Head Trauma

Kathryn Tomlin and Lana Liberto

Communication is the skill that allows us to perceive, analyze, formulate, express, and modify our ideas, needs, and emotions (1–5). Research (2–4,6–9) and clinical observation are showing that minor injury to the brain can disrupt the effectiveness of these processes. This disruption can then impair an individual's ability to function effectively on emotional, social, and vocational levels. Those who have survived a head injury frequently express that they know something is wrong but they cannot describe what it is. They frequently report that they are "mixed up" or "in a fog."

As therapists, it is our responsibility to identify these cognitive-communication impairments, to determine how they interrelate and affect functioning, to aid the client in his identification of what processes have been affected, and to assist him in the development of compensatory strategies.

In this chapter, specific cognitive skills will be reviewed; however, this does not imply that the brain functions in such an isolated manner. Difficulties are rarely specific to particular cognitive skill areas but, rather, lie in the capacity to integrate these skills in functional performance (1,2,7,9). A physical analogy for this would be learning to swim. Someone who is learning to swim can master the arm movements, the specific leg movements, and the breathing patterns; but it takes practice and integration skills for the person to be able to jump in the water and swim. Therefore, each area will also be addressed within the context of its relationship with the other areas of cognition, emotion, and behavior.

Assessment of Cognitive-Communicative Skills

There are no standardized measures that accurately assess the total integrative cognitive-communication styles of the minor head injured (6,9). Certain subtests of standardized measures (e.g., Detroit Tests of Learning Aptitude [2]) are helpful for gleaning information about specific target areas, but it is necessary to obtain information through various sources in order to have a comprehensive understanding of the person's level of function, both pre- and post-injury. These sources may include school records, work evaluations, and information from family and friends to assess pre-injury levels of function and current observations in structured (e.g., individual speech therapy sessions) and unstructured situations (e.g., interactions with peers at lunch) to assess post-injury levels. Reports from other professionals as well as family members are valuable sources of information when evaluating a person's performance in various contexts.

A comprehensive cognitive-communication skills assessment includes five basic areas:

1. How the person codes and retrieves information
2. How the person organizes information for processing and retrieval
3. How the person reasons and problem-solves
4. How previously learned material affects new learning
5. How language and cognitive deficits affect other areas of function

Area 1: Coding and Retrieving Information (Representational System)

Each individual will give different evidence of his preferred representational system, which will provide the professional with information about how the client processes, retrieves, and organizes information in order to produce an answer. The three primary styles are visual, auditory, and kinethetic (VAK), although the gustatory/olfactory system also influences processing in a more primitive way (10). Each client will exhibit use of all of the primary representational systems, although one will predominate. Clues for determining a person's predominant style can be gleaned from his eye movement while processing, mannerisms, and use of certain verbal predicates. A person with a predominant *visual representational system* tends to look up while processing as he is making pictures, manipulating features, and adding/subtracting components. Of the three systems, people who use the visual strategy tend to think the quickest, talk at a moderate rate, and are creative with visual imagery. The visual person uses predicates which reflect this imagery, such as I *see* what you are saying, I can *picture* that, *Looks* good to me, and That sure *paints a picture*. The person with a predominant *auditory representational system* tends to keep his eyes midline while processing and organizing the words and sounds. He tends to take a little longer to think than the visual person, and is much more methodical, organized, and regimented. The auditory person uses predicates such as That *sounds* right, That *rings* a bell, and It *reads* like . . . A person with a predominant *kinesthetic representational system* tends to look down when processing and focuses on the feelings, either motoric or emotional. Of the three systems, this is the slowest. The kinesthetic person tends to speak at the slowest rate, and uses predicates such as That *feels* right, I need to *touch* base with you, and That *shakes* me up. Although a person will have a predominant style, the other two systems will be present to a lesser extent. The professional watches, listens, and empathize with the client in order to determine his system. It is advisable for the professional to identify his own predominant style, and to familiarize himself with all systems, so that he can communicate with the client in the client's predominant pattern. This is the underlying basis for establishing rapport.

The professional will frequently observe a family member stating something like, "I just can't get him to see the picture, and I've made it as clear as I could." This is followed by the client stating, "I've explained it to her over and over, and she just doesn't seem to hear a word I am saying." It should be clear to the professional that as long as the family member communicates in the visual realm, and the client through his auditory system, there will be poor communication, incongruence, and misunderstanding.

Area 2: Processing and Retrieving Information

Once the client's predominant system is identified, the effectiveness of that system is analyzed to determine the areas of strengths and weaknesses. For many, the processing time is greatly lengthened because a client is jumping from system to system, and is diverging into tangential areas instead of converging on concise, well-formulated concepts; or the strongest system prior to the injury is no longer as efficient owing to the area of brain damage. It is helpful if the professional aids some clients with paced leaders in order best to utilize the predominant system, which assists topic maintenance. In addition, the professional needs to be very respectful of the client's processing, and needs to be careful not to interfere while the client is comparing, contrasting, and organizing information. Observe which strategies are most effective for a client. For example, when coding associated word pairs, an auditory person may benefit from auditory strategies such as mnemonics, embedding the pair into a sentence, or creating short stories; a visual person may benefit from creating a "snapshot" of the words or the image the words create; and a kinesthetic person may be able to code the words by associated what feelings are connected to the words. Observe whether a client utilizes a strategy automatically (and effectively), or tends to just assume that the information will be understood and coded.

Frequently, assessment reveals that the person's predominant system will no longer be as effective as it once was owing to the specific nature of the head injury. An aphasic client whose predominant pattern was auditory is going to find that his auditory strategies are no longer as effective because of the language impairments. An artist, who excelled in visual imagery pre-injury, may find the quality of his work is now very different if he is suffering from visual processing and visual motor deficits.

Observe what strategy appears to be the most efficient for the client and build on that in therapy. Utilize the strongest modality (VAK) to improve the weaker areas. For example, if a client excels in visual memory, but has difficulty with auditory, he will have difficulty learning in a classroom setting and benefiting from taped information. He will be much more successful if he is taught how to convert the information into pictures, graphs, and charts, because that is his strongest modality for storage and retrieval of information.

Area 3: Reasoning and Problem-Solving

It is important to note how a client processes information, retrieves, and organizes in order to produce a formulated answer. For example, when a client is asked a general information question, such as What is the Statue of Liberty?, many areas need to be observed and assessed. For example, Did the client verbally rehearse the question several times? Is there a time delay? Is the client giving evidence of processing, and in what system? Is the information provided in a concise, well-formulated answer, or are the thoughts expressed in a disjointed manner? Is there a paucity of information? Is the answer presented in a self-oriented, egocentric manner? Some suggested areas to observe are abstract versus concrete reasoning patterns, thought flexibility, egocentrism, and inhibition/disinhibition.

If a client answers a question correctly, it cannot be assumed that the process was efficient and logical. For example, when asked to determine what *flagpole*, *giant*, and *house* have in common, and then to add one similiar item, frequently the answer "tree" will be given. The professional must then ask why that was added. A client who has some abstract reasoning ability will explain, "Because they are all tall." Someone who is still reasoning concretely will be likely to state that he added "tree" because he pictured trees and a flagpole around the giant's house.

Problem-solving and reasoning styles can be assessed through various approaches. Does the client interpret proverbs concretely or abstractly? Frequently, a client will be able to interpret an idiom, which shows that abstract skills are returning, but will then have difficulty interpreting proverbs because the level of abstraction is higher. Is he able to find creative uses for objects, or does he fixate on their major functions? (e.g., What can you use a metal hanger for besides hanging up clothing?) Does he factor his physical and cognitive limitations into his solutions? For example, a client may be hemiparetic and wheelchair-bound, but still express that if he saw someone choking, he would get out of his wheelchair and administer the Heimlich manuver.

Area 4: Pre-Injury Learning Styles

It will also be beneficial to determine how much old learning styles interfere with the acquisition of new learning, as it is frequently apparent that the information recalled may include items from the client's remote memory interspersed with some of the new information provided. For example, when working with clients who are taking academic courses, prelearning knowledge and opinions tend to override the new information provided. This is also compounded by decreased thought flexibility and self-orientation, which causes the client to disregard new input or input which would cause him to modify his existing concepts.

Pre-injury skills also influence how new learning occurs. If the client had a tendency to be disorganized prior to his injury, that will be exacerbated. It is beneficial to be familiar with the client's pre-injury manner of interacting with peers, family, and authority figures. Determine what strategies the client was successful with prior to the injury and utilize them in the therapeutic program. Developing strategies around pre-injury styles will increase the client's success and motivation. Some suggested areas to assess are the following

1. Reading style—amount, what types of material were of interest.
2. How did the client retain information—rehearsal, lists, notes, systems of reminders, practice, etc.?
3. What kinds of instruction best suited the client—teaching, lectures, hands-on experience, trial and error, studying graphs and pictures, copying the information, etc.?

4. Communication style—speaker versus listener skills, follower versus a leader, interpersonal skills, ability to understand another person's viewpoint, non-verbal communication styles, etc.

Area 5: Effects on Other Areas of Function

The manner of assessment will affect the reliability and validity of data collected. For example, a client may be able to sequence, organize, and problem-solve verbally but then not be able to execute this process in behavior. One client who had suffered a mild head injury was able to state how he would write, organize, and send out memos at work but, in actuality, was calling his wife several times a day to ask her how to spell certain words and to confirm that the intent of the memo was actually conveyed in the manner in which he had written it. Another client was able to explain, in detail, how he would arrange to get his broken stereo fixed but then was not able to execute his plan owing to decreased ability to use the telephone book, make a phone call, communicate with the serviceman, disconnect the stereo to take it to the shop, or even to arrange to get it to the shop.

The interplay of different impairments with various cognitive abilities should be determined. Since non-standardized measures are used, it is crucial that assessment strategies be as closely related to the actual practical skills as possible, and that evaluation data be interpreted within the limitations of the testing situations. For example, a client may be able to perform complex tasks in a quiet setting but then have difficulty doing a simple task in a work situation because of attention/distractibility difficulties. Results can also be substantiated through neuropsychological testing.

Summary

In summary, the professional assessing the cognitive-communication skills of a client with minor head injury must use a combination of information gleaned from specific subtests of standardized tests and from observation in structured and in unstructured therapy and life situations. The evaluator should look at the processing/reasoning style, the effective strategies the client maintained, the strategies which are now proving ineffective, and the interplay of the integration of the various processes.

Intervention

Attention and Concentration

With all the energy the client is putting into integrating thinking and behavior, it is understandable that attention/concentration skills would show a marked decrease. A client may attend to some of the information presented in his primary representation system and disregard any information presented in his secondary systems. Since the ability to discriminate salient features is reduced, the person may attend to anything that catches the eye or ear. As a result, the person may neglect many of the relevant aspects of a situation because he or she is overwhelmed by the excess stimuli. Also, when abstract language skills are decreased or distorted, the client may tune out just because he does not understand or finds it "boring." Likewise, when processing speed is slowed, clients may be unable to keep pace with the information and may find it easier to turn to inner thoughts. If speaker/listener skills are poor, he may be totally unaware that there are many aspects of the interaction to attend to such as facial expression, voice tonality, or other persons' conversations.

There are many structured tasks and computer programs that focus on attention and concentration. The client is frequently aware of having difficulty with this area, because it is something he can recognize and gets feedback about. The significant others frequently report concern about this area and will structure the home and social life in such a manner that the distractions are greatly reduced. The professional should develop a hierarchy that meets the individual's specific needs. Usually it is best to start with minimal distractors and increase them slowly as skills are regained. It is then possible to address situations that require simultaneous attention, or on shifting focus from one activity to another and then back to the original task. The therapy, work, or home situation can be modified to meet the client's needs. Noise level can be varied. Visual distractors can be minimized initially and then slowly be reintroduced. Skills needed for attention and shifting can be taught, or compensation strategies can be instituted. In these ways, the professional works as the external manipulator and guide to the client, family, and employers or teachers.

New Learning

New learning is extremely difficult for a person with a head injury for a number of reasons. Previously learned information may interfere with the acceptance of new information (retroactive inhibition).

Attention deficits may cause loss or distortion of information, since stimuli not attended to fully may never be coded or may be coded only partially. Deficits in thought flexibility may cause the person to reject the acquisition of new information and skills because they do not fit into the rigid framework he has created for himself. Decreased reasoning skills may also cause the client to assume that he has learned the new skills or information when in actuality he has not. Clients and their significant others need to be made aware of these factors, how they may affect functioning, and how the environment can be structured to minimize their effects.

Identification of the person's primary style of learning is a major factor in utilizing that person's strengths for acquiring new knowledge and skills. The first step in this process is to determine the strongest way of assessing and retrieving information, that is, through the visual, auditory, or kinesthetic modality. Once that is identified, new information may be provided primarily through that modality. Professionals who assist the clients with new learning need to be familiar with these patterns and have the flexibility to teach in each modality. This will not insure that total new learning will occur, but it will help the client to utilize his residual skills best. For example, for our clients who are returning to college courses, they need to know how they will best learn and retain the information. As the majority of the classes are taught by lecture, a client with compromised auditory memory skills will need to learn how to create visual memory strategies, possibly record the lectures, diagram information, learn how to take notes that include salient information, and utilize various compensatory techniques. If the client had a predominant visual representational system, and has impaired visual memory, he is going to have difficulty making the mental pictures that he used to in order to code the information. He will have to be taught how to utilize his residual skills in conjunction with auditory strategies. He will need to be retaught some of the strategies that used to come naturally to him. Frequently, he will benefit greatly from first utilizing the strategies on an intentional basis then with transference to automatic use.

Organization Skills

In unstructured verbalizations and written skills, many clients with minor head injury reveal marked difficulty organizing their thoughts, even though in more structured activities they perform within normal limits. The following two examples illustrate this. The first was a verbal response to a question and the second was a written response.

Example 1 (verbal response):
I want to say yes, but . . . but it's probably no. Why do *I* think he did all these things? Well, actually now that I'm thinking about it . . . no, I'm . . . I don't think he, um, did it. He . . . well, I don't know why he would exaggerate to make it seem like he didn't like what he had.

Example 2 (written response):
About 4 years ago, my parents while at a garage sale in Lahaska, they noticed an old VW sitting in a hedgerow. Upon telling me about it, my curiosity running wild I grabbed my bike and rode 10 miles toting a pen + pad seeking information such as serial numbers, code numbers, options, and a general overall description.

This disorganization is one to the most devastating aftermaths of minor head injury, as it affects all levels of functioning and interaction. Thoughts come out uncensored and unorganized. Frequently verbal rehearsal precedes the response. Patients verbalize the incoming information until it makes sense and then chain the response onto the rehearsal. There is also an underlying uncertainty about the appropriateness of the response. They are to deal with feedback from others, such as, "Get to the point," "Don't ramble," or "What are you trying to say," but are still unable to modify their responses.

As with other areas, making the client aware of the characteristics of the behavior can make a major positive impact. Analyzing a spontaneous verbal or written language sample may help awareness and get the process of change well under way. Once the client identifies the problem, he is much better able to make modifications. If the client is not ready for this step, it is better to begin at a lower step on the hierarchy. For example, instruct the client to answer a question in one sentence, and mentally to rehearse what to say before actually saying it. You can also have the client analyze and correct unorganized written material, starting with shorter, easy material and progressing to the more complex. He may also practice with exercises that require convergent thinking or determining subjective from objective information. By creating the external structure and then slowly reducing this structure, the clients are able to internalize the compensatory strategies and use them automatically in functional situations.

Another area of intervention utilizes the significant others who can learn ways to give constructive feedback and structure to the client as skills are regained. This can be provided during observation of the sessions, during family conferences, or during conferences with the significant other and with whichever therapists and professionals are involved in the program.

The client frequently has an awareness of the disorganization but cannot seem to overcome it without external structure, guidance, and training. As one client stated, "My brain went to sleep. I forgot halfway through what I'm doing. I want to do things I used to do . . . depends if my mind is clear." One of the major thrusts of therapy for this client was to help her organize her thoughts and be able to build upon them in an orderly and hierarchical manner.

Thought Flexibility

Thought flexibility, that is, the ability to generate possible alternatives in various situations, is a necessary component in all forms of problem-solving and social interactions. Impairment in this area is a highly significant after effect of head injury. Often, a client may tend to generalize a conclusion to other situations that have at best a tangential relationship to the original situation. The person may also have difficulty modifying the conclusions to fit specific situations. An example of a structured therapy task that reflects this involved instructing the client to formulate three different sentences which include the words *over* and *talk*. One client who was having difficulty with thought flexibility produced the following three sentences:

I'm going to go over and talk to him.
I'm going to go over and talk to the teacher.
I'm going to go over and talk to my grandmother.

Another example of decreased flexibility was provided when a client was asked to name three different things that are usually green in color. He stated, "A tree, a bush, and a plant." This reflects the decreased ability to shift set and use flexibility skills.

Deficits in thought flexibility in social interactions are seen in the head-injured person's limited capacity to take the perspective of another. The egocentric behaviors that typically present with persons with brain injury reflect more cognitive dysfunction in the areas of thought flexibility and perspective-taking than personality factors. As such, interventions in social skills development need to include the prerequisite cognitive skills before interpersonal skills themselves can be changed.

Therapy interventions begin with education of the client about the deficit area and presentation of concrete, simple tasks that involve flexibility, such as providing two meanings for words, dividing items into two categories and then redoing the task with the focus on two different categories, viewing situations from two different viewpoints, or determining pros and cons for situations. As skills develop, complexity of the tasks, both cognitively and interpersonally, is increased until the client is able to engage in conversation and/or look at a situation or problem, deduce the salient features, modify any preconceptions, execute a possible solution, and then—most importantly of all—analyze the effects of the solution and make modifications if necessary.

Impulsivity—Inhibition

Initially, many clients will begin activities or engage in conversation in a manner which reflects difficulty with inhibition of verbalizations or actions. They initiate action before all necessary information has been received and processed adequately. Thus, they are frequently using a trial-and-error approach, which interferes greatly with the smoothness of activity or interaction. Much of their verbalizations contain their vocalized thought processing. They may also embed tangential or unrelated information into these verbalizations. For example, one client, when asked to provide a single sentence to complete this story—*Tom woke up with a fever of 102°. He took two aspirins, but still felt sick*—stated:

It didn't make his fever go down. That happened to me once. After night passes he called the doctor. He had to go see the doctor. The doctor discovered he has staph. Staph...strep throat...antibiotics. He had to take three days off work...I didn't go to work.

Once again, education as to the nature of this problem area is important. It is helpful at times for a client to analyze a language sample for conciseness and for the ability to stay on topic. Tasks that incorporate inhibition, such as responding only to certain visual or auditory stimuli, can aid in regaining this skill. Impulsive actions can be analyzed via videotapes, and then alternative methods can be tried and compared in their effectiveness. As with all other areas, as skills are regained, complexity is increased until the client is able to function in a manner that is consistent with socially acceptable behaviors and more efficient problem-solving strategies.

Memory

Memory impairments in the mildly head-injured client may be very subtle or very evident. The client may be able to recall items that had self-importance attached to them but not be able to recall less self-salient information. He may be able to report that he is aware of times when he had a memory loss, or he may be totally unaware of any instances. Frequently, he will be able to rationalize the instances of memory loss and attribute the cause to anything but the head injury.

The circumstances surrounding the incident will greatly affect the degree to which the memory loss is manifested. If the information is presented in a slow, stress-free manner, the brain-injured person will generally be able to process and code the information. But if distractors, stress elements, time delay, or time pressures are present, the chances of the information's not being coded will be greatly increased.

Intervention involves improving awareness and training the client to take sufficient time to code the information and to utilize a self-initiated approach to check to insure that the information has been coded in a manner that will reliably stimulate recall of the information when needed.

Evaluation of the memory, frequently by the neuropsychologist, will provide the therapist with valuable information as to the difference between visual and auditory skills. Frequently, one of the areas shows greater strength then the other. Coding strategies (or lack of using strategies) will be manifested during the testing. Observe the processes used and their level of effectiveness. Some clients will spontaneously use chunking for recalling serial items, when others will "assume" they will be able to recall the information, and utilize no overt strategy and recall a minimum of the information. Others will use imagery, paired associations, mnemonics, and so on, but with limited success because salient components of the process have been neglected. For example, some clients, when coding a paired association, will be able to report the two pieces of information but develop no association that will stimulate the recall. As an illustration, a client may report that she has to pick up a gallon of milk on the way home, but when asked how she will remember to do that, will state, "Oh, I'll just remember." At that point, the chances are extremely good that the milk will be forgotton, so training for various techniques will be reviewed. Some suggestions may include writing a note and taping it to her purse; planning a driving route home which will include passing the market which would provide a visual stimulus; or coding a tactile cue (e.g., when you touch the "cold" door handle you will be reminded of "cold" milk). Later in this section a multimodality triggering and recall approach will be reviewed.

The effectiveness of the client's ability to learn and utilize strategies will be affected by the individual's predominant representational system. If the client had a predominant auditory learning system, it will be advantageous if the auditory memory has retained some strengths and these can be built on in therapy; but if the "auditory" person has the greater impairment in his auditory memory, then new foundations need to be taught, and the client must be guided into developing, understanding, and using visual strategies to aid the impaired auditory channel.

It is recommended that new learning, whether for memory strategies or other cognitive-communication areas, be presented via the strongest channel, in the most effective manner, and that checks be made to determine whether material (part or in its entirety) is coded in a way that will lead to retrieval.

If it is discovered that only portions of the new learning have been coded, then the likelihood of distortion and incorrect assumptions is greatly enhanced. The therapist will then need to determine what and how the "lost" information can be retaught in a manner which minimizes distortion and assumption making.

Initially, these memory foundation skills are taught and used on an intentional basis. As speed and accuracy improves, note how well the skills are transferring to an automatic level. It may benefit the client to receive feedback on times when the therapist notes the effective use of a strategy, and for when it appears that there was an ineffective process which resulted in failure to retain all or part of the information.

It has benefited some clients to make a list (either an actual list or a mental list), and then to establish a system to insure that each item on the list was addressed at the proper time. For clients that exhibit impulsivity, this method will often reduce the frequency of memory-loss incidents. Such clients may benefit from a visual image of "stepping back and reviewing a mental list" in order to insure that all matters have been attended to. For example, one client actually "forgot" to get dressed for a wedding and attended it in very casual clothes. He was in such a rush with the rest of the family that it never occurred to him to get dressed in the clothes he had actually preplanned to wear. He had no awareness of his "error" until the service was in progress. This case illustrates how memory loss can be enhanced or actually caused by impulsivity.

The most effective means of retaining information appears to be coding with use of all three representational systems (visual, auditory, tactile/kinethetic); the stimuli that are being used to recall the information are also coded in all three systems. In the same example of the woman who needs to buy milk on the way home from therapy, coding could be done in the following manner (which encompasses all of the modalities):

	Triggering stimuli	Item to recall
Visual	When she goes out to her *white* car	Reminded of *white* milk
Auditory	When she *hears* idling of car engine	*Hears* the milk pouring
Tactile/kinesthetic	When she *feels* cold gear shift	*Feels* the cold milk

The strategy will require practice by the therapist, so that it can be taught effectively. In order to code accurately, the person will need to make a representation of the appropriate trigger in all three modalities, and then add on the visual, auditory, and kinesthetic aspects of what he wants to remember.

The nature of memory is extremely complicated and integrated into all areas of cognitive-communication. A client will benefit from knowing this, because it will answer questions, such as, "Why can I remember something in one situation, but not in another?" The therapist's role is to help him to build the foundations, and be his guide, so that he is then able to add the structure onto the foundation.

Abstract/Inferential Reasoning

Being able to use and/or interpret inferential abstract reasoning is greatly affected by pre-injury skills. It is highly beneficial if the therapist develops a picture of how the pre-injury skills were manifested. This can be gleaned from school or work records, from writing samples, and from reports from those who know the client on a more personal level. Ask what his humor was like—was he a punster, joke-cracker, producer of straight-faced dry humor, did he tend to not understand the punchline, etc. Information can also be gleaned from the kind of the reading material that was of primary interest. Did he prefer magazines (what kind?), the newspaper, novels, textbooks, etc.? The therapist must be careful not to make inaccurate assumptions from the information, but this knowledge will aid in determining reasoning style and selecting therapeutic materials.

Clients will benefit from various approaches to this area. Inferences can be determined about pictures, paragraphs, stories, math situations, life situations, and so on. As skills develop, areas can be overlapped, e.g., a paragraph under a picture, requiring information from each to be integrated in order to interpret it accurately; different levels of comic cartoons, ranging from purely visual one-frame cartoons to an integration of the punchline with the picture to multiple frames.

There will be situations in which the client has a basic idea of the inferential content but will be unable to explain the meaning in a cohesive manner. The following is an example of a client's attempt to explain why a man decided to dye his hair, which was explained in a metaphorical story:

Right, so doesn't that mean he would, he felt that it wouldn't be, it would be not such a drastic thing as it would be something like, like an accessory; you know, something like, . . . yeah.

Well, it, before he did it, like before he dyed his hair and got all this courage or whatever you call it. You know he would act the way he did in the first couple of paragraphs.

In many aspects, this example demonstrates how various cognitive-communication difficulties integrate and make communication ineffective. This client was demonstrating difficulties with thought organization, integration, verbal cohesiveness, maintaining train of thought, word-finding, relevancy, and with hierarchical building on sentences and content.

There will be a tendency for a concrete reasoning pattern to predominate at first, then a mixed pattern will emerge, followed by the ability to utilize abstract skills in a fuller range. For example, the next three samples are from the same client at various stages in her rehabilitation program. The task was for her to state her interpretation of the proverb An apple a day keeps the doctor away.

Response at time of initial evaluation (approximately one week post-injury):

Well, that's right. Well, if you eat an apple, the doctor will stay away—just what it says.

Response approximately eight weeks post-injury:

Yeah, I've heard that...it means if you eat an apple which are good for you, you won't need to see a doctor because you won't get sick as often.

Response approximately five months post-injury:

The apple stand for healthy food—so, let's see...if you eat healthy foods, you'll stay healthier and won't have to see the doctor because you won't get sick as much.

Here are some suggested activities for developing different levels of abstract reasoning:

Lower level	Interpretation of idioms, slang, expressions in our language
	Interpreting concrete-level jokes
	Paraphrasing idioms in sentences
	Making basic inferences about pictures (e.g., "I know it's winter because there's snow on the gound")
Middle level	Proverb interpretation
	Matching punchlines to jokes
	Putting the frames of comic strips in order
	Interpreting how voice tones and word accents change sentence meaning
	Stating opinions and explaining other people's opinions

	Labeling emotions conveyed in situations and pictures
	Determining consequences from specific actions/situation
Higher level	Interpreting cartoons and comic strips
	Reading and interpreting metaphoric stories
	Interpreting poetry
	Interpreting pictures and captions
	Analyzing other people's opinions and viewpoints
	Using humor and abstract language in structured situations and in conversation
	Analyzing how different actions will result from various approaches

Speaker/Listener Skills

The therapist involved will want to aid the client in developing an equal balance between listening and speaking skills. The client who has difficulties with initiation will need to develop "speaker" skills. The client who is exhibiting difficulty inhibiting verbalizations will need to develop "listener" skills. Training for being aware of and accurately interpreting the partner's nonverbal cues (facial expressions, hand gestures, body language, etc.), pitch, tone, word emphasis, stress, and so on is of primary importance, too. The progress achieved in establishing these skills will also be affected by pre-injury skills.

Therapy will initially focus on these areas at a highly intentional level. As each area is developed, the complexity can be increased, and the client can develop the skills with transference to automatic usage. As these skills are developed, the client can then be taught to focus on the rules of discourse and turn-taking.

Direct and indirect teaching of skills needed for communication may also be required. Such things may include teaching how to edit, how to listen, how to talk of things of interest, how to refrain from interrupting, how to avoid talking only about oneself, how to get to the point, how not to offend others, how to discuss things so an argument does not result, and how to include others in a conversation.

Integration

Each of the preceding areas was presented in a primarily isolated manner, but their effects on a person's ability to communicate manifest themselves in an integrated, compounded manner. Other areas also impinge upon communication, such as behavior, orientation to purpose, awareness of how deficits interfere with functioning, extra-linguistic features, pragmatics, insight, judgment, and so on. There are virtually no human actions that involve only one executive thinking function.

This chapter has given a very broad overview of many multifaceted areas. In actuality, an entire book could be written on each area. A metaphor that has proved useful for assisting the client or significant others in understanding what is transpiring is to compare the brain to a filing cabinet (or computer). The brain injury caused the effect of something dumping out all of the files on the floor and mixing them up. The initial phases of therapy focus on getting the files back into the drawers, followed by improving their organization so they can be used effectively. This is followed by establishing an efficient cross-referencing system. The integration phase of therapy, although addressed indirectly throughout the entire therapy course, focuses on specific training for and applications of integrating the executive thinking skills.

When the client progresses to this level, the therapist needs to utilize extensive creativity when devising therapeutic tasks. Actual community, life-experience situations are needed at this point, with mutual analysis of successes and failures. Structured therapy tasks will need to reflect a level of complexity and length that is suitable for the client's needs at the time and must be designed to complement the client's pre-injury style of functioning and capabilities.

Multifaceted tasks need to have varied executive thinking skills layered into them. For example, a memory task could be layered with abstract reasoning, sustained attention with noise and/or visual distractors present, and flexible problem-solving with a time constraint. This could mean that the client is provided with a metaphorical narrative to read during a limited period of time in a noisy, busy clinic, with instructions to recall the salient details and provide at least two ways the content could be interpreted and at least three suggestions for how the characters could use the situation in future life experiences.

There are endless possibilities for a therapist to meet each person's specific needs creatively. Initially, brain injury seems frustrating, if not hopeless. However, with patience, sensitivity, special training, and especially imagination, the therapist can make an invaluable contribution through recognition and remediation of cognitive-communication impairments in this exciting and gratifying client population.

References

1. Benton A: Behavioral consequences of closed head injury. CNS Trauma Res Status Rep, 1979; pp 221–231.
2. Condeluci A, Gretz-Lasky S: Social role valorization: A model for community reentry. J Head Trauma Rehabil, 1987; 2(1):49–56.
3. Lezak MD: Subtle sequelae of brain damage: perplexity, distractibility, and fatigue. Am J Phys Med, 1978; 57:9–15.
4. Mentis M, Prutting CA: Cohesion in the discourse of normal and head-injured adults. J Speech Hear Res, 1987; 30:88–98.
5. Sarno MT: Verbal impairment after closed head injury: Report of a republication study. J Nerv Ment Dis, 1984; 172:475–479.
6. Diller L, Gordon WA: Interventions for cognitive deficits in brain-injured adults. J Consult Clin Psychol, 1981; 49:822–834.
7. Liles BZ, Coelho CA, Duff RJ, Zalagens MR: Effects of elicitation procedures on the narratives of normal and closed head-injured adults. J Speech Hear Res, 1989; 54(3):356–366.
8. Milton SB: Management of subtle cognitive communication deficits. J Head Trauma Rehabil, 1988; 3(2):1–11.
9. Milton SB, Wertz R: Management of persisting communication deficits in patients with traumatic brain injury. Clinical Neuropsychology of Intervention. Boston: Martinus Nijhoff Publishing Co., 1986, pp 223–257.
10. Bandler R, Grinder J: Frogs into Princes—Neurolinguistic Programming. Moab, UT: Real People Press, 1979.

— 17

Cognitive Rehabilitation

Lana Liberto, Kathryn Tomlin, Karen Lutz, Lynn Nash,
and Sarita Schapiro

Medical and surgical advances during the past decade have improved the survival rates of persons with traumatic brain injury. Concurrently, the need for appropriate rehabilitation strategies to assist in the recovery of these individuals has increased (1). The traditional model of rehabilitation uses a *multi*disciplinary team approach to treatment management. Using discipline-specific modalities, this approach utilizes the special expertise of each discipline in addressing individual deficit areas—for example, mobility in physical therapy; activities of daily living, in occupational therapy.

The person with a traumatic brain injury, however, presents a unique challenge to the rehabilitation professional. Here the pattern of deficits and remaining abilities affects all levels of a person's functioning, requiring an *inter*disciplinary perspective, integrating all areas of expertise in a holistic treatment approach. Berrol (2) makes a useful distinction between cognitive retraining and cognitive rehabilitation. He sees cognitive retraining as a systematic approach to improve intellectual deficits that interfere with information processing. Cognitive rehabilitation aims at functional adaptation in activities of daily life. The distinction becomes clearer when we look at the typical deficits seen in those persons with mild brain injury and the effects these impairments have on emotional, social, vocational, and sexual functioning.

In the cognitive area, subtle attention/concentration deficits may interfere with processing incoming information, such as instructions from employers, family information from partners, or the plot of a movie. This inattention compounds general memory deficits. Impairments in abstract thinking and the ability to generate alternative solutions can limit the affected person's capacity to solve problems in daily living or at the job. This reduced thought flexibility is also related to difficulties in taking the perspective of others. The inability to understand how others have different feelings and opinions can have profound effects on interpersonal relationships and social skills.

The capacity to solve problems is further influenced by changes in emotional functioning, ranging from emotional lability to restricted affective response. Stress of any kind can reduce cognitive performance and elicit more intense emotional reactions than usual. Alternatively, some persons show reduced emotional response with limited facial expression. Both types of responses can alter relationships within family, work, and community. On a physical level, we can also see deficits in body integration, expecially when the person is stressed cognitively. Even an activity as simple as walking down the hall and talking simultaneously can present a major problem for a head-injured individual. This problem can have a significant impact on an adolescent who must navigate high-school halls between classes, for example. Moving one's body in space in a coordinated manner is also related to many vocations (e.g., mechanics) and recreational activities (e.g., dancing, sports).

As a result of these remediation challenges, we have developed a program of assessment, treatment, and follow-up that addresses not only the individual skills needed, but also how each skill relates to others and how they become integrated in functional living activities. In order to do this, professionals in each discipline spent a great deal of time learning about each other's areas of expertise, terminology, and methods. This resulted in negotiating a common language to assist all team members in communicating more effectively among themselves and with clients on a consistent basis. This process also forced team members to clarify their own thinking about what they observed, what theoretical models were useful, and what specific treatment strategies would be effective. Not only did this process foster stronger teamwork skills among professionals, but it also emphasized the need to develop a strong working partnership between the professional team and the patient in order to secure success in rehabilitation. Without respect for the patient's own goals and needs, no matter what cognitive deficits are present, the success of any intervention strategy is significantly limited.

Assessment

Applying the concepts of interdisciplinary teamwork and integration of cognitive/emotional skills, we arrive at the process approach to evaluation. The patient is assessed by all team members, including the following: physician/Physiatrist, physical therapist, occupational therapist, recreational therapist speech-language pathologist, psychologist, neuropsychologist, and social worker. Although each member is assessing areas specific to his/her discipline, each is also evaluating how these specific areas relate to all other areas of function. For example, the physical therapist may be evaluating strength, endurance, and coordination while he or she is assessing the patient's social skills, memory, attention, and problem-solving within a stressful situation.

The process approach to evaluation also requires the team members to observe *how* an individual proceeds with an activity—not just the end result or answer. For some disciplines, such as occupational therapy, this is a routine method, whereas the concept is relatively new to the field of neuropsychology (3). Using the process approach, a team member observes what strategies a person uses to code, retrieve, and process information and how this information is used to solve a problem or complete a motor activity. Since cognitive rehabilitation will address this process, it is important that the team members be aware of inefficient or inaccurate strategies even though at times the patient reaches correct solutions.

The assessment procedures also include the *Performance Progress Profile*, developed by the interdisciplinary team at Doylestown Hospital Rehabilitation Center (Table 17.1). This instrument was devised because there appeared to be no comprehensive protocol available that addressed specific cognitive areas within a developmental hierachy, integrating the lower-level skills with more complex skills involving emotional and social factors. The profile was created after addressing 15 areas of function from the most basic mental tracking skills to high-level perspective-taking skills required in complex social interactions. Each of these 15 areas is then evaluated within five to seven levels of functions, taking into consideration factors such as complexity of task, time required to complete a task, and the ability to function with or without stress factors. The fifteen areas include 1) attention, concentration, mental tracking; 2) visual-motor integration; 3) tactile-motor integration; 4) motor integration; 5) auditory perception; 6) visual and auditory memory; 7) processing speed; 8) thought organization; 9) oral expression; 10) written expression; 11) auditory comprehension; 12) reading comprehension; 13) independent living skills; 14) reasoning; and 15) social skills.

Treatment Planning

Once all team members have evaluated the patient, it is necessary to integrate the information from the various perspectives into one comprehensive treatment plan that all team members, including the

Table 17.1. Doylestown hospital rebabilitation center performance progress profile.

	Date of Team Review
Patient's Name:	

Ranchos Los Amigos Level of Cognitive Functioning:

Attention/Concentration/Mental Tracking
1. 1–5 minutes with maximum supervision and/or structure
2. 5–30 minutes with moderate supervision and/or structure
3. 5–30 minutes with minimum supervision and/or structure with some resistance to distraction and awareness of time limitations
4. 5–30 mins. with min. supervision/structure, despite distractions
5. able to complete structured tasks without supervision
6. able to attend to and complete unstructured tasks without supervision and independently adheres to time limits

Visual-Motor Integration
1. able to use isolated/foundation visual/perceptual skills for ADL's; direct assistance/supervision provided prn.
2. able to use isolated, foundation vis/per. skills for ADL's, s̄ assist/sup., although may require increased time and trial & error learning experiences
3. able to integrate and generalize foundation skills to a functionally simple task, consisting of 1–2 components
4. able to integrate and generalize foundation skills to a functional multistep task, with decreased speed
5. able to plan and execute highly integrative visual/perceptual skills for various tasks and settings, with normal speed.

Tactile/Motor Integration
1. able to discrim. bet. sim. objs. by texture, size and weight, c̄ vision occl.
2. able to manipulate objects in direct contact with one's body; vision occluded and extended time
3. able to manip. objs. in direct contact c̄ one's body vis. occl. & approp. speed
4. able to manip. objs/tools in relation to each other c̄ vis. occl. & ext. time
5. able to manipulate objects/tools, in relation to each other with vision occluded, in a safe and time efficient manner

Motor Integration
1. able to navigate in an uncoordinated, disorganized manner with decreased awareness of environment and people
2. able to coordinate self within a highly structured environment with intentional planning and with decreased speed
3. able to coordinate self in the environment without conscious effort when no cognitive stressors are present
4. able to coordinate & integrate motor patterns without conscious effort while processing cognitive & emotional stimuli—with increased time

Table 17.1. *Continued*

5. able to coordinate & integrate motor patterns without conscious effort while processing cognitive & emotional stimuli—no time constraints

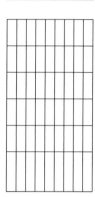

Auditory Perception
1. able to discriminate between environmental sounds & respond to the appropriate one
2. able to maint. attention to task and screen out low level non-essential sds
3. able to maint. attention to task and screen out high level non-essential sds
4. able to shift attention from task to distraction, & return attent. to task
5. able to attend to multiple auditory stimuli in social situations
6. able to use selective auditory perception in all environments and situations as relevant to the person's needs

Visual Memory   Auditory Memory

Visual Memory and Auditory Memory
1. does not use any perceivable memory strategies
2. able to use memory recognition strategies
3. able to use various memory strategies on an intentional basis with coaching for low to mid complexity stimuli
4. able to use various memory strategies on an intentional basis w/out coaching for low to mid complexity stimuli
5. able to use mem. strats. on an automatic basis for low to mid complexity stim.; carryover into incidental emerging
6. able to utilize intentional and incidental memory strats. automatically for mid to high complexity stimuli

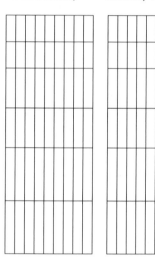

Processing Speed
1. able to complete a low cognitive challenge task with extended time period
2. able to complete a low cognitive challenge task w/in functional time frame
3. able to complete a mod. cognitive challenge task with w/in funct. time frame
4. able to complete a multi-factor complex task w/in functional time frame

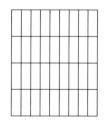

Thought Organization
1. able to organize and carryout basic self-care activities by following a structured routine
2. able to organize and perform daily activities c̄ consist. external feedback

Table 17.1. *Continued*

3. able to organize and perform familiar activities c̄
   intermittent feedback
4. able to organize and perform activities requiring new
   learning with intermittent feedback
5. able to analyze and store info. in an organized and flexible
   manner; & able to use the salient info. in the approp.
   context s̄ stress factors present
6. able to analyze and store info. in an organ. & flex. manner;
   & able to use the salient information in the appropriate
   context when normal stress factors are present

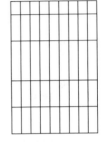

Oral Expression
1. able to verbalize in concrete, egocentric, disorganized manner
2. able to verbalize in more goal-directed fashion, but content
   remains concrete, egocentric and perseverative
3. able to verbalize in a more complex and less perseverative
   manner, with tendency to fixate, but content is concrete and
   egocentric
4. able to verbalize in a concrete manner with the emergence of
   abstraction
5. able to verbalize in a full range of concrete and abstract
   language

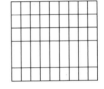

Writing
1. able to write words and phrases
2. able to write simple and compound sentences
3. able to write complex sentences &/or concrete paragraphs
4. able to write at paragraph level, using concrete and abstract
   language
5. able to write functional narratives

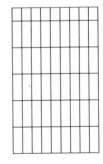

Auditory Comprehension
1. able to follow short concrete statements and simple
   instructions; needs frequent repetition and gestural or visual
   cues
2. able to follow concrete statements/instructions; needs
   occasional repetition and gestural or visual cues
3. able to process complex concrete stimuli but processing is
   slow, distorted and egocentric
4. able to process complex concrete and abstract stimuli but
   processing is slow and frequently distorted
5. able to efficiently and accurately process abstract complex
   input

Reading comprehension
1. able to comprehend written words and phrases
2. able to comprehend simple and compound sentences
3. able to comprehend complex sentences and/or concrete
   paragraphs
4. able to comprehend the literal and inferential meaning in
   paragraphs
5. able to comprehend the literal and inferential meaning in
   narratives
6. able to comprehend the literal and inferential/abstract
   meaning in books

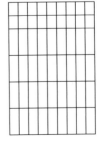

Table 17.1. *Continued*

ADL (Independent Living Skills)
1. requires frequent or constant supervision for organ. of self-care activs. with or without physical assistance to complete
2. requires occasional supervision for organization of self-care activities with or without physical assistance to complete
3. able to be left alone for a few hours & take care of immediate needs; may still need assistance for care
4. able to organize self-care & basic homemaking skills but needs supervision monitoring for community reintegration
5. able to live independently, with or without support services

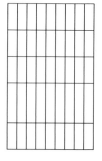

Reasoning
1. able to reason in a limited concrete random manner with no awareness of cause and effect
2. able to reason in a limited concrete manner with cause and effect related to immediate needs
3. able to reason in a highly egocentric manner with minimal awareness of external feedback
4. able to interpret & utilize abstract reasoning inconsistently and able to modify behavior by utilizing internal and external feedback
5. able to utilize flexible abstract reasoning within intellectual capacity

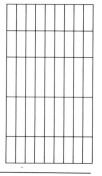

Social Skills
1. able to respond to environ. in an egocentric and undifferentiated manner
2. able to differentiate between others in the environment but with an egocentric and inappropriate manner
3. able to interact with others in a simplistic and egocentric manner, with no awareness of the effect of his/her behavior on others
4. able to recognize feedback and perspective of others, but has difficulty integrating the information in order to modify behavior to the situation
5. able to interact with others appropriately, use feedback, and demonstrates the ability to take the perspective of others

Education:
 Pre-injury Status:
 Discharge Status:

Employment:
 Pre-injury Status:
 Discharge Status:

Mobility:
 Pre-injury Status:
 Discharge Status:

Driving:
 Pre-injury Status:
 Discharge Status:

For intermediate status updates, please refer to chart and to treatment notes.
© 1992 Doylestown Hospital

patient, will use to develop and monitor treatment modalities. The professional team meets and formulates goals within five basic areas: 1) physical skills, 2) independent living skills, 3) cognition, 4) language, and 5) psychosocial/vocational skills. In a traditional model specific disciplines would be responsible for each area, for example, physical therapist for physical goals, occupational therapist for vocational and independent living skills, speech-language pathologist for cognition and language, and the psychologist for psychosocial skills. In contrast, with the brain-injury rehabilitation model, all team members may address all goals in some fashion.

An illustration of this process can be seen in the case of J., who had negotiated a goal for himself with the team to be able to participate appropriately in the high-school senior prom. In order to accomplish this goal, various deficits needed to be addressed: reduced balance and coordination, slowed processing speed, impaired thought organization, poor social skills in eating, reduced ability to process simultaneous stimuli, and poor self-confidence. As a result, multiple treatment modalities across disciplines were employed. The physical therapist scheduled two sessions per week to practice dancing to his favorite music. The speech-language pathologist continued to focus on increasing processing and thought organization and internalizing his verbal rehersal so conversation would be more appropriate. The occupational therapist and recreational therapist worked with J. on eating behaviors, giving him direct feedback from real situations, such as a trip to the hospital snack bar or a group picnic. The psychologist assisted J. in integrating his improvements in these areas to increase his self-confidence and self-esteem.

Once the treatment team has formulated the initial goals, a copy of the treatment plan is given to all team members and a copy is kept in the patient's medical chart for ongoing reference and modification. All team members sign this chart copy to verify their agreement with the plan. Also at this time, the Performance Progress Profile is reviewed and discussed so agreement is reached on the patient's current level of functioning. The patient may also receive a copy for his/her logbook. If the complexity is too great, a modified version may be prepared with the patient so it can act as a useful tool for the patient to assess his or her own progress and to understand the rationale behind the requests of the therapists.

Patient and Family as Team Members

Once the professional team members have developed a treatment plan from their assessment of and discussion with the patient, they present the plan to the patient and his or her significant others.

At this time, any feedback or modification can be incorporated to increase compliance by the patient and reinforcement and support from the significant others. The "significant others" may include not only family members, but also attorneys, insurance representatives, rehabilitation specialists, or educational/vocational persons involved with the patient's school or work. In this way, an integrated supportive network is created to enhance a consistent approach to the rehabilitation program.

The Comprehensive Cognitive Rehabilitation Program

Although the comprehensive cognitive rehabilitation model is applicable for all levels of brain dysfunction, it is particularly useful for those individuals who have sustained a minor head injury. Because most of these persons are functioning at a relatively high level, it is crucial that interventions be immediately relevant to daily life. This model presupposes integration of cognition and personality from the initial assessment on throughout the follow-up process.

Once the initial treatment plan is developed and accepted by the treatment team, including the patient and significant others, an intensive outpatient rehabilitation program begins, involving approximately six hours a day, five days a week. This schedule is based on the specific goals established and therefore varies with each individual. For example, for J., who plans to return to college, the schedule would include not only physical therapy, occupational therapy, speech-language therapy, and psychotherapy, but also social skills training and cognitive therapy with a tutor who incorporates cognitive skill training with study skills and academic tutoring.

In a different situation, a young woman, L., was to return to work as a billing clerk in an insurance company, as well as taken an evening college-level course. Her schedule included not only the cognitive/academic tutoring, but also job coaching sessions onsite to assist her in relearning premorbid skills and in adjusting the work environment to compensate better for her deficit areas, such as reduced attention and concentration. Thus, various types, formats, and locations of treatment are called for in order to optimize rehabilitation of individuals with minor brain injury.

One of the first tools supplied to the patient is a logbook, a three-ring notebook, to serve as an ancillary memory device and a vehicle of communication among therapists and significant others. If organizational deficits warrant it, the patient receives a notebook containing an outline of each day's schedule with space allotted to record a therapist's name and specific tasks accomplished in each session. If skills are on a higher level, the person may receive only a schedule for the week and blank notebook pages to organize his/her own daily routine and accomplishments. For those persons with significant short-term memory impairments, we encourage family members to record important events or activities so that the therapists can increase retention of these events as well as verify the input from the patient. The information in the logbook is reviewed with the patient on a daily basis within a group setting at the end of the day. During this time he/she gets to review and sequence the day's events, develop insight into areas of difficulty and of success, and set specific therapy goals for the following day. This group may be led by team members from any of the disciplines who have been trained in group format. This allows a view of the patient in a context different from the professional's specific skill area.

The choice of group and individual treatment permits a broader range of skills to be trained and integrated into functional behavior. All patients receive individual sessions to some degree. Here, specific one-to-one relations can develop and stimuli can be reduced to a manageable level for each person's needs. As the patient improves, the level of stimulation and complexity can be adjusted by the therapist to provide more challenge and closer simulation of real world situations. Here computer-assisted therapy is especially useful, but it requires that a professional be present to monitor progress and teach strategies for learning and compensation.

Group treatment, however, more closely approximates the world of school, work, and family. The head-injured person can develop higher-level abilities to screen out distractions; comprehend and process salient information; and perhaps most importantly, learn to utilize appropriate social behavior. In the comprehensive rehabilitation model being described, the person may be involved in various types of group interaction, including cognitive retraining (Cognitive Module), social skills training, recreation and leisure counseling, independent living skills, and physical therapy groups.

Before we discuss group treatment techniques in more detail, it is important to note the paucity of appropriate therapeutic materials available for remediating the higher-level cognitive deficits, whether on a individual or group basis. Many of the materials used in the program have been developed by team members to suit the specialized needs of each individual patient. As patterns have emerged in kinds of instruments and activities needed, the arsenal of therapeutic tools has increased. Most materials available traditionally in most rehabilitation disciplines address the more basic functions that are severely or moderately-to-severely compromised. However, individuals with a minor head injury require intervention at a more subtle level, concentrating on the capacity to integrate the intact functions (4). Also, because these persons are more aware of and involved in normal life situations than more severely injured persons, relevant and interesting tasks are essential to ensure compliance with treatment and generalization into the work, school, or home environment. Consequently, the treatment team members need to possess the skills they ask of their patients—flexibility, creativity, and commitment—in order to augment standard intervention strategies with original, relevant materials to address specific functions and their integration into activities of daily living. This includes using all sensory modalities, particularly visual, auditory, and kinesthetic, to facilitate learning. Examples of these types of tasks will be discussed as we look more closely at the use of groups in cognitive rehabilitation.

The Cognitive Module is a group process that focuses on multiple cognitive and language skills within the structure of specific exercises. The group meets daily for one hour, and each group member receives a booklet containing tasks to be completed for the week. A minimum of two group leaders is present within a group of five to eight. Because of the diversity of skill level in any group of persons with head injury, it is crucial that the leaders be available to monitor and assist each member at his or her own specific level of ability. Activities are led by either the group leaders or by individual members, depending on their skills. For those persons with higher-level dysfunction, the tasks of leading an activity allows them to work on simultaneous attention skills, perspective taking, leadership skills, memory, and organization in an integrated fashion.

The major objectives of this group are not only continued development of specific skills (language, attention, concentration, perceptual-motor skills, memory, reasoning, organization) but also increasing processing speed and acquiring flexibility of thinking and awareness of others. Therefore, members are asked to switch quickly from one type of task to another (e.g., verbal analogies to figure-ground discrimination task), and some tasks have specific time limitations. All members are expected to act socially appropriately and respect divergent points of views. Opinion questions are frequently used to assist members in learning to accept different perspectives as well as to learn to formulate their own opinion concisely and objectively. Exercises in comprehending verbal tonalities and nonverbal expressions are also included to increase the members' ability to relate more sensitively to others. Particularly for persons with minor head injury and high-level impairments, more difficult tasks may be assigned, such as observing behaviors within the group and analyzing the consequences of certain interactions between members or members and leaders.

The Physical Therapy group also emphasizes the integration of cognitive, physical, and personality functions. Persons involved in this group need to be relatively physically capable in terms of ambulation, but they may continue to struggle with deficits in coordination, body integration, and strength and endurance. Traditionally, it was not unusual for persons with minor head injury to be excluded from physical therapy unless an orthopedic injury was present. However, we have found that many head-injured people have subtle deficits in body integration, especially if cognitive tasks need to be performed simultaneously with a physical task, a situation typical of everyday life at work, school, or home. Therefore, activities are developed to address this process of thinking and doing simultaneously. An example of such an exercise is an obstacle course that can be constructed inside of outside and modified in complexity to suit the varying levels of the patients involved. Along the course a person is required to perform various physical activities requiring balance, strength, flexibility, and coordination while engaged in following specific instructions, performing mental tasks such as arithmetic, keeping track of number of repetitions of an exercise, and so on, depending on the complexity appropriate for each group. The ability to work in a competitive environment (number of errors of amount of time required to complete the course) creates an environment where social skills can be practiced or new ones learned.

A third group that is most closely related to the real world is the Social Skills group. Within this weekly group session, members have the opportunity to focus on specific interpersonal and communication skills while engaging in activities within the community. Issues like egocentrism, speaker/listener skills, and perspective-taking are discussed; and activities are planned by the group to use and understand these skills. Verbal and nonverbal communication skill are presented and practiced first within the safety of the group setting and then in the community in order to foster generalization. Many persons with minor head injury appear "normal" during superficial contacts. It is not until a more prolonged or intimate relationship is established that subtle difficulties such as mild attention deficits, inflexibility, or poor thought organization become evident. Through this process of ongoing group interaction and group cohesiveness, these areas can be identified in a supportive environment and new skills applied in daily activities. For example, the graduation of a group member from the rehabilitation program became the occasion for a group party. This event required various abilities, including planning the actual event in terms of time, place, food, who to invite; learning to share responsibilities for specific elements of the event; going out in the community to shop for needed materials; and finally communicating among members and guests in a social situation. Because of the complexity of skills addressed in this group, group leaders come from various disciplines, that is, occupational therapy, recreational therapy, and psychology.

Where therapy takes place can be as important as *how* it takes place. As was mentioned earlier, cognitive rehabilitation extends function to daily life; and as such not only activities within the community but also at the workplace are useful for intervention. This process also increases the likelihood of generalization and utilization of learned skills. Prevocational training and job coaching are major components in the comprehensive program. Initially patients may begin in volunteer positions within the rehabilitation facility, where learning to work with a supervisor, organizing and following through in a daily routing, or updating skills may be the goals. For a higher-functioning person, on-the-job evaluation and coaching is the treatment of choice. In this way the cooperation of the employer can be utilized to make any necessary modifications in job responsibilities and work environment, thereby increasing the likelihood of the patient's being successful. Also, specific skills needed for a job can be further developed within the therapy sessions and then transferred to the work environment.

Final components to the comprehensive rehabilitation program are counseling and education of the patient and significant others. All patients receive a minimum of a session a week of individual counseling with a clinical psychologist, and support groups for the survivors and for the significant others meet on a monthly basis. Family and couples counseling is also strongly encouraged throughout the rehabilitation process. As any rehabilitation professional knows, the consistent, supportive involvement of family is a crucial element for achieving positive gains in treatment. Also, trauma such as brain injury affects all persons who have a caring relationship with the survivor.

It is of particular importance in minor head injury that significant others be involved in education about the injury and its sequelae (5). This is crucial in order to facilitate treatment and prevent incorrect diagnosis, which frequently results in persons referred for psychiatric intervention rather than rehabilitation (6). One of the major stressors that persons with mild head injury experience is that others do not understand how their experience of the world has changed and how their emotional reactions have become unpredictable and at times overwhelming (7). Likewise, the survivors themselves need concrete information about how the injury has affected their functioning and what is a reasonable prognosis over time. Also, it is a necessary component of participation in treatment that the patient be made aware of both deficit areas and strengths and how they both relate to the therapeutic tasks presented. With this education comes increased insight into one's disability and a greater chance of a commitment to remediating the deficit areas.

It is also important to note that even though the clinical psychologist has responsibility for individual counseling or psychotherapy, all team members contribute to the education about brain injury and the learning of effective coping strategies to deal with the myriad of emotional and personality changes that can result from such an injury. Only through consistent feedback and successful experiences throughout the program can the person regain self-confidence and a strong sense of self.

Monitoring Progress

As with any therapeutic intervention, results and progress need to be monitored on a regular basis to evaluate completed goals, to modify goals based on the most current level of functioning, to problem-solve more effective intervention strategies, and to assist the team members in processing their own feelings and concerns about treating each patient. This is done every two weeks during "chart rounds." During this time all team members meet to review the individual treatment plan and Performance Progress Profile. Goals that have been reached are noted, new goals are formulated, and others are modified to reflect realistic expectations more accurately. The Performance Progress Profile is updated, giving information on what specific areas need more emphasis or different, more effective strategies. During this time, team members can voice their own frustrations or concerns and receive valuable suggestions for dealing with problem behaviors.

Since both patient and significant others are also team members, periodic conferences are held with the professional team to review the patient's progress and to modify goals. This serves as an excellent opportunity to get information about the patient's carryover of skills into family and community life. Frequently, significant others give a perspective that is rich in insight and observations about where treatment needs to be directed. These conferences are also important at the time of discharge from the formal structure of the rehabilitation program, to enable all members to focus on the application of the regained skills in the current situation and in future endeavors and to give information about the ongoing support available through the follow-up program.

As the current research shows, persons with brain injury of any severity may show changes in function, especially in psychosocial areas, for many months or years after discharge from a structured rehabilitation program (8). It is essential to monitor the transition back into the workplace or school, the family, and the community on an ongoing basis to assist the patient and family in preventing problems, or to intervene when concerns are still within manageable limits. Therefore, it is recommended that persons be scheduled for a follow-up visit at the rehabilitation center one month, three months, six months, and twelve months following discharge and on an annual basis thereafter, if needed. At the time of discharge the team decides who on the team would be most appropriate to see the patient in one month. Depending on the status of the person, only one or two members would be responsible for the follow-up evaluation. For example, a patient on seizure medication who has been placed in a modified work environment and has had a series of depressive episodes may be seen by the physiatrist, the occupational therapist, and the psychologist. Since all team members have been involved in the entire treatment process, a thorough evaluation can be completed without the unnecessary expense and use of time of all professional team members. At this time also the Performance Progress Profile is updated, providing an ongoing, concrete measure of change. This process is continued throughout the formal follow-up periods. Intervention on any level—cognitive, emotional, interpersonal, vocational, social—can then be made as needed.

Problems in Program Implementation

The comprehensive rehabilitation program presented is a complex one, involving many persons and many administrative procedures. Inevitably obstacles to program implementation and concerns among professionals arise. Three major areas will be discussed here: 1) securing funding, 2) receiving administrative support, and 3) managing, "turf" issues among diverse disciplines.

One of the most outstanding issues facing brain-injury rehabilitation today is the lack of available funding for ongoing cognitive rehabilitation. This is especially problematic with so-called minor head injury, where deficits are not obvious and are easily confused with psychiatric illness or "malingering" by professional persons not trained in subtle cognitive deficits. It is essential that a comprehensive neuropsychological evaluation be done by a person experienced in the kinds of deficits typical in minor heady injury, since test scores may be within normal levels yet still reflect significant impairment in the executive functions. Ongoing education of medical professionals and insurance representatives is an essential part of a rehabilitation facility's role as an advocate for the disabled population.

Because the treatment of brain-injured persons in staff intensive— that is, significant professional hours of perhaps eight team members are invested in one person—the need for administrative support and encouragement is acute. This is particularly true considering the funding issues mentioned above. Also, there must be the encouragement and funding for continued education in a field that is only beginning to develop a strong clinical and research base. Finally, management must endorse the interdisciplinary team spirit that is so essential to maintaining quality care, thereby helping to reduce the rivalry and "turf" issues so prevalent in some institutions.

It is essential that members of all disciplines acknowledge the expertise of each other, utilize each other's strengths, and respect each other as equally competent professionals. The process of developing a common language through the creation of the Performance Progress Profile has had a major impact on the quality of communication among experienced team members. The challenge now is to learn to communicate not only this common language but also the sense of mutual respect for each other's skills and insights to the new staff members as they join the treatment team.

Summary

In summary, we have described a comprehensive rehabilitation program for persons who have suffered a minor head injury. The main focus of this program is to facilitate the integration of basic cognitive skills into the capacity to function as a seeing, hearing, feeling person within the context of normal life activities. By working as a cohesive team, the professionals, the patient, and the significant others can achieve these goals. By fostering flexibility and creativity in both professionals and patients, the program at its best can enhance the quality of life and societal productivity of survivors of brain injury.

References

1. Rosenthal M, Griffith ER, Bond MR, Miller JD (eds): Rehabilitation of the Head Injured Adult. Philadelphia: Davis, 1983.
2. Berrol S: Issues in cognitive rehabilitation. Arch Neurol, 1990; 47:219–220.
3. Kaplan E: A process approach to neuropsychological assessment. Paper presented at the American Psychological Association Convention, New York, NY, 1987.
4. Lezak M: The problem of assessing executive functions. Int J Psychol, 1982; 17:281–291.
5. Mahon D, Elger C: Analysis of post-traumatic syndrome following a mild head injury. J Neurosci Nurs, 1989; 21(6):382–384.
6. Furst CJ: Head injury symptoms: Brain damage vs. neurosis. Framingham, MA: National Head Injury Foundation, 1984.
7. Liberto M: A phenomenological study of the experience of traumatic brain injury. Unpublished dissertation. Bryn Mawr College, 1989.
8. Oddy M, Coughlan T, Tyerman A, Jenkins D: Social adjustment after closed head injury: A further follow-up seven years after injury. J Neurol Neurosurg Psychiatry, 1985; 48:564–568.

— 18

Community and Vocational Re-Entry in Minor Head Injury

Karen Lutz and Lynn Nash

Minor head injury often has a significant impact on an individual's life-style as well as that of family members. The injury affects the areas that are crucial to an individual's definition of self, an individual's employment, activities of daily living, life skills, and social and leisure activities. Rimel's study (1) found that 34% of the patients who were gainfully employed prior to an injury were unemployed three months later. The same study revealed that 14% of the patients stated they had difficulty with household chores and activities of daily living. An additional 15% "complained of changes in transportation" such as "no longer feeling competent to drive."

Studies by Alves (2), Barth (3), Gronwall (4,5), and Kay (6) show that individuals with minor head injury demonstrate difficulties in the areas of concentration, memory, abstract reasoning, reaction time, and visual and verbal processing. Many individuals report an "inability to remember, concentrate, organize, handle a number of tasks at once, and get as much work done as efficiently" as before the accident (6). These studies do not correlate these limitations with specific functional deficits. Detailed discussion of cognitive limitations in this chapter highlights their effects on an individual's inability to carry out normal daily routines after minor head injury. Treatment programs geared to the individual with a minor head injury need to address these issues, as well as other changes noted by the individual or family.

As discussed in previous chapters, cognitive deficits are not always obvious in daily interaction or through standardized testing. "They emerge only under the rigorous demands of work, school, running a home or in the course of a well done neuropsychological examination. In addition, these deficits are more likely to occur under conditions of stress, fatigue, anxiety, or even moderate use of drugs and alcohol" (6).

Cognitive deficits may be noted first as decreased performance in the daily morning routine. These tasks frequently occur with a significant time pressure involved, as in preparing for work, school, or the coordination of household activities to coincide with the schedules of other family members. Performing such activities well at a relatively fast pace requires planning, execution and effective time management. Following head trauma, one's speed in carrying out a morning routine may be slower owing to difficulty handling normal interruptions such as a baby crying, the phone ringing, or other family members arguing. Premorbidly, these may not have caused problems, but given the patient's limited post-injury capacity to sustain attention to multiple tasks or to shift sets, deficits are frequently unmasked. Minor head injury also frequently alters the ability to carry out tasks within a given time frame in combination with other stressors, interruptions, or unexpected events such as a sick child or car problems.

Frequently a spouse may complain that the individual with a minor head injury can no longer budget the family income efficiently. He or she may need reminders that specific bills are due, or assistance in planning a budget to prepare for future larger bills such as house insurance or medical bills. These money management skills involve high-level problem-solving skills, including thought organization and planning ahead.

Driving is frequently viewed as a routine daily task. Actually, it is a complex, integrative, cognitive-perceptual skill. Such tasks can be significantly affected by a minor head injury. Driving simultaneously encompasses many of the areas that have been documented as problems for adults with minor head injury (1). To operate a vehicle, one relies strongly on the ability quickly and accurately to assess and process the ever-changing visual environment. Information must be integrated by the driver and coordinated with a physical response such as applying the brakes or avoiding an oncoming truck, all within a safe reaction time. At the same time the driver must attend to multiple tasks such as talking with passengers, listening to the radio, or monitoring the children in the back. This daily activity is complex for any driver and particularly for someone who has suffered a minor head injury who may present with limitations in reaction time, multiple attention, problem-solving, and information processing before even getting into the car.

Most often, the ultimate goal of an individual who has had a minor head injury is to return to previous work responsibilities, which frequently include home management, the care of others, and educational and vocational activities (7). These activities rely strongly on the component skills of memory, concentration, information processing, and thought organization.

A homemaker who has suffered a minor head injury may demonstrate difficulty with organizing the steps and timing involved with planning and preparing a family meal, completing household chores, and caring for children at home. In any home environment, the homemaker must be able to discriminate and screen out inappropriate distractions, such as the television or a dog barking, while concentrating on multiple household tasks. He or she must also maintain a mental list of priorities for daily and weekly activities such as doctor's appointments, food shopping, after-school activities, or repairman visits. The working spouse who would normally have come home to a calm and organized setting now returns to a disorganized and possibly stressful home situation.

Following minor head injury, many individuals return not only to responsibilities in the home, but also to those outside of the home which provide financial support. Productive job performance entails the integration of various components, including performance of job tasks in a timely and effective manner, incorporation of required work behaviors, demonstration of appropriate grooming and interpersonal skills, and adherence to safety procedures (7). An individual's work may require that he or she be efficient in the areas of motor speed, complex attention, learning, memory, and integrative thinking —the very areas that are impaired by a minor head injury (6).

Most occupations are not performed in a quiet or isolated environment; therefore, an individual must be able to perform in a distracting setting. An individual with a minor head injury often has difficulty in this area owing to limited thought flexibility and a decreased ability to filter out distractions and to concentrate on simultaneous tasks. Problems may be noted first in the clinic or in a social setting prior to the client's return to work. For example, the conversation of others in the room, or a telephone call, may provide enough distraction to disrupt the person's concentration and impede his or her ability to accomplish a task.

The effectiveness of job performance is influenced strongly by verbal and visual information-processing speed. In addition, this impacts on an individual's ability to assess a situation and make quick decisions. For example, a salesman with a minor head injury will often lose an account because he is no longer able to change his sales approach quickly in response to the verbal and nonverbal feedback he is receiving from his client.

Throughout each day, all jobs require frequent recall of verbal or visual information. This includes complex information that was presented minutes previously, as well as information from the morning or even the preceding day. Because of poor memory skills, an individual with a minor head injury may have difficulty recalling the information accurately. Often there are numerous interruptions between the time the information was presented and when it needed. These distractions further hinder an individual's already impaired ability to code, store, or retrieve the needed information unless an appropriate compensatory strategy is initiated.

In the area of vocational as well as life skills, the integration of cognition and motor skills is imperative. This is frequently foremost on the clinician's mind if the client is returning to a vocation that involved the use of machinery or motorized vehicles. However, executive office work and high-level leisure interests should not be overlooked as areas that also combine cognitive and physical skills at a fast pace. An individual who works in an office setting within a distracting environment is required to organize and problem-solve simultaneously while operating office equipment such as a type-writer, computer, or phone switchboard. Football, soccer, and skiing are a few examples of leisure interests that require quick problem-solving combined with a physical component. Most sports also require high-level attention for effective performance. When increasingly difficult cognitive demands are made on an individual who is only able to perform higher-level physical skills in isolation significant impairment becomes evident.

Physical endurance is an area frequently evaluated and often decreased after a minor head injury. However, cognitive endurance must also be evaluated. For example, an individual or his employer may note a decrease in performance towards midday or midweek. This presents as an increase in the number of errors or length of time needed to complete an activity. Initially upon return, the extra effort required of an individual with a minor head injury can be both physically and mentally exhausting. Anxiety, new learning, and multiple attention tasks all compound the problem within a distracting environment. Resultant fatigue may result in decreased mental performance. This should be taken into account when arranging a return to work schedule. Often, two or three half-days are better than two or three full days initially.

Assessment

In any minor head injury rehabilitation process, teamwork among the patient, the family, and the professionals is essential. The foundation for this process begins with a comprehensive evaluation of the cognitive areas. The formal neuropsychological test battery administered by a licensed neuropsychologist encompasses the spectrum of cognition and perception. All team members should be familiar with the test battery, including the occupational therapist who is dealing with community and vocational re-entry issues.

The data from neuropsychological testing provide the occupational therapist with an overall picture of the patient's strengths and deficits in relation to cognition and perception. It is important that within the individual occupational therapy evaluation, components of the neuropsychological battery are not duplicated. This will help eliminate the practice effect and avoid invalid data from poorly administered testing or misinterpreted results [8].

In addition to the information from the neuropsychological test battery, the patient's family provides valuable observations, which include the patient's performance and observed deficits. This information easily can be overlooked, but it is a necessary component of the assessment and treatment process.

It is important that the occupational therapist administer an individual evaluation to establish a functional performance baseline. As there are no standardized tests for the minor-head-injury population, it is necessary to rely on formal and informal testing for the areas related to community and vocational re-entry. The evaluation process that we have found to be most appropriate for this population involved the assessment of functional performance and specific cognitive skills. In addition to the end result of the specific skill evaluation task, one must accurately assess the process by which the patient achieves his end results [9].

Patient/Family Interview

An interview with the patient and family is used to establish the patient's baseline functional performance level. Questions address changes in the performance of daily living, work, and leisure skills: for example, Do you have difficulty taking phone messages? Is it hard to concentrate at family gatherings? Do you need more time to get ready in the morning? Is your handwriting of the same quality? Are you driving? Within the interview, the patient is also asked to identify and prioritize specific goals (i.e., What three activities do you want to perform again?). In addition, the patient is asked to give a verbal or written job description. This information is used to determine appropriate functional tasks to be evaluated in addition to evaluation of specific skill areas.

Functional Tasks

The functional tasks may be performed in a distracting environment which simulates the home or work environment. This is a crucial difference from the neuropsychological test procedure. Example of functional tasks include writing out checks, competing functional word problems, dictating a letter, using a telephone book, reading a map, calculating prices on a menu, fixing a small appliance, or cooking.

The forementioned tasks are graded to reveal possible deficits in the minor-head-injury patient. Grading may include changing the length and complexity of the task or of verbal or written directions. The amount or type of distraction may be varied, as well. While observing the functional task, the therapist must take note of the processing strategy that is used: Does the individual perform better with verbal or visual information? Does the individual use mental manipulation or trial and error to solve a problem? What other behaviors are displayed? One also must be aware of the physical status such as range of motion, gross and fine motor coordination, and balance.

Cognitive Skills

Attention/Concentration

An individual with a minor head injury may be able to complete a single task accurately. However, when asked to alternate attention between simultaneous multiple tasks which require decision-making skills, the person often demonstrates difficulties. Flexibility of thinking may also be affected as the individual is unable to develop alternate solutions (6). The area of complex attention and concentration can be accurately assessed by observing the individual's task performance. Observations should include the number of cues needed to refocus on a task after interruptions, the type of distractions tolerated, the length of time attending to the task (i.e., thirty minutes vs. two 15-minute periods), and the ability to attend to familiar versus unfamiliar task. An individual's concentration must also be avaluated in terms of presentation style, that is, verbal or visual information. The ability to concentrate may vary during the day depending on mental and physical exhaustion, as well as emotional stressors.

Memory

An individual's memory is evaluated for short-term, long-term, or delayed recall of visual, auditory, and tactile information. During the evaluation interview, it may be noted that the individual with a minor head injury has difficulty recalling the sequence of activities at home. For example, Was the baby shower on Saturday or Sunday? Do

I pass a MAC machine on the way to therapy? Did I wear the tan pants this week? Who is the therapist from the preceding session? What medications am I taking? Memory skills can also be assessed by presenting a list of five items needed at the store and then asking the patient to recall them later in the session. Information can be obtained by asking the individual to give directions or draw a map to a familiar location from memory. While assessing money management skills, for example, the individual may have difficulty recalling the given verbal directions to complete a blank check.

Processing Speed/Motor Integration

Individual's with minor head injury demonstrate decreased ability to process auditory, visual, or tactile information quickly, as well as react appropriately, especially with numerous choices (6). This area can be evaluated using observation and task analysis. The evaluation interview may reveal difficulty in processing directions quickly or responding to questions quickly. The injured individual may also mention activities that now seem slower such as completing his or her morning routine, doing housework, or locating items while shopping.

The speed at which the functional evaluation tasks are competed must also be noted. This is a crucial observation if the task is completed accurately, but not within a reasonable time frame for the home, community, or vocational setting. The processing speed and reaction time often vary depending on the level of complexity, as well as the mode of presentation, (visual or verbal). Variations in speed and reaction time may also be noted while processing information when combined with a physical activity such as walking, cooking, or operating machinery. Computer programs are available for determining an individual's speed of response to visual or auditory information. The Bracy Cognitive Rehabilitation Programs Foundations I & II assess this area (10,11).

Abstract Reasoning/Problem-Solving

Difficulties in the above-mentioned areas will result in a "decrease in complex problem-solving and creative thinking" (6). During the evaluation interview, the individual will report problem areas and his or her previously attempted solutions or strategies. Analysis of these strategies provides information regarding the individual's reasoning style (concrete or abstract), and the number of solutions attempted.

The individual's problem-solving process is also reflected in functional evaluation tasks. For example, What are three different routes from Doylestown to Philadelphia? What three separate meals can you have at the diner for under fifteen dollars each? What are three important areas to be included on a job resume?

The traditional method of evaluating spatial relations through reproduction of design will also assist in evaluating an individual's method of problem-solving. This can be assessed with or without the motor component involved. The use of paper-and-pencil tasks as well as those involving cubes or parquetry pieces will determine whether a trial-and-error approach or mental manipulation of the objects is used. The level of complexity may be increased to include only mental manipulation or covert problem-solving strategies. These tasks may include cube rotation, figure completion, or pattern sequencing.

Upon completion of the evaluation, the therapist must review all the test components. More importantly, they must be viewed as a whole in relation to the individual's ability to perform withing the community or vocational setting.

Treatment Methods

Treatment programs for the individual with a minor head injury must emphasize the integration of isolated cognitive subskills with everyday activities in order to achieve generalization of learned compensatory strategies. It is important that the individual's skills be brought to a level sufficient for this generalization. The following review of treatment for specific cognitive subskills highlights clinically important concepts.

Attention

The focus of a treatment program for attention deficits should include environmental stimuli and the individual's interest in the task (8). The level of task complexity that the individual is able to complete successfully in a quiet environment has been determined by the initial evaluation. Now distractions may be introduced and increased while maintaining the task complexity level. This may be done as easily as opening the door to a noisy hallway or clinic while the patient is working alone in a room. A further level of distraction may include having the patient listen to a radio or headset while working on the activity. Complexity can be increased, and strategies developed, until he or she is able to work in the clinic or office among other individuals.

The treatment program should then progress to include simultaneous attention and control of multiple tasks. An example is shifting from a visual perceptual task to a math task at regular intervals such as 30 seconds. This shift may also include visual versus verbal tasks, or motor versus non-motor tasks. Treatment examples at the functional level are cooking a complex meal or shopping at the grocery store.

Memory

The key to treating memory deficits effectively involves recognizing the individual's style for receiving, coding, and retrieving information. Styles include visual, auditory, tactile or a combination of cues. (8). Results from the occupational therapy, speech, psychology, and neuropsychology evaluations should be coordinated in order to determine deficit areas, memory style, and appropriate treatment methods. Through teamwork, this will provide consistency and thus enhance generalization of memory skills.

During a therapeutic activity, the therapist must assist the individual in recognizing and incorporating the individual's memory style. In order for this to occur, the therapist and patient must have an active rapport at a partnership level, as opposed to a therapist-dominant relationship. This allows the therapist to act as a role model for the thinking process until the individual can gradually incorporate the memory strategies independently. An example is the use of computerized memory tasks requiring visual or auditory memory. The therapist will assist the patient by providing strategy cues that will reinforce coding such as verbal rehearsal, visualization, writing, mnemonic devices, or chunking. The ability to break down information into smaller groupings is called chunking. To assist with recall or recognition, the therapist may provide cues such as asking questions, giving multiple possibilities, or providing the first sound of a word (8).

To assist the patient with memory deficits further, external compensatory techinques can be used. Post-It notes, lists, and Daykeepers are examples that can be incorporated into daily routines. Timers in the kitchen or notepads by the phone are techinques used daily even by individuals who have not had a head injury.

Processing Speed and Motor Intergration

Treatment of this deficit area will encompass auditory, visual, cognitive, and perceptual tasks, as well as gross and fine motor activities. One aspect includes increasing time restraints and demands on a task that an individual can complete successfully. The complexity may be varied by using a combined motor and cognitive task, or by increasing distractions.

Timed obstacle courses can provide a demanding situation for an individual, and external pressure is increased by videotaping. Computerized games, incorporating visual scanning and perceptual skills with a timed score and comparison, are also useful and provide internal competition for the injured individual. While working on a treadmill or an upper extremity ergometer, the patient can be quizzed with math problems. Card games that requires speed and competition among others are another valuable treatment tool. Any functional activity that is completed successfully can be used for improving processing speed and motor integration by including a time constraint.

Abstract Reasoning/Problem-Solving

This area of treatment incorporates a variety of levels from concrete planning and organizing to abstract reasoning. Treatment tasks can be varied according to the level of abstraction required. This may include situational problem-solving—what to wear to an interview, how to plan a route or how to plan a schedule within given time restraints. Computerized problem-solving tasks can also be used to master this skill (12). Workbooks, puzzles, and strategy games are used to develop the individual's reasoning and problem-solving ability.

The next treatment phase involves the group setting. Group activities can be planned and organized for various community outings—the mall, the theater, or a sports event. The amount of structure needed within the group will vary according to the social and cognitive skills of the group members. This allows the individual to interact within a more realistic environment than the sheltered clinic.

Vocational Re-Entry

As an individual progresses through treatment, the transition from deficit specific to task specific training is important. To accomplish this, the occupational therapist, or job coach, must be aware of the individual's job or home responsibilities. The process includes review and discussion of the job description with the individual, allowing him or her to clarify the written information and his or her responsibilities. Family members are also valuable resources.

Review of the job description and/or home responsibilities includes identification of cognitive, social, and physical demands. Consideration also must be given to quota requirements, time schedule constraints, work pace, work environment, and the level of supervision and structure. The therapist must be aware of the amount of new learning that is required. (i.e., changes in procedures, schedules, or techniques). After determining the job demands, the therapist can introduce task-specific treatment. Reviewing blueprints, taking menu orders, typing from dictation, or changing diapers are examples that can be performed in the clinical setting. At this time, the therapist should incorporate compensatory techniques as part of the problem-solving process in returning to the role of employee or homemaker.

The employer or spouse must become a key member of the team. His or her level of understanding, cooperation, and commitment will impact greatly on the success of the individual in returning to his or her previous vocational role. This lays the foundation for the job coach to begin observations at work or home, as discussed below.

Prior to returning to work, the therapist/job coach may complete an on-site analysis. This allows for clarification of job responsibilities and provides an opportunity to educate the employer and to address his or her concerns. Then, taking into consideration the individual's physical and cognitive endurance, the physician and the team will outline the physical restrictions and initial hours to be scheduled.

The role of the job coach is to observe the individual while performing in the work or home environment. At this time, the job coach will assist the individual in application of the learned compensatory strategies. The coach will give specific recommendations regarding observed social behavior and employer feedback. The job coach also encourages feedback from employer, fellow employees, or spouse directly to the individual.

As the individual's job performance improves, the hours and responsibilities can be increased. Simultaneously the role of the job coach will decrease. At this time, biweekly progressing to monthly observations or phone calls may be all that is needed to ensure successful re-entry at the community or vocational level.

Summary

Community and vocational re-entry may pose major problems following minor head trauma. However, successful re-entry can usually be achieved through careful assessment of the individual's problems and spontaneous solutions, progressive treatment with the evolution of effective compensatory strategies, and supported return to real-life challenges. Close communication and collaboration between the occupational therapist and all other members of the health care team, including the family, is essential for optimal results.

References

1. Rimel RW, Giordani B, Barth JT, Boll TJ, Jane JA: Disability caused by minor head injury. Neurosurgery, 1981; 9(3):221–228.
2. Alves WM, et al.: Understanding post-traumatic sysmptoms after minor head injury. J Head Trauma Rehabil, 1986; 1(2):1–12.
3. Barth JT, et al.: Forensic aspects of mild head trauma. J Head Trauma Rehabil, 1986; 1(2):63–70.
4. Gronwal D, Wrightson P: Delayed recovery of intellectual function after minor head injury. Lancet, 1974; Sept 14:605–609.
5. Gronwal D, Wrightson P: Memory and information processing capacity after closed head injury. J Neurol Neurosurg Psychiatry, 1981; 44:889–895.
6. Kay T: Minor Head Injury: An Introduction for Professionals. Framingham, MA: National Head Injury Foundation, 1986.
7. American Occupational Therapy Association: Uniform terminology for Occupational Therapy, 2nd ed. Am J Occupa Ther, 1989; 43(12):808–815.
8. Morse P: Brain Injury: Cognitive and Prevocational Approaches to Rehabilitation. New York: The Tiresias Press Inc., 1986.
9. Toglia J: Approaches to cognitive assessment of the brain injured adult: traditional methods and dynamic investigation. Occup Ther Practice 1989; 1(1):36–55.
10. Bracy OL: Cognitive Rehabilitation Program: Foundation I. Indianapolis: Psychological Software Services, Inc., 1987.
11. Bracy OL: Cognitive Rehabilitation Program: Foundation II. Indianapolis: Psychological Software Services, Inc., 1987.
12. Bracy OL: Cognitive Rehabilitation Program: Problem Solving. Indianapolis: Psychological Software Services, Inc., 1987.

— 19

Family Adjustment to Minor Traumatic Brain Injury

Paul R. Sachs

Families are recognized as an important part of the rehabilitation process for the survivor of severe traumatic brain injury (TBI). With this importance in mind, rehabilitation professionals have developed specific treatment approaches for families of these survivors [1–4].

For the survivor of minor traumatic brain injury the situation is different. Greater attention has been given recently to the sequelae of such injuries and the methods of assessment and treatment for survivors of minor TBI [5–9]. The impact of a minor TBI on the family of the survivor, however, is neither well documented nor understood.

Clinical experience suggests that there is not a simple linear relationship between family adjustment to the trauma and the severity of a trauma. That is, families of survivors of minor TBI do not necessarily have minor adjustment difficulties. Rather, it is more accurate to say that families of survivors of minor TBI face *different* adjustment difficulties when compared with families of severe TBI survivors. This chapter discusses the unique nature of the family's adjustment to the minor TBI and differentiates it from the adjustment difficulties of families of severe TBI survivors. Treatment interventions for families of minor TBI survivors are stressed.

The Impact of Minor TBI on the Family

The adjustment difficulties of the family of a survivor of minor TBI are primarily derived from the family's problems understanding the behavior of the survivor. When family members properly understand the causes of the survivor's behavior after a minor TBI, they are better able to develop adaptive means of responding to the survivor. When family members misunderstand or are unable to understand the reasons for the survivor's behavior, their reactions to the survivor are maladaptive, often resulting in increased family adjustment difficulties.

To elaborate on this position, the effects of minor TBI on the family will be briefly reviewed. The effects of minor TBI will be contrasted with those resulting from a severe TBI. For more detailed information on the clinical picture of a survivor of minor TBI the reader should refer to relevant chapters in the book.

Physical Sequelae

By definition (6,8) the clinical picture of a survivor of mild TBI is different from that of the survivor of a severe TBI. The survivor of mild TBI has a briefer and shallower period of unconsciousness. Survivors of mild TBI have fewer medical complications than do survivors of severe TBI (9). Examinations of brain structure or function (e.g., EEG or CT scan) may also be negative, although brain lesions may be detected with other procedures (i.e., MRI) (9).

Often the survivor of a mild TBI has few visible physical impairments. Normal range of motion in body parts is retained. Limitations in strength or speed of performance are usually not noted. Physical disfigurement as a result of the injury is not commonly reported. The most common physical symptom is headache pain (5). Pain and muscle weakness as the result of musculoskeletal injuries from the incident which caused the injury are also reported.

In contrast, a severe TBI often results in a variety of long-lasting physical difficulties, including limitations in gross and fine motor movements. Surgical intervention or special rehabilitation equipment may be needed by the individual to maintain his or her independence in some physical activities. Physical disfigurement or other physical evidence of injury such as fractures are frequently seen.

The relatively minor physical sequelae that accompany minor TBI have implications for family adjustment patterns. After severe TBI, physical difficulties of the survivor are often a focus of concern for families. These physical problems are concrete evidence of the survivor's injury. For example, limitations in mobility have a major impact on the survivor's ability to return to independent living and working. Physical disfigurement may also be distressing to the family as evidence of the abnormality of the survivor. The severity of these physical impairments provides a basis for the family's recognition of the less visible cognitive and behavioral impairments that the severe TBI survivor has.

To family members, the survivor of a minor TBI may appear to have no physical limitations or impairment. Even when the survivor has physical pain, it is not visible to others. As a result, physical sequelae are not a major focus of concern for family members of the minor TBI survivor.

Without concrete evidence of injury, the cognitive and behavioral changes that the survivor of minor TBI demonstrates may be hard for families to grasp. Families may expect that the survivor without obvious physical limitations will also have few if any cognitive and behavioral limitations. Conflicts may result between the expectations that the family members hold for the survivor and his/her actual capabilities post-trauma. Even when the survivor has physical symptoms such as pain, conflicts may arise with family members because they are unable to see the pain. They may even misinterpret the survivor's lack of physical activity as a result of poor motivation rather than inability to perform physical activity.

Cognitive Sequelae

Cognitive limitations after mild TBI are more subtle than those after severe TBI. The survivor of mild TBI usually has a briefer period of post-traumatic amnesia. Cognitive difficulties after the injury may include attention and memory impairments, slowed thought processing, and cognitive inflexibility (6). In many other respects, however, the survivor of mild TBI may show intact cognitive abilities, with language skills, familiar sequential skills (e.g., dressing and eating), and visual spatial orientation well-preserved. In contrast, the survivor of severe TBI shows a wider range of cognitive impairments and a greater severity of impairment that have been widely documented by clinicians (10,11).

The subtle cognitive difficulties reported in survivors of minor TBI pose a difficult adjustment problem for the family. Family members must adjust to the survivor's changed cognitive skills in specific areas rather than the broad, generalized changes in cognition noted after a severe TBI. The survivor of minor TBI may appear to function well in a wide variety of basic cognitive skill areas at home or in the workplace and have difficulty only with more complex, integrative cognitive activities. The survivor may perform well at a task one day and poorly at the same task on a different day because of the vagaries of his or her physical condition or increased sensitivity to fatigue as the result of the trauma. This variability in cognitive performance makes it difficult for the family members to understand the survivor's behavior and to gauge properly their expectations for the survivor. Family members may incorrectly explain the survivor's inability to perform cognitive activities as being the result of his or her unwillingness to do the activities rather than due to a genuine cognitive impairment.

Emotional and Behavioral Sequelae

Emotional changes that are reported after minor TBI include increased irritability, decreased frustration tolerance, lethargy, or flattened affect (12). As with the cognitive changes after minor TBI, these emotional changes may be inconsistent. A survivor may be irritable one day and calm the next. Many of the same emotional difficulties are seen after severe TBI, but the presentation of the symptoms is more extreme and often overshadowed by cognitive changes in the survivor. For example, survivors of severe TBI at the early stages of recovery do not show depressed mood because their cognitive status is so reduced that they are not sufficiently alert nor aware of their condition to experience depression. At later stages of recovery, when the survivor of severe TBI has increased awareness of cognitive impairments and has improved memory that allows his/her to reflect on his/her condition, depressed mood becomes more evident.

In the survivor of minor TBI the interaction among emotional, behavioral, and cognitive changes is seen almost immediately after the injury. For example, cognitive difficulties such as memory impairments may cause the survivor of a minor TBI to become depressed. The survivor's depressed mood may in turn intensify the attention and concentration impairments. Kay has further discussed this issue by distinguishing between primary and secondary effects of minor TBI (6). Primary effects of the trauma include those emotional changes listed above that result from the trauma, and the survivor's emotional reaction to the sequelae of the trauma. Secondary effects of the trauma involve the interaction of the primary effects with other life events, resulting in dysfunctional emotional adjustment patterns. For example, the survivor's initial anxiety may develop into a more generalized fear of failure. At times, psychiatric imbalance can occur after minor TBI. Though the injury itself may not cause changes in the brain that create the psychiatric difficulty, the disruption in life activities that follow the injury may be enough to destabilize the survivor, leading to the development of psychiatric symptoms.

The close interaction between the emotional and cognitive states of the survivor of minor TBI again poses potential adjustment problems for the family. The family may find the emotional changes that are observed in the survivor difficult to explain. The changes may be attributed to the brain injury itself, to acute emotional stressors, or to the individual's pre-injury personality. Secondary effects of the injury that may occur months after the injury itself may not be recognized by the family as being related to the injury. Furthermore, because the emotional changes are inconsistent, family members may not know when to expect the changes and have difficulty adapting to them. Table 19.1 summarizes some of the differences in family reactions to various sequelae of minor TBI.

The case example presented below clearly illustrates how the interaction among cognitive and emotional sequelae of minor TBI, and other life events can affect a survivor and his family.

Case Example

L.R. was a 29-year-old married man when he was involved in a motor vehicle accident. He sustained fractures of his right leg and facial lacerations. He was unconscious for a brief period after the accident. Prior to his injury, he had earned a bachelor's degree and had worked as a food service supervisor. His work activities involved supervision of other employees and some aspects of food preparation.

His wife was pregnant at the time of the injury. The couple described their marital relationship as a close and supportive one prior to the injury. L.R. returned home after a three-day hospital stay but he did not return to work immediately. He managed his personal care independently. He noticed, however, that he was more irritable and had some short-term memory difficulties within the home environment. After the baby was born, the wife was more aware of these problems and disturbed by them. She was uncertain about his ability to help her with the baby and felt upset that she had to return to work sooner than she would have liked to because her husband did not feel able to return to work himself. L.R.'s wife wondered to what degree his behavior was due to his inability to perform certain tasks or his lack of desire to perform them. L.R. did not seem to feel his problems were as bad as his wife did. This difference was another source of tension between them.

The couple sought the help of a psychologist for evaluation of L.R. and treatment recommendations. Neuropsychological evaluation of this man showed evidence of impairment consistent with self-report. In addition, it was clear that emotional stressors from the changes associated with the baby's birth contributed to difficulties in com-

Table 19.1. Sequelae of mild brain injury and their effects on families of the survivor.

Sequelae	Effects on family adjustment
Physical: Headache and musculoskeletal pain are prominant; physical disfiguration is infrequent; gross and fine motor skills generally unimpaired	Family has little outward evidence of the survivor's problems; may expect survivor to be able to perform home and work tasks without difficulty; conflict may arise between family's expectations and survivor's capabilities
Cognitive: Difficulties in attention and concentration underlying reported memory problems, difficulties in complex cognitive tasks; sensitive to fatigue	Cognitive difficulties may be inconsistent and thus appear confusing to family; family may attribute cognitive difficulties to emotional or motivational factors; survivor's cognitive impairments may be masked by family members who attempt to compensate for the survivor's difficulties by taking on survivor's responsibilities at home
Emotional: Mood changes with symptoms of anxiety or depression; level of emotional distress may depend on the degree to which the survivor is aware of his or her difficulties and attributes them to the brain injury rather than to other causes	Family may have difficulty differentiating the injury-related mood changes from those that might occur as the result of everyday life events; the lack of overt physical impairments and the presence of subtle cognitive impairments may lead families to invoke a halo effect and expect that the survivor's emotional troubles will also be mild or inconsequential

munication between the spouses and to L.R.'s mood change and cognitive difficulties. Cognitive remediation was recommended for L.R. Marital counseling was also recommended to improve communication and to help the couple to set realistic expectations for themselves in light of the baby and L.R.'s decreased abilities.

This case example illustrates several of the points previously described. 1) L.R. had few lasting physical difficulties post-injury. He looked well despite underlying cognitive and emotional problems. 2) He had subtle cognitive problems that interfered with his ability to perform complex tasks and reduced his endurance. 3) His wife found the subtle cognitive changes in the context of his good physical condition and independence in many skills to be confusing and distressing. 4) L.R.'s functioning post-injury was a function of the interaction between his cognitive difficulties, his emotional reaction to the trauma, and the birth of his baby. 5) The effect of L.R.'s injury on his family life was a function of how his wife understood and explained his behavior. Because she saw his behavior as the result of poor motivation (for example, an unwillingness to return to work or perform certain tasks around the home), she became upset and angry.

Although treatment interventions will be discussed later in this chapter, it can be briefly said here that treatment for L.R. focused on both his cognitive and emotional adjustment difficulties. Treatment for L.R. and his wife focused on education about the nature of minor brain injury and how it could affect L.R.'s abilities.

Effect of Minor TBI on Family Structure

The preceding section has focused on the family's adjustment to the survivor of minor TBI by examining the various sequelae of minor TBI and the family's interpretation of such sequelae. It is also important to examine the structure of the family and how the structure is changed by the survivor's injury.

Briefly, the structural approach (13,14) to understanding families conceptualizes the family as an organization which operates according to certain rules, guidelines, and lines of communication. In order to assess the family and to understand the impact of the minor TBI on the family, the clinician needs to understand the underlying organization of the family. Five components of family structure are briefly described in Table 19.2, with comments about how they are affected by a minor TBI to a family member. These components include cohesion, family values, communication, organization, and relationships with society (3).

As noted in Table 19.2, severe TBI results in radical changes to family structure. The cohesiveness of the family is disrupted because of the needs of the injured survivor. Changes in organization, communication, and division of responsibility are necessitated by the injury. Family members experience a loss of values or a sense of demoralization. They may withdraw from their contacts with other people in society or feel that extended family and friends withdraw from them (1,15,16).

The picture of family structure after minor TBI is not as well-described. Indeed, a valuable area for further clinical research concerns documenting the nature of changes in family structure after minor TBI.

Because the injury is minor, as defined earlier in the chapter, the family does not face the imminent death of the survivor in a way that family members of the severe TBI survivor do. Thus, the value system of the minor TBI survivor's family may not be as radically shaken as that of the severe TBI survivor's family.

The survivor of a minor TBI is not likely to require inpatient treatment. Rather, the survivor is sent home with the family. The constant contact between the survivor and the family may result in greater stress and conflict at home for the family of a minor TBI

Table 19.2. Effects of mild traumatic brain injury on the structural aspects of family functioning.

Structural component	Effect of brain injury on structural component
Cohesion: Degree of togetherness or other forces keeping family members together	Survivor's behavior leads to a disruption in family cohesion; family may experience an inconsistent sense of attachment and separation as the result of survivor's behavior
Values: Beliefs and important feelings of family that underlie their decisions and interactions	Family does not experience a sense of demoralization, but does question the methods and beliefs by which the family life is organized; the survivor's relatively mild difficulties suggest to family that complete recovery is possible and thus no change in family values is necessary
Communication and organization of responsibilities: Patterns of interaction and means by which family accomplishes its duties	Patterns and methods of communication change as the result of the survivor's changed cognitive status, yet the inconsistency in these cognitive changes makes it difficult for families to develop new communication patterns and organizational patterns
Relationship with society: Degree to which family is connected to outside community	Family has little exposure to the system of rehabilitation care because the survivor is usually not referred for extensive rehabilitation services; family may show less dependency on professional care but also finds less peer support in rehabilitation care community

survivor than for the family of a severe TBI survivor. It may also, however, provide greater opportunity to resolve conflicts and make changes.

The minor TBI survivor's family does not have to adjust to the rehabilitation care system, the team of rehabilitation professionals, and many of the financial and legal complications that ensue from the injury. On the other hand, the family does not have an extensive support system of rehabilitation professionals to assist them in handling the changed behaviors of the survivor.

The survivor's subtle and inconsistent cognitive and emotional changes may necessitate some changes in organizational structure and communication patterns in the family. These changes may, however, be minor compared to the changes in the family's structure after a member suffers a severe TBI. The family members may prefer that the survivor continue with the same activities and responsibilities he or she had before the injury, albeit at a slower pace and less effectively, rather than reorganize and have other family members take on these responsibilities. In this situation, the family's stress after the minor TBI may be the result of trying to maintain the same structure, rather than undergoing a forced change in structure as is seen after a severe TBI.

In addition to family structure, it is important to consider the family's stage of development in understanding the impact of minor TBI. For example, the effect of a L.R.'s minor TBI in the case example mentioned earlier at a time just before the birth of his first child had a different impact than it would have had if the injury had occurred to an older couple with grown children.

Assessment of the Family

Concepts of family structure and development are cornerstones of an assessment of the family. Prior to instituting any treatment with family members of survivors of minor TBI, it is important to have an assessment of the family's status. Since it is only recently that survivors of minor head injury began receiving attention in medical and rehabilitation settings, it is no surprise that their families may be overlooked in the course of treatment. Treatment for the survivor should include an assessment of the family.

The structure of the assessment process for the family should be directed to collecting information about the family as a whole, the family's understanding of the minor TBI, explanations about the survivor's behavior, and the family structure. A brief outline of the components of such an assessment is listed in Table 19.3. Some of this information could be collected in written data sheets that the family completes as part of the assessment process. It should be noted that development of a standardized format for assessment of the family of a survivor of minor TBI would be of great benefit to clinicians in the field. This task represents a valuable opportunity for clinical research.

There are similarities and differences between the assessment processes for families of survivors of minor and severe TBI. A basic similarity is that the family members did not anticipate the injury. Their involvement in rehabilitation treatment is initially involuntary. Therefore, the clinician evaluating the family after any TBI must be sensitive to the family's uncertainty about the evaluation process. The family of a survivor of minor TBI may be particularly uncertain about becoming involved in a psychological evaluation if it occurs immediately after the injury. At this stage the survivor's difficulties may not be apparent. Even if the problems are evident, the family may not see the connection between these problems in the survivor and the family's functioning. There often must be a strong educational component to the evaluation process. The clinician may need to explain to the family how the survivor's behavior can interact with the family as a whole to cause adjustment problems. The

Table 19.3. Outline for assessment of family of the survivor of minor TBI.

A. Identifying information
 1. Names and ages of family members
 2. Spouse and/or parents of survivor: history of their relationship and marriage, educational background, vocational history, medical and mental health history, socioeconomic status
 3. Children and/or siblings of the survivor: developmental milestones, educations and vocational history, medical and mental health history
B. Family's understanding of the trauma
 1. Family's description of the nature of the injury
 2. Family's level of understanding about the survivor's condition post-trauma
 3. Family's level of emotional control at this time and coping strategies
 4. Family's expectations for the survivor's recovery
C. Characteristic functioning of the family
 1. Description of typical family weekly activities
 2. Description of family decision making procedures
 3. Description of family communication methods and patterns
 4. Family involvement in community activities
 5. Role of the survivor in the family prior to trauma
 6. Description of how family organization has been changed since the trauma

clinician needs to modulate the depth and intensity of the questioning in an evaluation interview according to the family's willingness to consider and ability to understand these matters.

Another similarity in assessment of all families after TBI is that the initial interview is an opportunity to establish a trust between the clinician and the family. The clinician has the need to collect information about the survivor, about the family, and about the family's willingness to participate in treatment. The family has the need to get information about the family member's condition and to get to know the clinician. A trusting relationship between clinician and family is essential to further successful work in treatment. Thus, the assessment interview should not be conducted in an imbalanced question-and-answer format where the clinician fires questions at the family members about themselves or about the survivor. Rather, it should be a mutual discussion between the clinician and family. The clinician seeks to become involved in the family and its reactions to the trauma. The process of establishing a relationship with the family should occur simultaneously with the process of learning about the family predicament.

A major difference between assessments of families of survivors of severe and minor TBI concerns the family's overall level of distress and disorganization. After the survivor's severe TBI, families are under extreme distress. This distress is particularly evident if they are evaluated while the survivor is at the acute medical or acute rehabilitation stages of treatment. Regardless of their willingness to become involved in evaluation or treatment, these families may have difficulty focusing on the key questions or issues presented to them by the clinician because of their level of distress.

Families of survivors of minor TBI may be better able to engage in the evaluation interview because they are experiencing less structural disorganization. They may, concomitantly, have less motivation to participate in such evaluations. As noted above, if families are evaluated within a few days after the minor TBI occurs, they may be unaware of the changes that the survivor is experiencing. The clinician, in this case, should adapt the evaluation interview to the family's needs by using an initial brief interview with the family within one week after the injury. This interview may set the foundation for further contacts with the clinician in the future when the family discovers more adjustment problems.

Treatment Intervention

Treatment for families of survivors of TBI should focus on several levels of intervention. These include education, peer support, professional support, problem-solving, and structural intervention. Each of these treatment levels will be discussed and methods for applying them to families of survivors of minor TBI will be described.

Education

The greatest source of emotional distress for families of all survivors of TBI is uncertainty about the course of recovery and prognosis. Therefore, a key to handling this emotional distress is education. In this intervention the clinician attempts to answer the family's questions about the trauma and to provide information for family members.

One central area for family education is the understanding of the cognitive and behavioral sequelae of minor TBI, and the methods of differentiating these changes from changes that are the result of acute emotional stress. As noted above, it is also important to explain the connection between an individual family member's distress and the distress of the family as a whole. Unfortunately, it is unusual that the family or injured individual will have received much information about what to expect after the injury. Much educational information that is available about TBI is focused on severe rather than minor injuries. The clinician should not presume that the family has received information simply because they have had contact with other medical professionals.

Peer Support

In the field of brain-injury rehabilitation, self-help groups have developed through the National Head Injury Foundation as a way of having families assist each other in coping with the distress of the trauma. These groups provide education and emotional support. Very often family members of survivors of TBI are better able to respond to information and suggestions provided by family members who have faced similar circumstances than they would be to suggestions from professionals.

Peer support groups can be beneficial to families of survivors of minor TBI. The system of TBI peer support, however, tends to be focused on the needs of the families of survivors of severe TBI. Therefore, the family of a survivor of minor TBI may derive little benefit from a support group meeting dominated by families of survivors of severe TBI. The family members of a survivor of minor TBI may feel uncomfortable discussing some of their adjustment problems, which appear so minor in the context of a support group that is focused on the problems of severely injured survivors.

It is anticipated that the peer support system will develop further to meet the needs of the families of survivors of minor TBI. Until that time the clinician needs to be circumspect in advising families to attend support groups unless more information is obtained about the scope of the specific support group.

Professional Support

Families often need to ventilate their feelings of frustration and confusion about the minor TBI and the survivor's behavior. Psychological treatment sessions can be a supportive, nonjudgmental environment in which families may express their feelings. In a treatment session, the clinician facilitates the family's emotional expression by communicating to the family members that all feelings are acceptable reactions to the injury. Family members are allowed to express feelings that they might feel uncomfortable expressing to the survivor himself or herself or to other friends, without fear that the clinician will judge them for their feelings. For example, the frustration that families feel about the changes in the survivor and the uncertainty about how to communicate their frustration to the survivor are feelings that all families experience regardless of the severity of the injury.

Problem-Solving

The subtlety of the survivor's deficits may make identification of the problems to be resolved a difficult task for the clinician and family. Nevertheless, the survivor of minor TBI presents the family with practical problems that need to be addressed for the family to function well. For example, as noted earlier, the survivor's changed behavior may necessitate changes in the organization of the family responsibilities or changes in expectations for the survivor. A proper focus for psychological treatment, therefore, is to help the family to develop options for responding to the changes brought about by the minor TBI. The family must evaluate these options and decide on a course of action. Very often, the family's distress is the result of feelings of helplessness. If family members can generate ideas and decide on a course of action, they will be reassured regardless of the outcome of their decision. Because the survivor of minor TBI is usually at home with the family rather than in an institution, it is often easier for the family to implement a plan of action to remedy a problem situation. Families of survivors of severe TBI are often separated by the survivor's need for institutional care thereby complicating any implementation of treatment plans.

Structural Treatment Intervention

The minor TBI may highlight or create problems in the family's organizational structure. As a result, psychological treatment may focus on remediating problems that exist in the family's structure. The case example below illustrates how minor TBI resulted in changes in roles and household responsibilities for the survivor, spouse, and children that were stressful to the family. Psychological intervention focused, in part, on strengthening the family structure in such a way as to reduce this stress.

Case Example

E.M. was a 42-year-old married woman who was injured in the street when an object fell on her head from a nearby construction site. She fell down and injured her back but was not unconscious. Prior to her injury, E.M. was actively involved as a local school board official. She did not report any preexisting family adjustment problems. Her husband traveled frequently for business and relied on her to manage the three children's activities and the household. E.M. described herself as the "rock of Gibraltar" in the family. After the injury she experienced back pain, headache, and memory loss. She described difficulties in managing her household, finding her way while carpooling her children, and misplacing items in her home. Her youngest son, age 10, had begun to feel anxious when she was driving him because he was fearful that she would become lost and could not find her way back home. The teenaged children had begun to disregard E.M. in making decisions about their activities and found themselves giving her orders rather than taking orders from her. Since the injury, she felt she was unable to take such an active role in her school board. She resigned from her post and focussed on more assistance with behind-the-scenes work. She had lost confidence in her ability to speak persuasively about her work. She appeared to be saddened by this change because the school board work had been personally meaningful to her.

E.M.'s husband had become frustrated by the long duration of her symptoms. E.M. and her husband reported more frequent arguments, usually about E.M.'s work activities and about how well E.M. was monitoring the children. The husband felt that E.M. should cut back further on her community activities in order to concentrate on the home activities. E.M. felt that her husband was distressed because he had greater responsibilities for the children than he had had prior to her injury. E.M. felt that this tension in the household further intensified her headache pain and reduced her self-confidence. Both E.M. and her husband wondered if her memory difficulties would improve if she could reduce her headache and back pain. Consequently, she became involved in a pain management program but had little success.

E.M. then sought a consultation with a neuropsychologist. The neuropsychological evaluation indicated attention and concentration difficulties that appeared to underlie her memory problems. In addition, E.M. showed evidence of depression on a personality inventory. The results of this testing were helpful to E.M. and her husband in documenting her cognitive problems. The neuropsychologist suggested some methods of compensating for her memory problems and some cognitive remediation activities that she could practice to try to improve her cognitive performance. In addition, the neuropsychologist discussed how the changes in E.M. had changed the entire structure of the family. Patterns of organization and communication, particularly with the children, had changed. The boundaries between parents and children had been disrupted, resulting in the children treating E.M. like a child, and a rift between E.M. and her husband. Counseling was recommended for E.M. and her husband to focus on developing a closer bond between them in order to manage their children and to support each other.

E.M. and her spouse were encouraged to make joint decisions about household management without involving the children. This intervention was designed to strengthen the boundary between parents and children.

As in the first case example, this example illustrates how the structure of the family was affected by one family member's injury. Communication, boundaries, and relationships with those outside the family were all changed for E.M. after her minor TBI. The example also highlights the importance of considering developmental issues in understanding the stressors on the family. E.M. and her husband were parents to three children. Each partner had developed spheres of responsibilities and compentencies in work and family activities. Had the injury to E.M. occurred after the children had been grown or in a situation in which she were the primary breadwinner for the family, the stressors on the family as a whole would have been different.

In this case example the children of a survivor had emotional adjustment problems because of confusion about the changes that occured in the parent. The children reacted differently, depending on their level of cognitive and emotional development with the youngest child becoming fearful and the older children becoming more defiant. In considering the impact of any TBI on a family, the clinician must recognize that the effects will vary across family members. Assessment and treatment of the family should consider the reactions and needs of all family members.

Treatment for the family spanned the different levels of intervention described above. Education about the injury and its effects on E.M. and the family was provided to E.M. and to her husband. The couple also had the need for emotional support and the opportunity to ventilate their feelings of frustration about their changed family life after the injury. Simultaneously, however, there were practical problems that needed to be solved in how the family was to manage its responsibilities in light of E.M.'s changed abilities. Practical problem-solving discussions and more structural interventions were provided in this regard. By attempting to solidify the emotional bond between E.M. and her husband, the clinician sought to facilitate their ability to communicate and make decisions about management of family affairs. Though any one of these levels of intervention may have been helpful to the family, treatment is most effective when it is flexible enough to integrate several approaches.

Indeed, it would be a valuable contribution of clinical research to investigate the relative benefits of different types of treatment intervention to families of minor TBI survivors. Table 19.4 summarizes the different levels of treatment intervention and how they are utilized differently with families after minor and severe TBI.

Table 19.4. Comparison of treatment interventions for families of mild and severe brain injury survivors.

Treatment intervention	Severe injury	Mild injury
Education	Wide range of information available; team of professionals working with survivor	Less information available, maybe only one or two professionals working with survivor
Peer support	Well-established network of groups	Weakly established network of groups; families may feel uneasy discussing their problems in a group designed for families of severe brain injury survivors
Professional support and problem-solving	Identification of adjustment problems in survivor and family is relatively easy, but implementation of treatment is difficult because of diversity of problems and the high level of emotional distress in family	Identification of adjustment problems in survivor and family is relatively difficult; implementation may be easier because family is intact and it is easier to circumscribe treatment
Structural interventions	Structual changes very evident; degree of family disorganization may interfere with family's involvement in this modality	Structural changes may be inconsistent or less disruptive; lack of extended hospitalization for the survivor and fewer number of problems may make this intervention feasible and beneficial

Conclusions

The family of a survivor of minor TBI presents the clinician with unique psychological adjustment issues. The survivor of minor TBI manifests symptomatology that results from a combination of cognitive and emotional sequelae from the injury in the context of the survivor's premorbid personality. The family members of the survivor are baffled by the survivor's behavior. The family's misunderstanding or lack of understanding of the survivor's behavior post-injury is the major source of family distress.

The rehabilitation clinician must, therefore, be able to educate the family about 1) the relationship between the brain-injury sequelae and the survivor's behavior, and 2) the relationship between the survivor's behavior and the family's emotional reaction to the survivor. To accomplish these goals, the clinician must be flexible in his or her assessment and treatment of the family. Assessment should encompass several different spheres of analysis of the presenting problems, including the survivor's premorbid personality and the problems manifested post-injury, the family structure, and the difficulties in family adjustment post-injury. Treatment should span educational, supportive, problem-solving, and structural techniques. The clinician who is knowledgeable in these areas will be able to provide effective intervention for the family.

References

1. Rosenthal M: Strategies for intervention with families of brain-injured patients. In Edelstein BA, Couture ET (eds): Behavioral Assessment and Rehabilitation of the Traumatically Brain-Damaged. New York: Plenum, 1984; pp 227–245.
2. Muir C, Rosenthal R, Diehl LN: Methods of family intervention. In Rosenthal M, Bond MR, Griffith ER, Miller JD (eds): Rehabilitation of the Adult and Child with Traumatic Brain Injury. Philadelphia: Davis, 1990; pp 433–448.
3. Sachs PR: Treating Families of Brain-Injury Survivors. New York: Springer, 1991.
4. Williams JM, Kay T (eds): Head Injury: A Family Matter. Baltimore: Brookes, 1991.
5. Alves WM, Coloban ART, O'Leary TJ, Rimel RW, Jane JA: Understanding posttraumatic symptoms after minor head injury. J Head Trauma Rehabil, 1986; 1:1–12.
6. Kay T: Minor head injury: An introduction for professionals. Southborough, MA: National Head Injury Foundation, 1986.
7. Ruff RM, Levin HS, Marshall LF: Neurobehavioral methods of assessment and the study of outcome in minor head injury. J Head Trauma Rehabil, 1986; 1:43–52.
8. Mandel S: Minor head injury may not be 'minor.' Postgrad Med, 1989; 85:213–225.
9. Miller JD, Jones PA: Minor head injury. In Rosenthal M, Bond MR, Griffith ER, Miller JD (eds): Rehabilitation of the adult and child with traumatic brain injury Philadelphia: Davis, 1990; pp 236–247.
10. Malkmus D, Hagen C, Durham T: Rehabilitation of the head injury adult: Comprehensive physical management. Downey, CA: Los Amigos Research and Education Institute of Rancho los Amigos Medical Center, 1979.
11. Brooks N: Cognitive deficits. In Rosenthal M, Bond MR, Griffith ER, Miller JD (eds): Rehabilitation of the Adult and Child with Traumatic Brain Injury. Philadelphia: Davis, 1990; pp 163–178.
12. Lezak MD: The walking wounded of head injury: When subtle deficits can be disabling. Trends Rehabil 1988; 3:4–9.
13. Minuchin S: Families and Family Therapy. Cambridge, MA: Harvard, 1974.
14. Minuchin S, Fishman HC: Family Therapy Techniques. Cambridge, MA: Harvard, 1981.

15. Romano MD: Family response to traumatic head injury. Scand J Rehabil Med 1974; 6:1–4.
16. Lezak MD: Psychological implications of traumatic brain damage for the patient's family. Rehabil Psychol 1986; 31:241–250.

Appendix: The Glasgow Coma Scale

Robert T. Sataloff

The Glasgow Coma Scale was developed in response to the need for a reproducible, consistent system for neurological assessment of patients following head injury. A universally accepted method of describing precisely a patient's initial status permits consistent monitoring of the individual, comparison of presentation and outcome characteristics in patients with similar degrees of injury, and assessment of the value of various treatments at multiple medical centers. The Glasgow Coma Scale is used most widely for these purposes.

In 1974, Teasdale and Jennett suggested that the degree of coma after severe head injury is the most reliable clinical indicator of the severity of brain damage (1). They proposed a scale to assess the depth and duration of coma. Coma was defined as the inability to obey commands, speak, or open the eyes. These three behavioral aspects were incorporated into the Glasgow Coma Scale. The scale was revised in 1977, adding another motor response level (2,3) (Table A.1). The sum of the $E+M+V$ values was called the responsiveness score; and coma was defined as all combinations which added up to 7 or less. A score of 9 or more precluded the diagnosis of coma. Teasdale and Jennett believed that correlations among the responsiveness score and pupillary reactions, breathing patterns, and eye movements were limited. Therefore, they did not include brainstem reflexes in the coma scale. This led to later criticism and the proposal of several other scaling systems (4–6). Nevertheless, the Glasgow Coma Scale has been studied most thoroughly and widely accepted. In 1978,

Table A.1. Glasgow Coma Scale.

Parameter	Score
Eye opening (E)	
Opens eyes spontaneously	4
Opens eyes to voice	3
Opens eyes to pain	2
No eye opening	1
Best motor response (M)	
Obeys commands	6
Localizes to pain	5
Withdraws to pain	4
Abnormal flexor response	3
Abnormal extensor response	2
No movement	1
Best verbal response (V)	
Appropriate and oriented	5
Confused conversation	4
Inappropriate words	3
Incomprehensible sounds	2
No sounds	1

Table A.2. Glasgow Outcome Scale.

Good recovery—resumption of normal life-style
Moderate disability—disabled but independent
Severe disability—conscious but dependent
Persistent vegetative state—unresponsive and speechless
Death

Langfitt reported an extensive review of head injury data and concluded that the Glasgow Coma Scale "should be adopted by neurosurgical units throughout the world to evaluate their patients with head injuries" (7). In general, it has been.

The Glasgow Coma Scale is helpful for initial assessment and monitoring, but it provides no parameters to describe the clinical outcomes of patients following head injury. Consequently, the Glasgow Outcome Scale was introduced in 1975 to be used in conjunction with the Glasgow Coma Scale (8) (Table A.2). Detailed descriptions of the clinical characteristics of each level were provided in order to avoid improper usage of the terminology. The value of the Glasgow Coma Scale and Glasgow Outcome Scale was studied initially through a collaborative investigation involving neurosurgical services in Glasgow, Groningen, Rotterdam, and Southern California universities (9). The Glasgow Coma Scale was found to be an excellent predictor of outcome. For example, a best Glasgow Coma Scale score of 3 or 4 was associated with a 97% incidence of death or persistent vegetative state (PVS); and a best Glasgow Coma Scale score of 8 was associated with only a 25% incidence of death or PVS and a 61% incidence of moderate disability or good recovery. The Glasgow Coma Scale and Glasgow Outcome Scale have remained the most standard, simple, repeatable, and widely used guidelines for evaluation of patients following head trauma.

References

1. Teasdale G, Jennett B: Assessment of coma and impaired consciousness: A practical scale. Lancet, 1974; 2:81–89.
2. Jennett B, Teasdale G: Aspects of coma after severe head injury. Lancet, 1977; 1:878–881.
3. Jennett B, Teasdale G: Management of Head Injuries. Philadelphia: Davis, 1981; pp 95–151.
4. Ommaya AD, Sadowsky D: A system of coding medical data for punched-card machine retrieval: Part II. As applied to head injuries. J Trauma, 1966; 6:605–617.
5. Bouzarth WF, Lindermuth JR: Head injury watch sheet modified for a digital scale. J Trauma, 1978; 18:571–579.
6. Yen JK, Bourke RS, Nelson LR, Popp AJ: Numerical grading of clinical neurological status after serious head injury. J Neurol Neurosurg Psychiatry, 1978; 41:1125–1130.
7. Langfitt TW: Measuring the outcome from head injuries. J Neurosurg, 1978; 48:673–678.
8. Jennett B, Bond M: Assessment of outcome after severe brain damage: A practical scale. Lancet, 1975; 1:480–484.
9. Jennett B, Teasdale G, Braakman R, Minderhoud J, Heiden J, Kurze T: Prognosis of patients with severe head injury. Neurosurgery, 1979; 4:283–289.

Index